ITCH

ITCH
Mechanisms and Management of Pruritus

Editor

JEFFREY D. BERNHARD, M.D.
Professor of Medicine
Director, Division of Dermatology
Department of Medicine
Associate Dean for Admissions
University of Massachusetts
Medical School
Worcester, Massachusetts

McGraw-Hill, Inc.
HEALTH PROFESSIONS DIVISION

New York St. Louis San Francisco Auckland Bogatá Caracas Lisbon
London Madrid Mexico City Milan Montreal New Delhi Paris
San Juan Singapore Sydney Tokyo Toronto

ITCH
Mechanisms and Management of Pruritus

1234567890   DOC DOC   9876543

ISBN 0-07-004935-1

This book was set in Korinna by J. M. Post Graphics,
     division of Cardinal Communications Group, Inc.
The editors were J. Dereck Jeffers and Lester A. Sheinis;
the production supervisor was Richard C. Ruzycka;
the project supervision was by Tage Publishing Service, Inc.;
the cover designer was José Fonfrias;
R. R. Donnelley & Sons Company was printer and binder.

Library of Congress Cataloging-in-Publication Data

Itch : Mechanisms and management of pruritus / [edited by] Jeffrey D.
  Bernhard.
       p.   cm.
    Includes bibliographical references and index.
    ISBN 0-07-004935-1
    1. Itching.   I. Bernhard, Jeffrey D.
    [DNLM: 1. Pruritus—etiology, 2. Pruritus—physiopathology.
    3. Pruritus—therapy.   WR 282 188 1994]
    RL721.183 1994
    616.5—dc20
    DNLM/DLC
    for Library of Congress   93-21008
                                                                   CIP

This book is printed on acid-free paper.

TO

ANNE

CONTENTS

III Systemic Aspects of Pruritus

IV Psychologic and Psychiatric Aspects

V Treatment

CONTRIBUTORS

Jeffrey D. Bernhard, M.D. [3, 4, 6, 12, 13, 18, 22, 23, 26]*
Professor of Medicine
Director, Division of Dermatology
Department of Medicine
Associate Dean for Admissions
University of Massachusetts
  Medical School
Worcester, MA

Susan J. Adams, M.B. FRCPEd FRCP [17]
Consultant Dermatologist
Royal Devon & Exeter Hospital
  (Wonford)
Exeter, ENGLAND

Andrew J. Carmichael, M.B. B.S. MRCP [15]
Consultant Dermatologist
South Cleveland Hospital
Middlesbrough
Cleveland, UK

Clay J. Cockerell, M.D. [20]
Associate Professor of Dermatology
  and Pathology
University of Texas Southwestern
  Medical Center
Dallas, TX

Thomas B. Fitzpatrick, M.D. Ph.D., D.Sc. (Hon.) [14]
Wigglesworth Professor of
  Dermatology, Emeritus
Department of Dermatology
Harvard Medical School
Massachusetts General Hospital
Boston, MA

C. N. Ghent, M.D. FRCPC [16]
Associate Professor of Medicine
Department of Medicine
Section of Gastroenterology
University Hospital
London, CANADA

Barry D. Goldman, M.D. [21]
Resident in Dermatology
Department of Dermatology
State University of New York at
  Buffalo Medical School
Buffalo, NY

Lori E. U. Herman, M.D. [10, 29]
Assistant Professor of Medicine
Division of Dermatology
Department of Medicine
University of Massachusetts
  Medical School
Worcester, MA 01655

Gary R. Kantor, M.D. [5, 24]
Associate Professor
Chief, Section of Dermatopathology
Division of Dermatology
Hahnemann University
Philadelphia, PA

Caroline S. Koblenzer, M.D. [25]
Clinical Associate Professor of
  Dermatology and Dermatology in
  Psychiatry
University of Pennsylvania
Philadelphia, PA

* The numbers in brackets following the contributors' names refer to the chapters written or co-written by the contributors.

Howard K. Koh, M.D. [21]
Associate Professor of Dermatology
Medicine and Public Health
Department of Dermatology
Boston University Schools of
    Medicine and Public Health
Boston, MA

Mark Lebwohl, M.D. [28]
Professor of Dermatology
Department of Dermatology
Mt. Sinai School of Medicine
New York, NY

Ethan A. Lerner, M.D. Ph.D. [2]
Assistant Professor of Dermatology
Department of Dermatology
Harvard Medical School
Boston, MA

Jerome Z. Litt, M.D. [27]
Assistant Clinical Professor of
    Dermatology
Case Western Reserve University
    School of Medicine
Cleveland, OH

Marilynne McKay, M.D. [11]
Associate Professor of Dermatology
    and Gynecology
Department of Dermatology
Emory University School of
    Medicine
Atlanta, GA

Karen F. Rothman, M.D. [8]
Assistant Professor of Medicine and
    Pediatrics
Division of Dermatology
Department of Medicine
University of Massachusetts
    Medical School
Worcester, MA

**C.M.E. Rowland Payne,
MRCP [7]**
Consultant Dermatologist
Cromwell Hospital
London, Great Britain

Anna M. Sarno, M.D. [23]
Resident in Dermatology
Department of Dermatology
University of Rochester
    School of Medicine and Dentistry
Rochester, NY

Mark Jordan Scharf, M.D. [9]
Assistant Professor of Medicine
Director Dermatology Laser Center
Division of Dermatology
Department of Medicine
University of Massachusetts
    Medical School
Worcester, MA

Jeff K. Shornick, M.D. [19]
Group Health Cooperative of
    Puget Sound
Division of Dermatology
Seattle, WA

Robert P. Tuckett, Ph.D. [1]
Department of Physiology
Research Associate Professor
University of Utah
    School of Medicine
Salt Lake City, UT

PREFACE

Most of what we know about itch has not, until now, been put together in one book. Dermatologists, internists, pediatricians, family physicians, and allergists need a single comprehensive text on itching that will help them at the bedside, and researchers need one to help them put itching in clinical perspective.

Research and progress in the understanding and treatment of itching have been slow for several reasons. First, it is difficult to study a subjective sensation for which no particularly good animal model exists. Second, itch is not a leading cause of death, although it is *on occasion a sign of serious underlying disease,* and it sometimes makes life so miserable that it can lead to suicide. Third, itch has been traditionally considered a variety of pain. At least as far back as 1942, Thomas Lewis argued that "itch and pain are separate phenomena,"* but the view that itch is merely "subthreshold" pain has persisted nonetheless. Although there may be some relationships and similarities between itch and pain, the itch/pain paradigm has not even led to any treatment for itching as simple or effective as aspirin is for pain. (The mounting evidence for the newer view that itch is a separate, primary sensory modality and not a form of pain is presented in Chapter 1.) Despite these impediments, the amount of what is now known about itching is substantial, and this book is the first to attempt a comprehensive, clinically oriented treatment of the field. Future editions will address more topics in even greater detail. In the meantime, I hope that the abundant citations will make it easy for readers to access the primary sources of additional information.

The first section of this book covers the basic neuroanatomy, neurophysiology, and chemical physiology of itching. The second section covers its dermatologic aspects and most of the skin disorders in which itching is especially important. It also includes chapters on strange skin sensations and pruritic curiosities. ("Who lives without folly is not so wise as he thinks," according to La Rochefoucauld.) The third section deals with itching as a manifestation of systemic diseases and also addresses the evaluation of the patient who presents with generalized pruritus. The fourth section covers the

---

* *Lewis T: Pain.* New York, Macmillan, 1942, p 113.

psychologic and psychiatric aspects of itching, and the fifth section covers treatment. Many subjects overlap several sections.

There are not many clinical pictures in this book. Excellent color atlases are available for those readers less familiar with the diseases discussed here. Some of the atlases and newer general dermatology textbooks have truly superb clinical color photographs. In any event, it is ironic that the quintessential symptom in the most visual of medical specialties should be invisible.

A WORD ON "ITCH" VERSUS "PRURITUS"

> Faced with two terms for the same thing, one tends to cast about for a distinction.
>
> W.V. Quine*

Some writers use *pruritus* to signify itching without visible skin lesions. Others use the terms *essential pruritus, pruritus sine materia,* or *generalized pruritus* to describe itching without a rash as well. But such terms can be misleading when a patient with itching caused by renal failure or another underlying systemic disease has excoriations or a non-specific rash created by rubbing and scratching. And doesn't a patient with extensive, severe atopic dermatitis also have *generalized pruritus?* Although distinctions can be drawn, and many have been, *itch* and *pruritus* are synonymous. *Prurigo* presents some additional and controversial semantic problems of its own; these are discussed in Chapter 4. I prefer (and suspect that it is safer) to use a few extra words to describe different clinical situations whenever pruritus, prurigo, or itching is present. Casting distinctions away, the editor and contributors will use *itch* and *pruritus* interchangeably throughout this book.

J.D.B.

---

* Quine WV: *Quiddities. An Intermittently Philosophical Dictionary.* Cambridge, MA, Harvard University Press, 1987, p 24.

ACKNOWLEDGMENTS

I am grateful to the secretaries of the Division of Dermatology at the University of Massachusetts Medical School, Cynthia Hough and Maria Snell, for their many efforts in the preparation of this book. The library staffs at the University of Massachusetts Medical School and the Marine Biological Laboratory in Woods Hole were helpful in all of the usual ways, but most importantly in providing wonderful environments for writing. I am also grateful to the University of Massachusetts for sabbatical time, which permitted me to complete this work.

I am grateful to my many teachers for their inspiration and help along the way. I must particularly mention Gerald Cohen (deceased), my ninth-grade science teacher who helped me set my sights; Edmund Klein, who gave me my first introduction to the skin when I was a high school student in the National Science Foundation summer program at Roswell Park Memorial Institute in Buffalo, New York; and Thomas B. Fitzpatrick, who showed me how much fun it could be to eat, sleep, and breathe dermatology (and still does). I honor the memory of my late parents, Iris and Wilbert Bernhard, who were my first teachers and much more.

I would like to thank Walter B. Shelley for giving me his collection of books about pain, and for his perpetual demonstration of just how vibrant medical writing can be.

I am greatly indebted to colleagues who contributed chapters in their special areas of expertise: one of the additional ironies of itching is that, despite how little I have claimed is known about it, the field is sufficiently large and specialized enough to force the confession that it would be difficult for one person to master all of it. Nonetheless, I shall retain responsibility for errors and omissions, in the hope that readers will let me know how I can improve what I hope will be a second edition of this medium-sized book on such a big little subject. Work now underway at several itch centers around the globe, in Stockholm, London, Erlangen, New Haven, Salt Lake City, and elsewhere, must inevitably lead to a most welcome expansion of the "mechanisms" section. That, of course, is also our best hope for expansion, if not simplification, of the "treatment" section as well.

I am grateful to Dereck Jeffers at McGraw-Hill for his confidence and support, to Lester Sheinis at McGraw-Hill for his editorial assistance, and to Maria and Tony Caruso for putting up with a lot of changes in the galleys.

I am most grateful to my wife and sons, who quite cheerfully put up with my itch to write.

J.D.B.

PATHOPHYSIOLOGY

NEUROPHYSIOLOGY AND NEUROANATOMY OF PRURITUS

Robert P. Tuckett

Itch can be defined as an unpleasant sensation that provokes the desire to scratch.[1] This definition is meant to exclude sensory qualities, such as tickle, which in most instances evoke a motor response such as light rubbing. The response of the nervous system to pruritogenic stimuli is complex. The purpose of this chapter is to give the reader an overview of major issues in the neurophysiology and neuroanatomy of pruritus.

BACKGROUND INFORMATION

Cutaneous sensory neurons terminate in specialized endings that are sensitive to specific kinds of stimuli (e.g., mechanical, thermal, chemical). When activated, the nerve terminal generates action potentials that travel along the axon toward the central nervous system. The concept of labeled lines or specific "sensory channels" has a long history.[2] According to this theory, the neural activity that is related to each type of sensation (referred to as a sensory modality) travels along a defined neural pathway from the receptor in the skin, along spinal relays, to the higher centers in the brain (Fig. 1-1). When activated, these centers give rise to information about the nature, intensity, and location of cutaneous stimuli.

The peripheral nervous system consists of individual neurons, the cell bodies of which are clustered into ganglia located in close proximity to the spinal cord (Fig. 1-2). From the ganglia, axons extend toward their target tissues. These axonal projections are organized into nerve fascicles. Fascicles

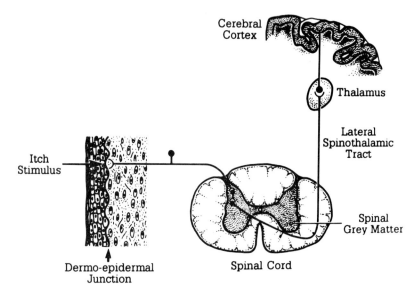

Figure 1-1 A simplified diagram of a hypothesized neuroanatomical pathway for itching, in which spinothalamic relay axons cross to the contralateral ventrolateral quadrant rostral to the level at which the sensory neurons enter the spinal cord. In addition to the spinothalamic pathway shown, there may be propriospinal (interneuron) and other pathways (Fig. 1-11) that are involved in signaling information related to irritant sensory experience.[36] (Reprinted with permission.)

innervating the skin run subcutaneously, extend into the lower dermis, and eventually terminate in receptive endings throughout the dermis and epidermis.

Techniques for Neural Recording

As can be seen from Fig. 1-2, to record from single neurons in peripheral nerve there must be some method to obtain the signal from individual fibers as action potentials generated in the receptive nerve terminals travel toward the central nervous system.

One method is to impale the nervous tissue with a microelectrode that has a sharpened tip and preferentially records electrical activity in adjacent tissue. For human recording, the peripheral nerve is palpated and held in place while the microelectrode is manually pushed through the skin and into a nerve fascicle. The experimenter then releases the electrode, allowing it to be anchored by the skin and subcutaneous tissue, and then stimulates the subject's skin to determine whether the electrode is in a position to record activity from single neurons. If not, the electrode is repositioned in the nerve and the process repeated. Microelectrodes are also used extensively for recording within the central nervous system.

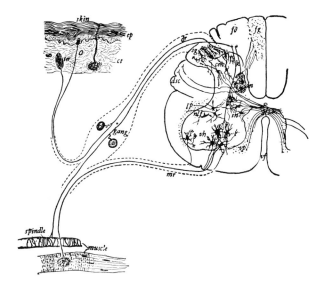

Figure 1-2 Diagram of the peripheral innervation of sensory neurons. Individual neuronal cell bodies reside in the dorsal root ganglia and project through the dorsal roots to connections within the central nervous system. Also shown are efferent motor fibers traveling from the ventral roots to the muscle.[37]

cen: central nucleus of dorsal horn
dn: dorsal nucleus of cord
dr: dorsal root
dsc: dorsal spinalo cerebellar tract
ep: epithelium
fc: fasciculus cuneatus
fg: fasciculus gracilis
in: intermediate nucleus
k: collateral

lp: lateral fasciculus proprius
mr: motor or ventral root
nlf: nucleus of lateral fasciculus
sg: substantia gelatinosa
ter: nerve terminal
vf: ventral fissure
vh: ventral horn
vp: ventral fasciculus proprius

For recording from peripheral nerve in animals, microdissection is the preferred technique. The peripheral nerve is isolated through a subcutaneous incision in the anesthetized animal and covered with oil. Under high magnification, a fine filament of nerve is dissected free and wrapped around a fine-wire recording electrode that is placed in the oil. When a receptive field is activated, the action potentials travel through the nerve filament. Because a ground electrode is attached to the animal and the oil layer is electrically nonconductive, the recording electrode measures the electrical voltage produced as the action potentials travel along the nerve filament (Fig. 1-3). The experimenter searches the skin for receptive fields of neurons in the recorded filament. If too many neurons are activated, the experimenter must split the filament into finer strands, place one strand at a time on the recording electrode, and repeat the search procedure.

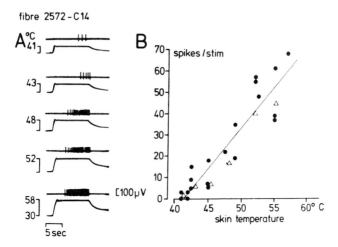

Figure 1-3 Response of a C-polymodal nociceptor to noxious thermal stimuli (**A**) which showed a (**B**) linear relationship between discharge rate and cutaneous temperature.[38] (Reprinted with permission.)

With both microelectrode and dissection techniques, the experimenter must be able to distinguish the firing of a single neuron (i.e., single-unit recording). As long as recording conditions remain constant, the fibers being recorded from will generate action potential signals of constant height and shape. Most laboratories distinguish single units on the basis of the amplitude of the recorded action potential. Hence, the art of single-unit recording is to ensure that the action potentials from a neuron being studied can be distinguished from all other active units. Fortunately, most cutaneous sensory neurons are quiet when not being stimulated; and hence, unless receptive fields are overlapping, it is often possible to distinguish single units in nerve filaments with several active fibers.

Classification of Cutaneous Sensory Neurons

Neurons can be categorized as either myelinated (Fig. 1-4) or unmyelinated (Fig. 1-5). The coating on myelinated neurons allows action potentials to travel at a higher speed than on unmyelinated fibers. Because the conduction velocity of action potentials on individual axons remains constant and conduction velocities of myelinated and unmyelinated fibers do not overlap, conduction velocity is a useful tool in the classification of sensory neurons.

Myelinated cutaneous sensory neurons have traditionally been divided on the basis of conduction velocity into rapidly conducting (A-beta) and slowly conducting (A-delta) subcategories. The most rapidly conducting populations are mechanoreceptive. Some mechanoreceptors are slowly adapting and continue to respond for extended periods of time during skin indentation.

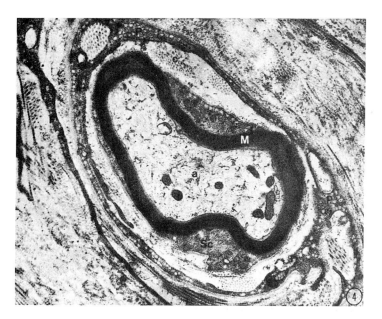

Figure 1-4 Electron micrograph of an isolated small myelinated (M) axon and its Schwann cell (Sc) in subpapillary dermis surrounded by perineurial sheath (P), fibroblasts (F), and endoneurial collagen (c). These and other myelinated axonal processes were found to correlate closely with discrete points on the skin surface from which an A-delta nociceptive neuron could be mechanically activated. X12,700.[39] (Reprinted with permission.)

These include the type I/Merkel cell complex, which is located in the epidermis. In hairy skin, rapidly adapting populations contain hair receptors that include the more rapidly conducting guard hair receptors as well as a slowly conducting population (d-hair receptors). Rapidly conducting mechanoreceptive neurons also include field receptors that have a spectrum of response characteristics that is similar to the hair-receptor population. The Pacinian corpuscle is located in subcutaneous tissue and is sensitive to vibratory stimuli applied to the skin surface. In addition to the myelinated mechanoreceptors, a C-mechanoresponsive population has been reported in several species. Because of its preferential response to extremely light, slow movement over the skin's surface and its ability to continue firing after cessation of the mechanical stimulus, this neuron is uniquely positioned to encode "tickle" sensations. Recent reports of the discovery of this receptor in human peripheral nerve[3] have renewed enthusiasm for such a possibility.

Thermal reception is encoded by separate warmth and cooling neurons the combined response of which spans the entire range of non-noxious temperatures. At noxiously high temperatures, pain-signaling neurons (see following) are activated and continue to fire with increased frequency as the temperature extends to levels that can cause extensive cutaneous injury (Fig.

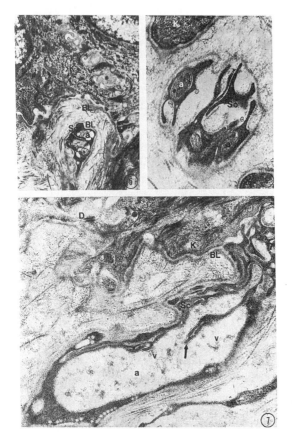

Figure 1-5 Electron micrograph of a typical dermal unmyelinated nerve bundle with numerous axons (a) surrounded by single Schwann cell (Sc), endoneurial collagen (c), and thin layer of perineurium (P). X11,800.[39] (Reprinted with permission.)

1-3). The ability of these heat-activated neurons to signal cold-induced pain has been less convincing; however, in recent years a population of neurons that is responsive to noxious cold has been reported.[4]

Neurons that signal pain and irritation exist in both the myelinated and unmyelinated populations and have been given the name "nociceptors" to indicate their responsiveness to noxious stimuli. Myelinated nociceptive neurons tend to have slow conduction velocities that fall within the A-delta range. Human psychophysical studies have shown that the painful sensation evoked by activating myelinated neurons is different in quality (e.g., stinging, pricking) from the dull, aching pain evoked by the recruitment of unmyelinated neurons.

In general, it has been found that nociceptive neurons can be activated by mechanical, thermal, and chemical stimuli, and these neurons have been subgrouped on the basis of (a) conduction velocity, (b) mechanical threshold, (c) responsiveness to thermal stimuli and (d) activation by specific chemicals. Some respond only to mechanical stimuli, some to mechanical and thermal stimuli and some to mechanical, thermal, and chemical stimuli. The latter are often referred to as chemosensitive nociceptors.[5] Although in many species myelinated, chemosensitive nociceptors appear to be rare, they may be more common in humans.[6]

Some nociceptors that respond to chemical stimuli are responsive to different types of chemical compounds. For example, preliminary studies in our laboratory suggest some neurons that respond to itch-producing chemicals might not be activated by chemicals thought to produce pain. A fundamental barrier to this research is a lack of chemicals that exclusively produce either itch or pain in human subjects. For example, histamine can produce both itch and pain depending on the route of administration and the subject being tested, and cowhage (see following) produces stinging and burning sensations as well as intense pruritus.

Human psychophysical experiments have given consistent evidence that neurons responsible for signaling pruritus are present in the unmyelinated sensory population. Whether they also exist in the myelinated population remains controversial. As acute pruritus is most commonly evoked by chemical stimuli (e.g., histamine), two alternatives appear to be most likely for a peripheral itch-encoding mechanism: Either itch-signaling neurons belong to a chemosensitive subpopulation of pain-signaling sensory neurons (i.e., nociceptors), or they belong to a previously undocumented system of sensory neurons as discussed at the end of this chapter.

MECHANISMS OF ACUTE PRURITUS

When pulses of electrical current are applied to the skin and the pulse amplitude is gradually increased, the threshold sensation in a majority of human subjects is pruritus. The observation that sensations of pain are only elicited at higher current levels suggests either that the nerve terminals of neurons signaling pruritus are located more superficially in the skin than those signaling pain or that differences exist in the electrical thresholds of itch- and pain-signaling sensory neurons. In addition, pressure at discrete points on the skin surface with fine-tipped mechanical probes can often produce a faint but unambiguous sensation of pruritus. [The itch induced by wool in some individuals may be due to mechanical stimulation.[7]] Hence, although chemical stimuli are a major cause of itch in many experimental and clinical conditions (see following), it is possible to induce experimental pruritus with nondamaging stimuli that presumably stimulate itch-signaling nerve terminals directly. Consequently, the ability to produce pruritus with innocuous mechanical stimuli should be taken into account in any model for generation of pruritic sensation.

Early investigators recognized that many types of mildly damaging stimuli (e.g., mechanical, electrical, thermal) caused pruritus whereas more intense injury evoked pain.[8] These mildly damaging stimuli might (a) directly excite itch-signaling sensory neurons, or indirectly produce pruritus through (b) the release of pruritogens from injured tissues, or (c) an axon reflex mechanism.

In most models of the axon reflex (Fig. 1-6), nerve-terminal activation produces action potentials that travel along the nerve fiber to a branch point in the skin. From this branch point, action potentials travel along the parent axon toward the central nervous system and also travel in the opposite direction along a branched network of neuronal processes that terminate in close proximity to dermal blood vessels and cause the release of Substance P from nerve endings. Substance-P release results in cutaneous flare directly through vasodilation of local arterioles and indirectly through mast cell degranulation. Mast cell degranulation results in the release of a variety of substances including histamine, which is (a) vasoactive, (b) increases capillary permeability (thus contributing to localized edema and wheal formation), and (c) can contribute to increased pruritus or to a peripheral mechanism of itchy skin. Furthermore, mast cells can be degranulated through a variety of additional mechanisms such as direct mechanical injury and IgE-mediated allergic reactions.

A number of chemicals are known to evoke pruritus.[9] In addition to histamine[10] and mast cell degranulators such as Substance P and compound

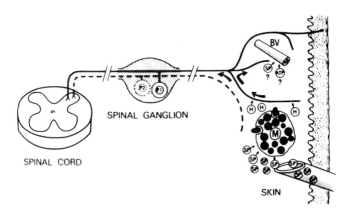

Figure 1-6 Hypothetical scheme of events caused by intradermal Substance P (SP) injection. SP stimulates mast cells (M) to exocytotically release histamine (H). H stimulates sensory nerve terminals to produce action potentials that travel in two directions at the branch point: (1) In the periphery, action potentials travel along a branching network of peripheral nerve processes that terminate near blood vessels (BV). These action potentials are thought to cause a flare response, possibly via release of SP. (2) Action potentials travel to the central nervous system by the central branch of the primary sensory neuron, which likely terminates in the dorsal horn of the spinal cord and ultimately results in generation of the sensation of pruritus.[40] (Reprinted with permission.)

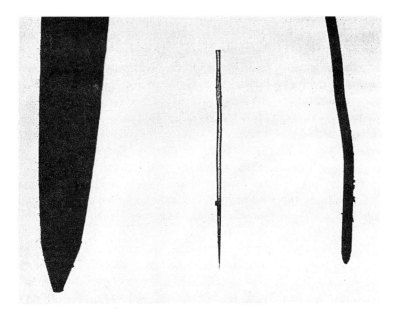

Figure 1-7 Size comparison (reading from left to right) of a common pinpoint, a cowhage spicule, and a copper wire electrode (about 100μ in diam.). Because of its sharp tip, the cowhage spicule permits micropenetration of the skin surface.[41] (Reprinted with permission.)

48/80, substances such as kallikrein, bradykinin, papain, trypsin, and the classical itch-producing substance cowhage (*Mucuna pruriens,* Fig. 1-7) have been shown to produce experimental pruritus. Presumably there are specific molecular receptors on the surface of itch-signaling nerve terminals to which primary pruritogenic agents (such as histamine) bind and thereby cause the generation of action potentials. The finding that antagonists to specific pruritogens can inhibit pruritus supports this concept. For example, the experimental pruritus produced by intradermal histamine injection is effectively blocked by systemically administered H_1-histamine antagonists. Because the intense pruritus produced by even small amounts of cowhage is reported to be unaffected by antihistamines, it is interesting to speculate that the active molecule in this botanical substance might have a specific binding site on itch-signaling sensory neurons that is independent of histamine membrane receptors.

The linkage between endogenous chemicals that are known to produce experimental pruritus and those that are involved in chronic pruritus is unclear. Although some types of itching dermatitis are histamine mediated, other types of chronic pruritus (e.g., dermatitis herpetiformis, atopy) are not effectively treated by antihistamines. Intriguingly, this list includes mastocytosis, suggesting that not all mast-cell pruritogens are histaminergic. Some forms of clinical pruritus may not be chemically mediated. For example, pruritus often follows severe burn injury and subsequent split thickness grafting procedures. Itching occurs frequently during the healing of superficial cutaneous wounds (see Chap. 10). On the other hand, some types of chronic pruritus appear to be related to changes in systemic physiology, such as pregnancy, biliary obstruction, renal dialysis, and Hodgkin's disease. In such cases itching might result from circulating pruritogenic factors that excite either peripheral nerve terminals or an itch-related nucleus within the central nervous system, as discussed in the following section.

NEUROANATOMY OF PRURITUS

Most, if not all, rapidly conducting neurons are mechanoreceptive and many have specialized receptive endings that can be identified histologically. In contrast, most slowly conducting myelinated fibers and all unmyelinated fibers form "free nerve endings" without obvious morphological characteristics by which to distinguish different receptor types.

Early investigators reported that pressing discrete points on the skin with small mechanical probes would produce sensations of itch and that these points were separable from those that produced pain. Reports of histological changes in human unmyelinated nerve terminals after experimental and chronic pruritus are intriguing and await confirmation by other investigators.[11] Some authors have suggested that itch is a "superficial" sensation and have speculated that scratching may temporarily interrupt pruritus by mechanically removing or otherwise affecting the terminals of itch-signaling sensory neurons.[1] For many years it was difficult to confirm with electron microscopy the light microscopy observations of free nerve endings within the epidermis. However, more recent studies have shown evidence of intraepidermal innervation.

To date, the use of conventional light microscopy has not revealed convincing differences in the structure of free nerve endings by which different types of neurons can be identified. Although electron microscopy might reveal such differences,[11] obstacles remain: (a) Because of the thinness of histological sections used in electron microscopy, a great deal of time and effort is required to serially reconstruct the terminals of individual neurons; (b) it appears that cutaneous sensory neurons often terminate in a complex plexus through which it is difficult to trace individual axonal processes; and (c) both myelinated and unmyelinated neurons are unmyelinated at their termination and hence difficult to distinguish under high magnification.

Recent technical advances are likely to further our understanding of cutaneous innervation and the generation of pruritic sensation. First, the advent of immunocytochemical staining shows great promise for enhancing

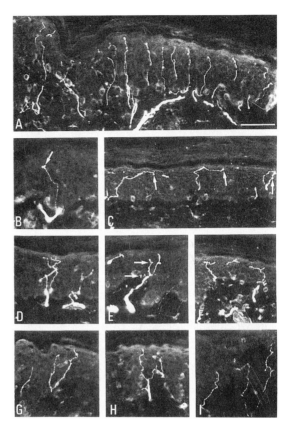

Figure 1-8 PGP 9.5-immunoreactive nerves in human epidermis (indirect immunofluorescence technique). (**A**) Back; (**B–E**) lower leg; (**F**) chest; (**G, H**) upper arm; (**I**) fingertip. Arrows in (**B**) and (**C**) show "knob"-like figures. Arrows in (**E**) show "claw"-like endings. Bar: 50μm.[42] (Reprinted with permission.)

our ability to trace individual cutaneous fibers (Fig. 1-8). A variety of neuropeptides have been discovered in cutaneous nerve fibers such as Substance P, calcitonin gene-related peptide, and vasoactive intestinal peptide.[12–15] Furthermore, neuropeptides seem to exist in different combinations in different nerve fibers, raising the possibility that different populations of sensory neurons might contain different neuropeptide profiles. In the future, immunohistochemical staining techniques may allow subpopulations of unmyelinated neurons to be distinguished reproducibly and hence allow identification of free nerve endings associated with transmission of different sensory qualities (mechano-, thermo-, pain-, and itch-related). For example, recent work from Johansson's lab has shown evidence of proliferation of intraepidermal fibers in patients suffering from pruritus as a consequence of renal dialysis (Fig. 1-9).

Because unmyelinated fibers often form a plexus of neurons (Fig. 1-5), individual neurons are difficult to distinguish and trace in three-dimensional space. Such three-dimensional reconstruction of individual neurons is

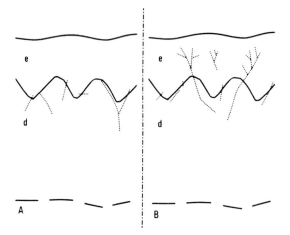

Figure 1-9 Schematic presentation of the NSE-immunoreactive nerve fibers seen in normal (**A**) and uremic (**B**) human skin. In B, the nerve fibers are found sprouting throughout the epidermal layers, but, not penetrating the stratum lucidum. e, epidermis; d, dermis.[43] (Reprinted with permission.)

time-consuming and for the most part is beyond current technologies. Hopefully new digital processing techniques such as confocal microscopy will allow three-dimensional imaging of neural plexes and tracing of individual cutaneous fibers.

Location of Itch-Signaling Nerve Terminals

It is tempting to speculate that the endings of itch-encoding neurons terminate more superficially in the skin than those that signal pain. To review: (a) Low threshold electrical pulses induce itch, while higher intensities produce pain; (b) mild, superficial injury to the skin tends to produce itch, while more intense stimuli of the same type produce pain; (c) some chemicals when applied superficially seem to evoke pruritus-related sensations more frequently than when more deeply administered (e.g., bradykinin, histamine); (d) there was an early report that scotch-tape stripping could eliminate pruritus,[16] however, to my knowledge these results have not been reproduced (Fig. 1-10).

To some extent, these arguments remain unconvincing. To my knowledge, no obvious differences in the physiological characteristics of pruritogen responsive and unresponsive receptors have been observed (such as their mechanical threshold or latency of response to a pulsed thermal stimulus[17]) that might correlate with the depth at which their nerve terminals innervate cutaneous tissue.

Before convincing evidence on the relative depth of pain- and itch-signaling nerve terminals can be obtained, significant problems must be overcome. In addition to the previously discussed difficulties of finding stimuli that produce exclusively itch or pain, there are problems of delivery. For example, although preferential delivery of chemicals to superficial layers of

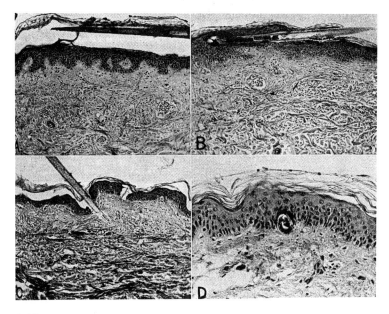

Figure 1-10 Histological estimation of the depth of an itch point in the skin. A cowhage spicule was inserted to a controlled depth and any pruritic response was recorded. Serial sections were then made of a biopsy specimen to determine the depth of spicule penetration. (**A**) Subcorneal insertion of the spicule produced no pruritus, (**B**) intraepidermal insertion produced pruritus, (**C**) superficial vertical insertion of a spicule produced pruritus only at an itch point, and (**D**) insertion of a spicule at the dermoepidermal junction produced maximal pruritus. Deep insertion in the corium was without effect.[41] (Reprinted with permission.)

the skin is attainable, delivery to deeper layers without exposure of superficial layers is difficult to guarantee. For instance, following intradermal injection, fluid is likely to flow out of the needle track to superficial layers. Perhaps it will someday be possible to differentiate itch from pain-signaling neurons histologically and thus answer this question.

ITCH AND PAIN

In response to painful stimuli, cutaneous sensory neurons can evoke a reflex response at the spinal level (i.e., ipsilateral flexion, usually accompanied by contralateral extension) mediated by polysynaptic connections in the spinal cord. Reflex reactions increase with increases in the intensity of painful stimuli.[18] In contrast, itch does not provoke a spinal reflex, suggesting that involvement of suprasegmental neural structures is necessary to generate scratching movements.

In all probability, the sensory information concerning itch is transmitted

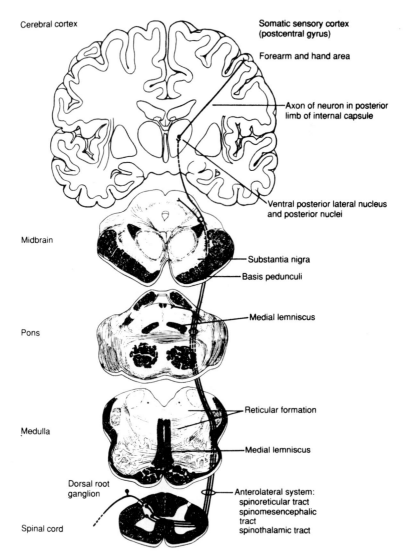

Cerebral cortex

Somatic sensory cortex
(postcentral gyrus)

Forearm and hand area

Axon of neuron in posterior
limb of internal capsule

Ventral posterior lateral nucleus
and posterior nuclei

Midbrain

Substantia nigra

Basis pedunculi

Medial lemniscus

Pons

Reticular formation

Medulla

Medial lemniscus

Dorsal root
ganglion

Anterolateral system:
spinoreticular tract
spinomesencephalic
tract
spinothalamic tract

Spinal cord

Figure 1-11 The anterolateral system, the spinothalamic, spinoreticular, and spinotectal pathways travel through the ventrolateral quadrant of the spinal cord and convey information about pain to several regions of the brain stem and diencephalon.[44] (Reprinted with permission.)

to higher neural centers through pathways similar to those that transmit pain-related information to the sensory cortex (Fig.1-11). Observations of relief of pruritic symptoms[19] and inhibition of experimentally induced pruritus[20] following contralateral ventrolateral cordotomy suggest that in humans the spinothalamic tract (Fig. 1-1, 1-11) is involved in transmission of itch-related information. There is also evidence from our laboratory of cat ventrolateral neurons that are responsive to active cowhage.[21] Because of evidence that spinal pathways outside the ventrolateral quadrant transmit nociception-related information in nonprimate models,[22] the possibility that such pathways might also relay itch-related information in humans cannot be excluded. As with pain, these pathways probably transmit relatively imprecise information about the location of the pruritic stimulus. Execution of the scratching movement may be coordinated by the motor cortex. It would be of interest to investigate whether the motor cortex and other cortical regions involved in generating complex voluntary movements (i.e., the supplementary motor area, premotor cortex, and posterior parietal cortices) are necessary for the generation of efficient scratching behaviors.[23]

Itch has sometimes been regarded as a subquality of pain, especially by investigators who thought sensations resulted from patterning of activity in nerve fibers rather than activation of specific labeled lines of communication within the peripheral and central nervous systems. Gradually, a number of persuasive arguments have accumulated in favor of itch and pain being independent sensory modalities.

1. They evoke unambiguously different motor responses: scratching for itch and withdrawal for pain.
2. An opiate analgesic (morphine) and its antagonist (naloxone) have dichotomous effects on itch and pain. Morphine inhibits pain but can promote itch; in contrast, naloxone is reported to inhibit itch in some subjects while having the ability to lower pain threshold.
3. As discussed in the following section, thresholds for eliciting itch and pain differ. While weak stimuli often promote itch, the same types of stimuli at greater intensity will produce pain.
4. Some authors have suggested that itch-signaling neurons innervate more superficial layers of skin than pain-signaling neurons.[24]
5. Itch and pain reportedly can be felt simultaneously in the same area of skin while varying independently in intensity;[25] or alternatively, itch and pain can be felt in isolation.
6. Gradual reduction in the magnitude of a painful stimulus has been found to reduce, or eliminate, pain without inducing itch.
7. Studies that have directly recorded from peripheral nerve fibers in awake human subjects suggest that itch and pain are encoded by different peripheral receptors.[26]
8. There is no evidence that itch- and pain-related information are transmitted as different patterns of neural activity along the same sensory channel.[26,27]

In summarizing the preceding discussion, it can be seen that there is considerable evidence that the mechanisms for processing of itch- and pain-related information differ. Hence, it is likely that itch and pain are transmitted to higher neural centers by independent sensory channels. This independence is not meant to imply that sensations of itch and pain cannot be modified by one another. For example, it has been known for many years that pain will effectively diminish, or fully inhibit, pruritic sensations.[28] Such inhibition may be similar to counter-irritant mechanisms that have been popularized in the gate control theory of pain (Fig. 1-12). Although it has not been adequately studied, a reciprocal mechanism may exist by which itch can inhibit sensations of pain or irritation. For example, a common experience is the pleasurable sensation of scratching a mosquito bite: The

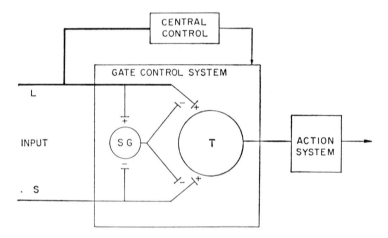

Figure 1-12 Schematic diagram from the original article by Melzack and Wall[48] describing the gate control theory of pain mechanisms in which large diameter (L) and small diameter (S) axonal processes were proposed to project to the substantia gelantinosa (SG) and to a hypothesized central transmission (T) cell population. SG was thought to exert an inhibitory effect on the primary afferent terminals as a result of increased activity in L and/or decreased activity in S. Output from T was to activate neural mechanisms that cause perception and response (+ = excitation; − = inhibition). Hence, SG was to act as a gating mechanism to control the level of afferent input before reaching T[2]. The gate theory proposed that activity in L inhibits synaptic transmission in a system otherwise activated by small afferents carrying the signal for pain. Note that L also projected through the dorsal columns to higher centers, which were thought to act as a "central control trigger" to influence central control mechanisms. These central control mechanisms would in turn project back to the gate-control system through descending pathways. Although the gate-control theory has led to several important clinical applications that are based on the stimulation of large afferent fibers to relieve chronic pain (and which may be of some use in treatment of pruritus[45]), experimental evidence has challenged the basic details of the gate-control circuitry.[2,46] Wall[47] has discussed the need to revise the theory's wiring diagram on the basis of recent neurophysiological evidence.[48] Because "it is doubtful that the gate model continues to be a satisfactory basis for future experiments,"[2] it may not be an appropriate foundation on which to design future experiments on central mechanisms of pruritus.[48] (Reprinted with permission.)

scratching can inflict cutaneous injury which in other circumstances might have been uncomfortable.

For the treatment of pruritic dermatitis, it is important to appreciate that the major differences between chronic itch and pain are to some extent a direct result of the differences in how the central nervous system reacts to these two sensory inputs. For example, a complication of chronic pain can be atrophy of an extremity as a result of the patient's unwillingness to use a limb when movement results in discomfort (e.g., sympathetic reflex dystrophy). On the other hand, in chronic pruritus the incessant desire to scratch can directly lead to significant, mechanically induced injury and to the consequent release of inflammatory mediators that are thought to produce (e.g., histamine) or enhance (e.g., prostaglandins) pruritic sensation. This continued cycle of pruritus and inflammation is often referred to as an itch–scratch cycle. It is one important component of the mechanism by which itch can result in extensive cutaneous injury (e.g., excoriation, secondary eczematization, and lichenification).

MECHANISMS OF CHRONIC PRURITUS

In addition to counter-irritation, there are other parallels between the systems that signal itch and pain. For example, in the pain system the sensitization that occurs in an area of cutaneous injury is referred to as primary hyperalgesia. In this area, the threshold is lowered such that stimuli that were felt as nonpainful prior to injury become algesic. In addition, the area of injury becomes more sensitive to above-threshold stimuli. The area of primary hyperalgesia is surrounded by an area of secondary hyperalgesia that also exhibits lowered threshold and is thought to be produced by mechanisms within the peripheral and central nervous systems.[29]

In an analogous manner, spontaneously itching skin has been reported to be surrounded by an area of "itchy skin."[28] Although itchy skin does not exhibit ongoing pruritus, light brushing evokes pruritic sensations. The mechanism of itchy skin has not been adequately studied but is of theoretical importance in the etiology of chronic pruritus. For example, mild mechanical, and perhaps thermal, stimuli might generate pruritus in an area surrounding a pruritic lesion, causing the pruritic sensation to spread and thereby enlarging the area of scratch-induced injury. In turn, the enlarged area would be surrounded by itchy skin, resulting in a "cascading" spread of itch-related injury. As with painful secondary hyperalgesia, itchy skin is probably due to a combination of mechanisms within the peripheral and central nervous systems.

It is known from the theory of control-system design that without adequate inhibitory feedback, systems often oscillate and become unstable. To state this concept in a different manner, there must be inhibition in order to regulate biological systems. Such inhibition is admirably maintained in the control of biological processes such as arterial blood pressure and plasma hydrogen ion levels. The nervous system participates in these autonomic processes as well as more "conscious" tasks such as the control of motor performance. However, the "motor performance" task of scratching often lacks adequate inhibitory feedback and often results in significant cutaneous injury. Patients sometimes compensate for this lack of inhibition by substituting stimuli such as heat or cold. Even stinging, painful sensations produced by chemicals such as alcohol are often preferable to ongoing pruritus. Of these types of counter-irritation, cold can be argued to be theoretically preferable because it is less likely to produce secondary inflammatory reactions.[30] In addition, sensitization within either the peripheral or central nervous systems could override inhibitory feedback mechanisms and make a significant contribution to the generation of chronic pruritus. Through sensitization, stimuli that are normally nonpruritic, or only mildly itchy, can cause intense pruritus.

It has been often hypothesized that some forms of chronic pruritus could be "cured" if scratching could be continuously inhibited. Such an inhibition could occur at *any point* on the feedback control circuitry responsible for scratch movement: by blocking the input (pruritic sensation), by increasing the inhibition in the system (perhaps through increased levels of pain or irritation), by decreasing the sensitization processes that might occur in either the peripheral or central nervous system, or by making the scratching movement less forceful and thereby less injurious.

AN ITCH CENTER WITHIN THE CENTRAL NERVOUS SYSTEM

Early experiments on animal models suggested that activation of an area within the central nervous system could evoke itch-related behavior. Furthermore, reports over the years of generalized, intractable pruritus as a consequence of tumors or lesions within the central nervous system have tended to support this possibility.[31] More recently, intense pruritus following the use of opiates in epidural anesthesia has been reported.[32] These observations (in combination with reports of pruritus associated with morphine analgesia) support the concept of a central center that can be activated by chemicals transported in either the cerebrospinal fluid or the blood. These observations also reintroduce the concept of divergence in the neuropharmacology of itch- and pain-related neural pathways. The possibility of inducing an antipruritic state by blocking or inhibiting this hypothesized center is intriguing.

CONCLUSION

Most, if not all, neurons that signal pruritus are chemosensitive. At present, animal experiments suggest that the neurons most likely to transmit itch-related information belong to a subpopulation of C-polymodal nociceptive neurons. As shown in Fig. 1-13, cowhage application activates a *subset* of C-polymodal nociceptive neurons in cats. Direct recordings from human C-polymodal neurons have demonstrated that some, but not all, are cowhage sensitive.[33] As discussed earlier, some C-polymodal neurons also respond with greater and greater levels of discharge as the magnitude of noxious thermal (Fig. 1-3) or mechanical stimulation is increased, and hence it is likely that they are involved in signaling pain-related sensations. In this signaling paradigm, the central nervous system would interpret the incoming signal as pruritic when only the pruritogen-responsive subpopulation of

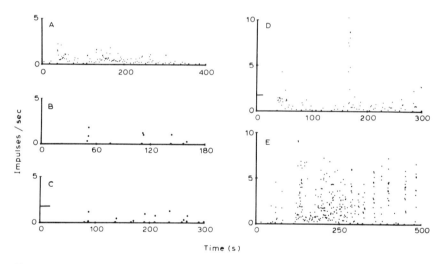

Figure 1-13 Response of two C-polymodal nociceptors to cowhage, with instantaneous frequency (i.e., the reciprocal of the time interval between consecutive action potentials) being plotted versus time. **A** shows the response to active cowhage of a receptor that was silent before stimulation and had no response to inactive cowhage. **B–E** illustrate the behavior of another C-polymodal nociceptor that had some ongoing activity before stimulation (**B**), no significant change in discharge following application of inactive cowhage (**C**), and reactivity to active cowhage (**D**). **E** shows an enhanced response to a second application of cowhage about 7 min. after first group of spicules was removed. The horizontal lines in **C** and **D** represent the time during which cowhage was being applied. Peak instantaneous frequencies evoked while cowhage spicules were being pressed into the skin were 55–63 impulses/sec (not shown in the figure). In **A**, number of spikes (n) = 119; in B, n = 15; in C, n = 20; in D, n = 91; in E, n = 317.[49] (Reprinted with permission.)

polymodal nociceptors is activated. In contrast, when the total population of C-polymodal nociceptive neurons fires, the signal would be experienced as painful. As discussed earlier, there is strong experimental evidence that pain can inhibit sensations of pruritus,[28] which is consistent with this subpopulation hypothesis.

An alternative mechanism for signaling itch postulates the existence of an as-yet undocumented receptor population that is chemosensitive and responds to itch-producing stimuli.[34,35] Because of its insensitivity to mechanical stimuli, these postulated receptors would have been missed in previous studies because they are, by definition, insensitive to mechanical stimuli and hence the receptive field was overlooked when the skin was searched with mechanical stimuli. In fact, the receptive fields of such neurons would be extremely difficult to locate using traditional searching techniques. Investigations are now proceeding in several laboratories to determine whether such an undocumented receptor population might exist.[34,35] Although such receptors might contribute to signaling the sensation of pruritus, it must be remembered that discrete mechanical stimuli when properly administered can also evoke unambiguous sensations of pruritus. Hence, any complete model for encoding pruritus should include recruitment of a mechanically sensitive neuronal population.

REFERENCES

1. Rothman S: Physiology of itching. *Physiol Rev* 21:357–381, 1941.
2. Willis WD, Coggeshall RE: *Sensory Mechanisms of the Spinal Cord,* 2d ed. New York, Plenum Press, 1991.
3. Nordin M: Low-threshold mechanoreceptive and nociceptive units with unmyelinated (C) fibres in the human supraorbital nerve. *J Physiol* 426:229–240, 1990.
4. Saumet J-L, Chery-Croze S, Duclaux R: Response of cat skin mechanothermal nociceptors to cold stimulation. *Brain Res Bull* 15:529–532, 1985.
5. Bessou P, Perl ER: Response of cutaneous sensory units with unmyelinated fibers to noxious stimuli. *J Neurophysiol* 32:1025–1043, 1969.
6. Adriaensen H, Gybels J, Handwerker HO, et al: Response properties of thin myelinated (A-δ) fibers in human skin nerves. *J Neurophysiol* 49:111–122, 1983.
7. Kenins P: The functional anatomy of the receptive fields of rabbit C polymodal nociceptors. *J Neurophysiol* 59:1098–1115, 1988.
8. Lewis T, Grant RT, Marvin HM: Vascular reactions of the skin to injury. Part X: The intervention of a chemical stimulus illustrated especially by the flare. The response to faradism. *Heart* 14:139–160, 1927.
9. Heyer G, Hornstein OP, Handwerker HO: Skin reactions and itch sensation induced by epicutaneous histamine application in atopic dermatitis and controls. *J Invest Dermatol* 93:492–496, 1989.
10. Simone DA, Ngeow JYF, Whitehouse J, et al: The magnitude and duration of itch produced by intracutaneous injections of histamine. *Somatosens Mot Res* 5:81–92, 1987.
11. Cauna N: Fine morphological changes in the penicillate nerve endings of human hairy skin during prolonged itching. *Anat Rec* 188:1–12, 1977.

12. Johansson O, Vaalasti A, Tainio H, et al: Immunohistochemical evidence of galanin in sensory nerves of human digital skin. *Acta Physiol Scand* 132:261–263, 1988.
13. Weihe E, Hartschuh W: Multiple peptides in cutaneous nerves: Regulators under physiological conditions and a pathogenic role in skin disease? *Semin Dermatol* 7:284–300, 1988.
14. Brain SD, Williams TJ: Neuropharmacology of peptides in skin. *Semin Dermatol* 7:278–283, 1988.
15. Ishida-Yamamoto A, Senba E, Tohyama M: Distribution and fine structure of calcitonin gene-related peptide-like immunoreactive nerve fibers in the rat skin. *Brain Res* 491:93–101, 1989.
16. Shelley WB, Arthur RP: Studies on cowhage (Mucuna pruriens) and its pruritogenic proteinase, Mucunain. *Arch Dermatol* 72:399–406, 1955.
17. Meyer RA, Campbell JN: Evidence for two distinct classes of unmyelinated nociceptive afferents in monkey. *Brain Res* 224:149–152, 1981.
18. Carew TJ: The control of reflex action, in Kandel ER, Schwartz JH (eds): *Principles of Neural Science*, 2d ed New York, Elsevier. 1985, Chap. 35.
19. White JC, Sweet WH, Hawkins R, et al: Anterolateral cordotomy: Results, complications and causes of failure. *Brain* 73:346–367, 1950.
20. Hyndman OR, Wolkin J: Anterior chordotomy. Further observations on physiologic results and optimum manner of performance. *Arch Neurol Psychiat* 50:129–148, 1943.
21. Wei JY, Tuckett RP: Response of cat ventrolateral spinal axons to an itch-producing substance (cowhage). *Somatosens Mot Res* 8:227–239, 1991.
22. Hammond DL: New insights regarding organization of spinal cord pain pathways. *NIPS* 4:98–101, 1989.
23. Ghez C: Voluntary movement, in Kandel ER, Schwartz JH (eds): *Principles of Neural Science*, 2d ed New York, Elsevier. 1985, Chap 38.
24. Graham DT, Goodell H, Wolff HG: Neural mechanisms involved in itch, "itchy skin" and tickle sensations. *J Clin Invest* 30:37–49, 1951.
25. Keele CA, Armstrong D: *Substances Producing Pain and Itch.* Baltimore, Williams and Wilkins, 1964.
26. Torebjörk HE, Ochoa JL: Pain and itch from C-fiber stimulation. *Soc Neurosci Abstr* 6:428, 1980.
27. Tuckett RP: Itch evoked by electrical stimulation of the skin. *J Invest Dermatol* 79:368–373, 1982.
28. Bickford RG: Experiments relating to the itch sensation, its peripheral mechanism and central pathways. *Clin Sci* 3:377–386, 1938.
29. Raja SN, Meyer RA, Campbell JN: Peripheral mechanisms of somatic pain. *Anesthesiology* 68:571–590, 1988.
30. Fruhstorfer H, Hermanns M, Latzke L: The effects of thermal stimulation on clinical and experimental itch. *Pain* 24:259–269, 1986.
31. King CA, Huff FJ, Jorizzo JL: Unilateral neurogenic pruritus: Paroxysmal itching associated with central nervous system lesions. *Ann Int Med* 97:222–223, 1982.
32. Scott PV, Fischer HBJ: Spinal opiate analgesia and facial pruritus: A neural theory. *Postgrad Med J* 58:531–535, 1982.
33. Torebjörk HE: Afferent C units responding to mechanical, thermal and chemical stimuli in human non-glabrous skin. *Acta Physiol Scand* 92:374–390, 1974.
34. Meyer RA, Campbell JN: A novel electrophysiological technique for locating cutaneous nociceptive and chemospecific receptors. *Brain Res* 441:81–86, 1988.
35. LaMotte RH, Simone DA, Baumann TK, et al: Hypothesis for novel classes of chemoreceptors mediating chemogenic pain and itch, in Dubner R, Gebhart GF, Bond MR (eds): *Proceedings of the Vth World Congress on Pain.* New York, Elsevier Science Publishers BV, 1988, pp. 529–535.

36. Bernhard JD: Cutaneous sensation and the pathophysiology of pruritus, in Soter NA, Baden HP (eds): *Pathophysiology of Dermatologic Diseases,* 2d ed New York, McGraw-Hill, 1991, Chap 6.
37. Papez JW: *Comparative Neurology.* New York, Thomas Y. Crowell, 1929.
38. Beck PW, Handwerker HO, Zimmermann M: Nervous outflow from the cat's foot during noxious radiant heat stimulation. *Brain Res* 67:373–386, 1974.
39. Kruger L, Perl ER, Sedivec MJ: Fine structure of myelinated mechanical nociceptor endings in cat hairy skin. *J Comp Neurol* 198:137–154, 1981.
40. Hägermark Ö, Hökfelt T, Pernow B: Flare and itch induced by substance P in human skin. *J Invest Dermatol* 71:233–235, 1978.
41. Shelley WB, Arthur RP: The neurohistology and neurophysiology of the itch sensation in man. *Arch Dermatol* 76:296–323, 1957.
42. Wang L, Hilliges M, Jernberg T, et al: Protein gene product 9.5-immunoreactive nerve fibres and cells in human skin. *Cell Tissue Res* 261:25–33, 1990.
43. Johansson O, Hilliges M, Ståhle-Bäckdahl M: Intraepidermal neuron-specific enolase (NSE)-immunoreactive nerve fibres: Evidence for sprouting in uremic patients on maintenance hemodialysis. *Neurosci Lett* 99:281–286, 1989.
44. Kelly DD: Central representations of pain and analgesia, in Kandel ER, Schwartz JH (eds): *Principles of Neural Science,* 2d ed New York, Elsevier, 1985, Chap 26.
45. Ekblom A, Fjellner B, Hansson P: The influence of mechanical vibratory stimulation and transcutaneous electrical nerve stimulation on experimental pruritus induced by histamine. *Acta Physiol Scand* 122:361–367, 1984.
46. Nathan PW: The gate-control theory of pain. A critical review. *Brain* 99:123–158, 1976.
47. Wall PD: The gate control theory of pain mechanisms. A re-examination and re-statement. *Brain* 101:1–18, 1978.
48. Melzack R, Wall PD: Pain mechanisms: A new theory. *Science* 150:971–979, 1965.
49. Tuckett RP, Wei JY: Response to an itch-producing substance in cat. II. Cutaneous receptor populations with unmyelinated axons. *Brain Res* 413:95–103, 1987.

CHEMICAL MEDIATORS OF ITCHING

Ethan A. Lerner

INTRODUCTION

Mediators of pruritus presumably act on nerve fibers or lead to a cascade whose final common pathway of nerve stimulation is interpreted in the central nervous system as itching (Fig. 2-1). Knowledge of chemical mediators has changed over time reflecting the different classes of molecules that have been discovered. While histamine was described in the 1920s, the role of proteinases in biology in general and pruritus specifically gained attention in the 1950s with advances in biochemistry. The 1960s and 1970s saw the rise of leukotrienes and prostaglandins, the products of arachidonic acid metabolism. In the 1970s and early 1980s the endorphins and enkephalins received substantial attention. With the techniques of molecular biology, the 1980s and 1990s have become the era of signal transduction, cytokines, and growth factors. Studies in all of these areas provide new molecules and concepts. Combined with advances in the cell biology of eosinophils, mast cells, nerves, and other components of the dermis and epidermis, ideas concerning the physiology of pruritus abound.

It is simple to define a mediator of itch: An itch mediator is a substance the introduction into the skin of which induces the sensation of itching and the urge to scratch. While a number of substances satisfy this definition, which of these, other than histamine, is physiologically relevant is not known. Complexity and difficulty arise because experimental systems to investigate itch are extremely limited and because no acceptable animal or in vitro models exist. While it may be convenient to test putative mediators by injecting them into the skin of a laboratory animal, we do not know how to

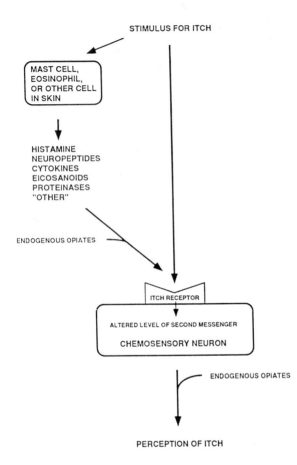

STIMULUS FOR ITCH

MAST CELL,
EOSINOPHIL,
OR OTHER CELL
IN SKIN

HISTAMINE
NEUROPEPTIDES
CYTOKINES
EICOSANOIDS
PROTEINASES
"OTHER"

ENDOGENOUS OPIATES

ITCH RECEPTOR

ALTERED LEVEL OF SECOND MESSENGER

CHEMOSENSORY NEURON

ENDOGENOUS OPIATES

PERCEPTION OF ITCH

Figure 2-1 Chemical mediators of pruritus. Some molecules may act directly on the itch receptor (vertical arrow). Most pruritogens act indirectly by inducing the release of substances from cells in the skin which then act on the itch receptor. Endogenous opiates may modify peripheral and central sensations of pruritus. The itch receptor is depicted on an unmyelinated chemosensory neuron. Stimulation of the receptor, which is coupled to a signal transduction pathway, presumably leads to an alteration in the level of a second messenger with resultant activation of the neuron.

ask the animal if it has an urge to scratch and scratching may be a reflex response provoked by "irritation" rather than "itch." In addition, not all itching need involve chemical mediators in the periphery; it is possible that mechanical irritants, such as wool, may lead to direct stimulation of itch-perceiving nerve fibers without the involvement of a chemical mediator.

Two independent observations indicate that the epidermis is important in itch. First, its removal abolishes the sensation of itch.[1] Second, experiments performed in the 1950s revealed that spicules of the legume *Mucuna pruriens,* the active component of itch powder, induced the most itching when inserted into the epidermis rather than into the dermis.[2] These observations suggest that itch receptors are located superficially in the skin—consistent with the location of free nerve endings in the epidermis. It is thus reasonable to consider the epidermis as one source of mediators. Substances can also diffuse or be carried from the dermis and stimulate nerve endings in the

Table 2-1 Potential chemical mediators of pruritus

Amines
  histamine*
  serotonin
  adrenaline
  noradrenaline
  melatonin
  dopamine

Proteases
  tryptases
  chymases
  carboxypeptidases
  papain
  kallikrein

Neuropeptides (including tachykinins)
  Substance P*
  Substance K
  calcitonin
  calcitonin gene-related peptide (CGRP)
  endothelin*
  vasoactive intestinal peptide (VIP)
  neurotensin
  cholecystokinin (CCK)
  α-melanocyte stimulating hormone
    (α-MSH)
  γ-melanocyte stimulating hormone
    (γ-MSH)
  neurokinin A
  neurokinin B
  eledoisin
  physalaemin
  bombesin
  bradykinin
  somatostatin
  corticotropin-releasing hormone

Opioids
  met-enkephalin*
  leu-enkephalin*
  β-endorphin*
  morphine

Eicosanoids
  LTC_4
  LTD_4
  LTE_4
  LTB_4
  PGD_2
  PGE_1
  PGE_2*
  $PGF_{2\alpha}$
  PGH_2*

Growth Factors and Cytokines
Growth factors
  epidermal growth factor (EGF)
  acidic and basic fibroblast growth factors
    (FGFs)
  nerve growth factor (NGF)
  platelet-derived growth factor (PDGF)
  transforming growth factors α and β
    (TGF-α, TGF-β)
  insulin-like growth factors (somatomedins)
  erythropoietin
  Colony stimulating factors (CSFs)
    granulocyte-macrophage-CSF (GM-CSF)
    granulocyte-CSF (G-CSF)
    macrophage-CSF (M-CSF)

Cytokines

  Interleukins
    IL-1 to IL-11

  Tumor necrosis factors (TNF)
    TNF-α (cachectin)
    TNF-β (lymphotoxin)

  Eosinophil products
    major basic protein (MBP)
    eosinophil cationic protein
    eosinophil-derived neurotoxin
    eosinophil peroxidase

  Platelet activating factor (PAF)

A (*) indicates substances for which a role in pruritus has been strongly suggested. This list gives the reader an idea of the kinds of molecules in the skin that biologists are studying. In the future, it is likely that some of these substances will be proven to be mediators or modulators of itch.

epidermis. Chemical mediators could also stimulate areas of the central nervous system in such a way that the sensation of itch occurs in the absence of peripheral stimulation. The remainder of this chapter focuses on potential itch mediators individually. The known or suspected chemical mediators of pruritus are listed in Table 2-1 with selected descriptions in the text.

BIOGENIC AMINES—HISTAMINE

In 1927, histamine was shown to be a natural constituent of tissue, hence the name from the Greek word for tissue, histos.[3] Histamine is released during mast cell degranulation and mediates its effects in the skin via H_1 receptors. H_2 receptors have not been demonstrated in skin. The effects of histamine, either from mast cell degranulation or injection, include the triple response described by Lewis in 1927:

1. Localized red spot around the injection site due to local dilatation of capillaries, venules, and terminal arterioles.
2. Brighter red flush or flare extending one or more centimeters beyond the red spot arising from widespread dilatation of arterioles mediated by a local axon reflex.
3. Wheal developing within 1 1/2 minutes at the site of the red spot, resulting from histamine-induced vascular permeability.

Histamine is considered the prototypic chemical mediator of itch. While intradermal injections cause pain, intraepidermal injection of less than 10ug in a volume of 0.1ml produces itch within 30 seconds. The reason for the delayed response is not clear.[4] It either takes time for histamine to diffuse to the nerve endings or histamine induces the release of another substance that leads to nerve stimulation.

The main argument in favor of a direct role for histamine in itching is the effectiveness of antihistamines (H_1) on pruritus associated with urticaria. Against a direct role for histamine in itching is the poor clinical response to antihistamines in patients with pruritus who do not have urticaria. For example, aside from their soporific effect, antihistamines are not effective in patients with underlying systemic diseases such as biliary cirrhosis, renal failure, or in patients with nonurticarial skin diseases such as psoriasis and lichen planus. A recent report demonstrated a decrease in both plasma histamine levels and pruritus in renal failure patients treated with erythropoietin but this correlation does not prove a relationship between histamine levels and pruritus.[5] From the laboratory standpoint, as decreasing doses of histamine are injected into skin, the sensation of itch is lost before wheal formation is lost. The combination of these clinical and laboratory observations argue against an important role for histamine as a direct chemical mediator of itch. Nonetheless, it will be noted that the majority of compounds discussed in this chapter, and implicated as itch mediators, are associated with wheal and flare responses, suggesting that they are not primary itch mediators but inducers of histamine release.

The injection of serotonin produces a painful, pricking itch only in some people and the sensation is not as marked as that from histamine.[6] This result suggests that serotonin, by itself, is not a significant pruritogen. Other amines, including adrenaline, noradrenaline, and melatonin, have been demonstrated to affect pain fibers in cutaneous tissues but their effect on pruritus has not been thoroughly examined (Table 2-1).

PROTEINASES AND KININS

The itch-inducing capacities of a number of proteinases have been examined (Table 2-1). Investigations during the 1950s suggested that endopeptidases, which cleave peptide bonds within proteins, as opposed to exopeptidases, which cleave at the ends of proteins, were mediators of pruritus. The injection of trypsin or chymotrypsin produces intense itch associated with a triple response. These effects are inhibited by antihistamines, suggesting mediation by histamine release. The painful, pricking effect from papain, a proteinase, and kallikrein, a kinin, is not associated with a triple response and not affected by antihistamines. This observation suggests that they could be important itch mediators. However, as heat inactivates the proteolytic properties of papain, while the itch-inducing property remains, itch induced by proteolysis may not be a tenable hypothesis.[7] If proteinases are mediators of pruritus, it is possible that they function by damaging nerve terminals, resulting in nerve stimulation and the subsequent sensation of itch.

Interesting observations have been made from studies of the source of "itching powder." Itching powder is derived from spicules of *Mucuna pruriens,* or cowhage. The spicules produce intense itching on insertion into the skin. In the 1950s, Shelley and Arthur experimented with spicules of this tropical plant, showed that insertion to the level of the dermal–epidermal (D–E) junction was critical for itch production, and suggested that the itch-inducing component was an endopeptidase which they named mucunain.[2] (See Figs. 1-7 and 1-10.) Given the limitations of the time, mucunain was not isolated in pure form nor thoroughly characterized. While not an endogenous mediator of pruritus, mucunain may be a direct mediator of pruritus: There is no associated erythema or edema, and the spicules function at the level of the D–E junction. Additional studies using this plant could shed light on the mysteries of pruritus.

NEUROPEPTIDES

As the sensation of pruritus is carried by nerves it is reasonable to consider the role of neuropeptides as itch mediators. With the growth of neurobiology, new neuropeptides have been discovered and some previously known peptides have come to be considered part of the neuropeptide family. For example, cholecystokinin and vasoactive intestinal peptide, both associated with the gastrointestinal tract, also function as neurotransmitters and play roles in the central nervous system. Table 2-1 lists a representative selection of neuropeptides, some of which are discussed in more detail later.

Substance P was discovered in 1931 by Von Euler who identified it as a hypotensive and smooth muscle contracting *Substance* in *P*reparations of brain and intestine. It is a member of the tachykinin family, which consists of structurally similar peptides originally identified in frog skin. The distribution of Substance P is widespread, including dorsal root ganglia, substantia gelatinosa, cornea, dental pulp, sympathetic ganglia, adrenal medulla, papillary dermis and possibly the epidermis. As Substance P is a potent itch and triple response inducer, its itch effects are probably mediated by the release of histamine. This conclusion is consistent with the observation that the pruritic effect of Substance P can be blocked by the prior administration of oral antihistamines.[6]

The importance of Substance P in neurophysiology and pain has been examined extensively in studies beginning in the 1960s using capsaicin, the substance that causes the hot taste of pepper plants of the genus *Capsicum*.[8] It was noted that topical or oral administration of capsaicin in a variety of animal models led to alterations in the neurophysiology and biochemical processes of sensory neurons. Close examination revealed that neonatal administration of capsaicin resulted in the degeneration and loss of type C sensory fibers. Administration of capsicum to adult animals results in the depletion of Substance P from nerve endings and or damage to unmyelinated type C fibers with eventual decreased sensitivity to capsicum and other noxious stimuli. Topical application of capsicum to humans causes burning, pain, and itching. Repeated application results in decreased sensation of pain but not pin prick, touch, or temperature. Itch, following the injection of histamine, remains but the axon reflex vasodilatation or flare disappears. While it is reasonable to believe that the application of capsicum depletes Substance P from nerve endings, little is known of its effects on calcitonin gene-related peptide (CGRP), endothelin or other neuropeptides (see next section). Substance P may not be "the" mediator of itch but studies with capsicum and its effects on neuropeptides in skin provide an approach to the pathophysiology of pruritus.

CGRP and endothelin are two recently discovered peptides that may have a role in pruritus. CGRP is a peptide the existence of which was predicted by molecular biologists studying transcripts of the calcitonin gene.[9] Downstream of the calcitonin gene was a piece of DNA that "looked" like it would code for an as yet undiscovered peptide. Biochemical analysis led to the discovery of CGRP and its presence in various tissues including the central nervous system, where it functions as a neurotransmitter. CGRP is also present, together with Substance P, in unmyelinated sensory nerves of the skin. CGRP is a potent endogenous vasodilator the release of which is linked to or controlled by Substance P.[10] Intradermal injection of CGRP creates a macular area of long-lasting erythema associated with pseudopods but no itching. Recent studies reveal that CGRP is also an immunomodulating agent capable of preventing the activation of macrophages and, by analogy, Langerhans cells in the skin.[11] Given that this 37 amino acid long peptide can affect the nervous, cardiovascular, and immune systems a possible role in pruritus would not be surprising.

Endothelin is a 21 amino acid peptide discovered in 1988 and shown to be both a neurotransmitter and a potent vasoconstrictor.[12] It appears that a major function of endothelin and CGRP is the regulation of peripheral vascular tone. In addition, the injection of endothelin into skin has been associated with mild itching in the absence of other clinical findings, indicating a potential role in pruritus.[13] In clinical conditions such as Raynaud's phenomenon blood vessels are constricted while in other conditions vessels may be dilated. These phenomena may result from alterations in the levels of CGRP or endothelin. Thus, it would be of interest to determine if itching is altered in these conditions.

The effects on inflammation of other neuropeptides, including somatostatin and Substance P, is now being investigated. The developing field of neuroimmunocutaneous biology should provide new insights in the area of pruritus.

OPIOIDS

Morphine has long been known to relieve pain and one might have expected that morphine would have a beneficial effect on itch. Ironically, morphine does not relieve pruritus and in some patients induces intractable itching. Although morphine induces histamine release from mast cells, it does not induce a triple response. Antihistamines, which work by blocking the interaction of histamine with its receptor, do not prevent or relieve morphine-induced itch. How to reconcile the combined observations of itching, histamine release, lack of a triple response, and lack of effectiveness of antihistamines is not clear. Perhaps the morphine-induced release of histamine from mast cells is physiologically irrelevant and the pruritus induced by morphine results from a modulatory effect on peripheral nerves or the perception of sensation in the central nervous system.

In an effort to examine these phenomena, the effects of endogenous opioids, the enkephalins and endorphins, as well as opiate antagonists such as naloxone, have been examined[6,14] (Table 2-1). Endogenous opioids are felt to be involved in the control of pain. When injected into skin they are mildly, if at all, pruritogenic, but they potentiate histamine-induced itch.

Systemic injection of naloxone has been reported to relieve intractable itch.[14] In addition, histamine-provoked itch is diminished or abolished by prior injection of naloxone. However, the intradermal administration of naloxone does not relieve the opioid-induced potentiation of itch from histamine. To further complicate this confusing picture involving opioids, it should be noted that there are different classes of opiate receptors. As different opiates or antagonists interact differentially with these receptors, a variety of effects might be predicted. Once opiate receptors are cloned, it should be possible to examine individual classes of such receptors in isolation in vitro, or in animal models and decipher the relationship between opiates, opiate antagonists, and histamine.

EICOSANOIDS

Eicosanoids are the biologically active products of arachidonic acid metabolism and include prostaglandins, leukotrienes, thromboxane, and prostacyclin. Because these compounds are important in allergic, immune, and vascular phenomena, it is reasonable to assess their role in pruritus (Table 2-1). A number of prostaglandins produce mild itching on injection, probably from histamine release. Potentiation of histamine-induced itch has been demonstrated for PGE_2 and PGH_2.[6] The leukotrienes B_4, C_4, D_4, and E_4 produce erythema and wheal formation following injection into skin but itching has not been described.[15] Thromboxane and prostacyclin have not been specifically studied as potential itch mediators. As mast cells are known to produce many components of acachidonic metabolism and these cells may be important in the biology of pruritus, it is possible that these components synergize with other pruritogens. The fact that inhibitors of prostaglandin synthesis, such as salicylates and indomethacin, do not alter the sensation of pruritus argues against a major role for these compounds in pruritus.

GROWTH FACTORS AND CYTOKINES

A nonexhaustive list of peptide growth factors, cytokines, and interleukins is included in Table 2-1. As of yet, none of these peptides has been shown to induce or prevent pruritus.[6] The reason to include them is that with molecular, biochemical, and immunologic advances, an ever increasing number of molecules are being found in the skin.[16] Some of these molecules individually or in combination may turn out to be important mediators of pruritus. A developing concept of sensory neurons stimulated by chemical mediators, as opposed to touch or stretch, leads to the suggestion that some of the numerous molecules associated with the inflammatory cascade could be mediators of pruritus, in the absence of overt inflammation.

BILE SALTS

Pruritus associated with cholestasis has long been recognized clinically. Patients who have cholestasis include those with primary biliary cirrhosis and some pregnant women who itch. Reviews of pruritus invariably discuss the possibility that bile acids or bile salts present in the skin mediate this itch but no correlation exists between bile salt levels in skin and the degree of pruritus.[17] Ghent has suggested that bile salts lead to itching indirectly by damaging hepatocyte membranes and causing the release of a pruritic substance (discussed in detail in Chap. 16).

It is time for a new theory and mediator to explain the pruritus of cholestasis. Recent studies suggest that the endogenous opiate agonists metenkephalin and leu-enkephalin accumulate in cholestasis. It is also known that opiates induce pruritus and a few studies have shown that opiate antagonists can precipitate an opiate-like withdrawal state and reduce pruritus in patients with primary biliary cirrhosis. Perhaps the pruritus of cholestasis, and perhaps many other conditions, is caused by elevated levels of endogenous opiates.[18]

EOSINOPHILS

Previous sections have focused on molecules without regard to the cells that produce them. The eosinophil is singled out here because of its products and because, in a variety of conditions in which pruritus is often a prominent feature, including drug allergies, bullous pemphigoid, and certain parasitic diseases such as onchocerciasis and scabies infestations, a peripheral eosinophilia is noted and eosinophils are found in skin biopsies. To the consternation of some physicians, the number of eosinophils present in skin biopsies has not been correlated with the degree of pruritus. Recent investigations suggest an explanation for the sometime paucity of tissue eosinophils: The eosinophils may no longer be visible because of degranulation.[19] Deposition of major basic protein (MBP) and other eosinophil products from secretory granules occurs in atopic dermatitis, urticaria, and other conditions. Elevated serum levels of MBP have been found in patients with peripheral eosinophilia. Platelet activating factor (PAF), produced by many cells, is a potent eosinophil chemoattractant. Eosinophils also produce PAF and its release could function in a local autocrine loop to recruit more eosinophils. Interleukin 5 (IL-5) and the complement components C3a and C5a are additional eosinophil chemoattractants. Perhaps PAF, IL-5, complement components, or one of the eosinophil products is a mediator of pruritus.

POTENTIAL CELLULAR SOURCES OF MEDIATORS OF PRURITUS

Keratinocytes, Langerhans cells, Merkel cells, melanocytes, mast cells, basophils, lymphocytes, endothelial cells, and fibroblasts are all either resident in the skin or attracted to the skin by a variety of chemoattractants and adhesion molecules. They are sources of a vast number of molecules, including most of those listed in the table of this chapter. While listed for completeness, undoubtedly one or more of these types of cells, in addition to eosinophils, produce products that singly or in combination cause itching (Fig. 2-1). For example, mast cells are present in the advancing edge of lesions of scleroderma or morphea and lesions of scleroderma and morphea often itch.[20] Does a mast cell product other than histamine cause the pruritus? Likewise, are mast cells, sometimes prominent in healing wounds, responsible for the pruritus that sometimes occurs during the healing phase of a wound?

PRURITIC MEDIATORS FROM THE OUTSIDE WORLD

Itching induced by contact with plants and insects results in much morbidity but has generated little scientific study.[21] Decades-old work on the spicules from cowhage was described earlier in this chapter. Few investigations have been performed on insect products to determine which may mediate pruritus or how they do it.

There are four ways insects may impart trouble to us: (1) direct contact via urticating hairs, wing scales, feces, or silk; (2) bite, with injection of digestive or salivary juices; (3) stinging, with resultant venom injection; (4) active projection of defensive secretions. Lepidopterism is the general term used to describe the ill effects that larval and adult butterflies and moths can have on us. Larva of the browntail moth *Eupterotidae chrysorrhoea* contain two million setae per caterpillar and are a source of a major pruritic problem in Europe for which no treatment exists. Chemical analysis of nettling hairs has revealed proteolytic activity but more detailed analyses are lacking. Caterpillars of the gypsy moth (family: Lymantriidae) caused thousands of cases of pruritic dermatitis in New England in the spring of 1981.[21a] The Hylesia moth (family: Saturniidae) is the source of "Caripito itch." A variety of flies (order: Diptera), mites, such as *Sarcoptes scabii* (family: Acari) and other insects have long been associated with pruritus, usually associated with delayed type hypersensitivity (DTH), or urticaria, presumably from histamine release—but few of the details of the reactions have been defined. Many of the chemicals ejected by insects have been described and include alcohols, aldehydes, alkaloids, carboxylic acids, esters, lactones, hydrocarbons, phenols, quinones, steroids and other miscellaneous compounds.

SIGNAL TRANSDUCTION AND PRURITUS

The first chapter of this volume discussed the neurophysiology of itch and the associated neuroanatomical pathways. This chapter has focused on potential itch mediators with no discussion of the physiological mechanism of action. The past decade has witnessed an explosion of information on the mechanisms through which chemicals and cells communicate. Typically, a chemical or ligand binds to a cell surface receptor which in turn transduces a signal to the inside of the cell, initiating a cascade of events. Hormone action and vision are two of many physiological processes that are coupled to such receptors. A number of receptor classes have been recognized, including G-protein coupled receptors, those coupled to inositol triphosphates and calcium, and those associated with tyrosine kinases. It is likely that the final common pathway of pruritus is triggered via one of these receptors present on afferent nerves. Support for this hypothesis comes from the recent identification of primary afferent nerves that respond to inflammatory and chemical signals[22] (Table 2-1). A mediator of pruritus could thus be a substance that directly affects a receptor on nervous tissue or leads to the release of a substance that does. Perhaps proteinases exert their effects by damaging a cell-surface receptor such that the conformation of the receptor is altered in a fashion analogous to being bound by its normal ligand.

THEORETICAL RELATIONSHIP OF PRURITUS TO DISEASE

Any disease, be it associated with infection, inflammation, tumor, or metabolic abnormalities, involves the generation and interaction of a large number of substances from exogenous and cellular sources. It is likely that some of these substances, acting singly or in combination, initiate or take part in a cascade that leads to stimulation of unmyelinated fibers in the skin with the resultant sensation of itching (Fig. 2-1). For example, the intense inflammatory infiltrate observed in lichen planus is a rich source of locally acting potential pruritic mediators. As some patients with lichen planus or other inflammatory diseases do not itch the balance of mediators in such patients must differ from that of a pruritic patient. An alternative explanation is that the response to the same balance of mediators differs between the pruritic and nonpruritic patients. This response may be genetically determined or it may be that the perception of itch simply differs between people. Consider also the observation that rashes appear where they do, typically sparing large areas of skin. Only the involved areas itch, presumably the result of a local alteration of mediators. In contrast, in systemic diseases, such as renal, liver, or other metabolic disorders, pruritus is generalized, consistent with a diffusible or long-lived mediator of pruritus. Such mediators may act at any level from the skin to the brain. In the pruritus associated with iron deficiency, perhaps a substance that suppresses pruritus is lacking, such as iron (see Chap. 17). If this hypothesis regarding itching in systemic disease is correct, then it should be feasible to develop a laboratory test for levels of pruritogens in systemic disease which may lead to therapies that affect patient comfort, and, it is to be hoped, the disease process.

CONCLUSIONS

Inquiries into the nature of chemical mediators of pruritus have been few. This statement may sound disappointing but must be viewed within the context of exciting advances in biomedical science in recent decades. Scientists in diverse fields have only recently begun to find and sort the myriad molecules that interact to make the human body work. Some of these compounds, or soon to be described compounds, are mediators of pruritus. We have barely scratched the surface of a problem for which the time is ripe to find an answer.

REFERENCES

1. Rothman S: Pathophysiology of itch sensation, in William Montagna (ed.) *Advances in Biology of Skin,* vol 1. New York, Pergamon Press. 1960, pp 189–201.
2. Shelley W, Arthur R: The neurohistology and neurophysiology of the itch sensation in man. *Arch Dermatol* 76:296–323, 1957.
3. Lewis T: *The Blood Vessels of the Human Skin and Their Responses.* London, Shaw & Sons. 1927.
4. Simone DA, Alreja M, LaMotte RH: Psychophysical studies of the itch sensation and itchy skin ("alloknesis") produced by intracutaneous injection of histamine. *Somatosen Mot Res* 8:271–329, 1991.
5. Marchi SD, Cedchin E, Villalta D, et al: Relief of pruritus and decreases in plasma histamine concentrations during erythropoietin therapy in patients with uremia. *N Engl J Med* 326:969–974, 1992.
6. Hagermark Ö: Peripheral and central mediators of itch. *Skin Pharmacol* 5:1–8, 1992.
7. Monash S, Woessner J: Pruritus and proteolytic enzymes. *Arch Dermatol* 78:214–217, 1958.

8. Buck SH, Bruks TF: The neuropharmacology of capsaicin: Review of some recent observations. *Pharmacol Rev* 38:179–226, 1986.

9. Amara SG, Jonas V, Rosenfeld MG, et al: Alternative RNA processing in calcitonin gene expression generates mRNAs encoding different polypeptide products. *Nature* 298:240–244, 1982.

10. Brain SD, Williams TJ: Substance P regulates the vasodilator activity of calcitonin gene-related peptide. *Nature* 335:73–75, 1988.

11. Nong Y, Titus RG, Ribeiro JMC, et al: Peptides encoded by the calcitoinin gene inhibit macrophage function. *J Immunol* 143:45–49, 1989.

12. Yanagisawa M, Kurihara H, Kimura S, et al: A potent vasoconstrictor peptide produced by vascular endothelial cells. *Nature* 332:411–415, 1988.

13. Ferreira SH, Romitelli M, Nucci G de: Endothelin-1 participation in overt and inflammatory pain. *J Cardiovasc Pharmcol* 12:S220–222, 1989.

14. Bernstein J, Swift R, Soltani K, et al: Antipruritic effect on an opiate antagonist, naloxone hydrochloride. *J Invest Dermatol* 78:82–83, 1982.

15. Soter NA, Lewis RA, Corey EJ, et al: Local effects of synthetic leukotrienes (LTC$_4$, LTD$_4$, LTE$_4$, and LTB$_4$) in human skin. *J Invest Dermatol* 80:115–119, 1983.

16. Luger TA, Schwarz T: Therapeutic uses of cytokines in dermatology. *J Am Acad Dermatol* 24:915–926, 1991.

17. Herndon JH: Pathophysiology of pruritus associated with elevated bile acid levels in serum. *Arch Intern Med* 130:632–637, 1972.

18. Jones EA, Bergasa NV: The pruritus of cholestasis: From bile acids to opiate agonists. *Hepatology* 11:884–887, 1990.

19. Leiferman KM: A current perspective on the role of eosinophils in dermatologic disease. *J Am Acad Dermatol* 24:1101–1112, 1991.

20. Claman HN: On scleroderma. Mast cells, endothelial cells, and fibroblasts. *JAMA* 262:1206–1209, 1989.

21. Henwood BP, MacDonald DM: Caterpillar dermatitis. *Clin Exp Dermatol* 8:77–93, 1983.

21a. Sharma SK, Etkind PF, Odell TM, et al: Gypsy-moth-caterpillar dermatitis. *N Engl J Med* 306:1300–1301, 1982.

22. McMahon S, Koltenberg M: The changing role of primary afferent neurones in pain. *Pain* 43:269–272, 1990.

DERMATOLOGIC ASPECTS
OF PRURITUS

THREE
PRURITUS IN SKIN DISEASES

Jeffrey D. Bernhard

Itching is the most characteristic and distressing symptom of diseases of the skin. "Itchy red rashes" and "itchy red bumps" provide dermatologists and primary care physicians with major diagnostic and therapeutic challenges on a daily basis. While it is well known that itching is a characteristic feature of atopic dermatitis, psoriasis, dermatitis herpetiformis, and scabies, it is clearly a prominent feature of many other primarily cutaneous disorders as well. Many of the most important of these are listed in Table 3-1.

What makes this area particularly intriguing and clinically difficult is that the characteristic lesions of a specific disease may or may not be present: Early lesions may be scratched, infected, secondarily eczematized, or absent altogether. Bullous pemphigoid, for example, can present without blisters months before the characteristic vesicles or bullae appear.[18,19,20] To make matters even more challenging, scabies can present with a vesicular eruption that is clinically indistinguishable from bullous pemphigoid.[21] Similarly, cutaneous mastocytosis can present without clinically obvious skin lesions.[22] At the other extreme is the patient with merely red or red and scaling skin all over—the erythroderma/exfoliative dermatitis syndrome—in which the skin changes can be dramatic but in which it can be extremely difficult to establish the precise diagnosis.

The physician evaluating a patient who complains of generalized pruritus *even without a rash,* or of a widespread, itchy eruption *with or without apparent diagnostic skin lesions,* must, therefore, consider a wide range of primarily cutaneous disorders in the differential diagnosis. Sometimes a recognizable and perhaps even pathognomonic skin lesion will be found on careful, scrutinizing physical examination of the skin. Sometimes a skin biopsy of an affected area, even if the clinical changes are not diagnostic, may yield a definitive diagnosis. Pemphigoid, dermatitis herpetiformis,

Table 3-1 Dermatologic disorders in which pruritus may be especially notable[a]

Infestation
  scabies and other mites
  pediculosis
  insect bites; papular urticaria (especially flea and bedbug; see Chap. 4 and 9)
  schistosomal cercarial dermatitis (swimmer's itch)

Inflammatory
  dermatitis herpetiformis[1,2]
  pemphigoid
  mastocytosis
  atopic dermatitis
  lichen simplex chronicus[3]
  prurigo nodularis
  allergic contact dermatitis (e.g., poison ivy)
  irritant contact dermatitis (e.g., fiberglass)
  psoriasis (especially on scalp and genitalia)
  lichen planus (inconstant)
  miliaria
  urticaria (often, inconstant)[4,5]
  dermographism and other forms of physical urticaria
  pityriasis rosea
  pityriasis rubra pilaris
  parapsoriasis
  aquagenic pruritus
  drug hypersensitivity
  polymorphic light eruption & its variants
  Grover's disease (transient acantholytic disease)[6]
  persistent acantholytic dermatosis
  pruritic urticarial papules and plaques of pregnancy (see Chap. 19)
  folliculitis[7]
  perforating folliculitis[8]
  acquired peforating dermatosis[9]
  eosinophilic pustular folliculitis[10]
  infundibulofolliculitis[11]
  Fox–Fordyce disease (apocrine miliaria)

Infectious
  varicella
  dermatophytosis
  bacterial folliculitis
  candidal folliculitis[12]
  pityrosporum folliculitis[13]
  impetigo (inconstant)

Hereditary or congenital
  Darier–White disease (keratosis follicularis)[14]
  Hailey–Hailey disease (benign familial pemphigus)
  inflammatory linear verrucous epidermal nevus (ILVEN)[15]

Neoplastic
  mycosis fungoides (cutaneous T-cell lymphoma)

Table 3-1 Continued

Miscellaneous, pharmacologic, or idiopathic
  xerosis[1]
  asteatotic eczema, eczema craquele
  "winter itch" (xerosis and asteatotic eczema may be detectable)
  exanthematous drug eruptions
  aquagenic pruritus
  aerogenic pruritus (atmoknesis)[51]
  anogenital pruritus
  sunburn
  exfoliative dermatitis
  senile pruritus
  contact pruritus[17]
  cholinergic pruritus (see Chap. 18)
  adrenergic pruritus (see Chap. 18)
  flushing
  lichen amyloidosus
  macular cutaneous amyloidosis (?notalgia paresthetica) (see Chap. 12)
  "itchy red bump disease"/prurigo simplex subacuta (see Chap. 4)

[a] Many skin disorders that may itch at one time or another are not included in the interest of some degree of selectivity. The categorization is not iron-clad, either, as the etiology of many of these conditions is not known and some could fall under several different headings. Finally, whether some of the conditions listed in this table can be considered "primarily dermatologic" is debatable; mastocytosis may be considered a skin disease, a mediator disease, and a proliferative disease. It, and others such as senile pruritus, the cause of which is unknown, are included because they present first to dermatologists with some regularity.

mastocytosis, and scabies incognita are frequently diagnosed this way. Chapter 5 provides a histologic differential diagnosis of some of the disorders most likely to be recognized in this way.

The most dangerous diagnostic trap in the evaluation of a patient with a "non-diagnostic" itchy eruption is the assumption that it must be the result of a primarily dermatologic disease such as "eczema" or "neurodermatitis." (See Fig. 3-1.) As the entire fourth section of this book makes abundantly clear, many significant and some potentially fatal, systemic diseases can lead to itching. That itch often leads to scratching, to excoriations, to secondary eczematization, and to secondary infection. The physician's attention may focus too narrowly on the skin, and an underlying problem such as Hodgkin's disease or thyrotoxicosis will be missed. "Eczema" and "dermatitis" are not definitive diagnoses: They beg the questions, "what kind of eczema?" and "what is causing it?"*

* Many authors believe that "eczema" and "dermatitis" can be used interchangeably. We consider "dermatitis" the broader of the terms, such that "eczema" may be considered a form of dermatitis. The critical clinical and intellectual issue is to specify what kind of eczema or dermatitis one is talking about, e.g., atopic, allergic contact, irritant, endogenous, exogenous, etc.

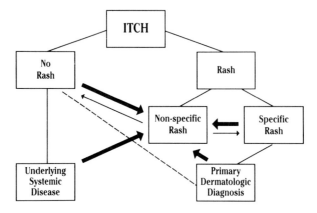

Figure 3-1 Connections and pathways between the causes and manifestations of itching. The broad arrows represent transitions created by rubbing and scratching. The narrow arrows represent transitions that may occur after spontaneous or therapeutic improvement. The most important implication of this figure is that both underlying systemic and specific dermatologic diseases may present with nonspecific cutaneous changes, or with no detectable cutaneous changes at all. Furthermore, a rash that is not diagnostic at one point in time may have diagnostic features at a later date. Re-examination over time is, therefore, a critical aspect of the approach to the patient with generalized pruritus or an undiagnosed pruritic eruption.

This chapter will focus on itching in several selected dermatologic disorders in which it is an especially important problem. To discuss in detail every skin disease that may itch at one time or another would wastefully reduplicate what is readily available in general textbooks of dermatology. We will not discuss definitional or other basic aspects of every disorder mentioned in this chapter, either; for these we refer the reader to any of the several general textbooks of dermatology as well. Several important external causes of itching are listed in Table 3-2. Several special skin disorders will be discussed in separate chapters in this section of the book (Table 3-3).

Table 3-2 External causes of itching

fiberglass[23] (industrial and remodeling exposures; curtains, draperies, plastic furniture)
low ambient humidity (winter itch, xerosis, and air-conditioner itch[24])
allergenic or irritating chemicals
connubial exposure to contactants
excessive bathing (especially in heavily chlorinated hot tubs; whirlpool or hot tub folliculitis; pseudomonas folliculitis[25])
arthropod and parasite contacts (birds, dogs, cats, farm animals, human contacts, vegetables, cheese [food mites], clothing, straw, horsehair mattresses; old offices and homes, fields, streams)
glochids (barbed cactus spines invisible to naked eye)[25a]

Table 3-3 Special pruritic skin
disorders discussed in separate
chapters

Disorder	Chapter
itchy papular eruptions	4
prurigo nodularis	7
bites	9
scars	10
anogenital pruritus	11
neurogenic itches	12
strange skin sensations	12
curiosities	13
other localized itches	13
HIV-related itches and rashes	20

THE UTILITY OF ITCHING, AND ITS FEATURES, IN DIFFERENTIAL DIAGNOSIS

[DOCTOR] KNOCK: What's the matter with you?
CRIER: Let me think! (*laughs*) Well, sometimes after I've eaten I feel a kind of itch here. (puts hand on upper part of stomach) It tickles . . . or scratches.
KNOCK: (*deep concentration*) Let's be clear about it. Does it tickle or does it scratch?
CRIER: It scratches. (*thinks it over*) But it tickles too, sort of.
  (from *Knock* by Jules Romains, translated from the French by James B. Gidney. Woodbury: Barron's Educational Series, Inc. 1962, pp 26–27.)

The utility of itching in diagnosis was recognized by Hippocrates, who, in one of his aphorisms, stated "Broad exanthemata are not very itchy."[26] Unfortunately, we do not know what Hippocrates meant by "broad exanthemata." Adams indicates that it may have been a pustular disease, and possibly even scabies when it has small pustules, supposedly because "the kind of itch in which the pustules are small, is known to be attended with more tingling than when the pustules are broader."[26] If we attach a modern meaning to exanthemata, and assume that the "broad" ones may be measles, the aphorism may still apply.

Certain disorders, such as prurigo nodularis, itch by definition. In others, such as atopic dermatitis, dermatitis herpetiformis, and lichen simplex chronicus, the presence of itching is so characteristic that most dermatologists would not make the diagnosis in its absence. In other settings, the presence or absence of itching may be helpful, but will not be enough on which to rest a diagnosis. For example, pityriasis rosea usually itches, small plaque parapsoriasis sometimes itches slightly, and large plaque parapsoriasis often itches intensely. It is said that the rash of secondary syphilis does not itch—but it can. It is said that cutaneous lupus erythematosus does not itch, but we have encountered several cases that did, although itching was not the chief complaint. The presence of itching may be important in the evaluation of a changing mole. Lesional itching is noted in one out of four melanomas.[27] The presence of itching may be an indicator of poor outcome in long-term hemodialysis patients,[28] and perhaps, in Hodgkin's disease (see Chap. 21).

As in the evaluation of pain, which can be characterized by a variety of descriptive features, distinguishing aspects of pruritus should also be sought. Unlike pain, in which features such as location, radiation, and provocative factors may point to a specific diagnosis, such as angina, appendicitis, or nephrolithiasis, itching is much more difficult to characterize and describe. Nonetheless, some features may be helpful in differential diagnosis, and every effort should be made to describe the patient's symptoms in terms of the descriptive features listed in Table 3-4.

Sometimes the character of the itch can be helpful. The itch of dermatitis herpetiformis is famous for its burning or stinging or "firey" character, especially on the scalp. The itch of aquagenic pruritus and of phototoxic drug eruptions can have a prickling, "irritating" quality. Pins and needles, tingling, numbness, and formication (the sensation that something is crawling under the skin) may have several different important causes, such as schizophrenia, drug addiction, peripheral neuropathy, parasitosis, and delusional parasitosis (monosymptomatic hypochondriacal psychosis). It is also important to distinguish itching from sensations with which it may be confused, such as pain, tactile dysesthesias, and thermal dysesthesias. As discussed in Chap. 25, complaints of tactile dysesthesias such as burning may have a psychiatric basis in some cases. Finally, K. Frank Austen has observed that, "If a *positive systems review* includes itching of the teeth, the sedimentation rate will probably be within the normal range."[29]

In the last analysis, so many pruritic skin diseases have similar appearances that the presence or absence of pruritus by itself does not have very much sensitivity or specificity in differential diagnosis, with certain notable exceptions. No tool comparable to the McGill Pain Index has been developed for pruritus; one we have been working on at the University of Massachusetts at Worcester (The Worcester Itch Index, called WITCH), has yet to measure up to the task. Nonetheless, the partial adaptation of it in Table 3-4 may be helpful in the initial evaluation of the itchy patient.

SCRATCHING—see Chap. 5.

ITCHY PAPULAR ERUPTIONS AND PRURIGOS—see Chap. 4.

Table 3-4 Pruritus: descriptive features[a]

I. Location: 1) localized vs. generalized? 2) Does normal looking skin itch, or does it itch only where there is a rash?

    [Comment: Pruritus restricted to one anatomic region usually points to specific local causes, but may point to a systemic illness (e.g., diabetes in the case of anogenital pruritus). More generalized itching, especially when skin that looks normal also itches, may point to an underlying systemic disease.]

II. Sequence of events: does itching occur before the rash, or does the rash precede the itch? Is the rash merely the consequence of scratching and rubbing?

    [Comment: In most primarily cutaneous disorders, the rash precedes the itch. In others, such as polymorphic light eruption, itching may precede the rash. In itch caused by an underlying metabolic disorder, itching clearly precedes the appearance of skin changes caused by scratching, and the patient tends to itch all over.]

III. Provoking and relieving factors

    [Comment: Itching after a bath may point to polycythemia vera or aquagenic pruritus. Failure to obtain relief from usual symptomatic measures indicates severity. Itching from wool may point to atopy; from exercise, to cholinergic pruritus; from stress, to adrenergic pruritus; from other contactants, to contact pruritus.]

IV. Character

    [Comment: burning, prickling, deep, superficial, tingling, other? Burning itch, especially of the scalp, is a clue to dermatitis herpetiformis. Prickling is a clue to aquagenic pruritus and phototoxicity.]

V. Severity; effect on normal daily activities; does it waken the patient from sleep?

    [Comment: Skin diseases and other "organic" causes of itching are said to waken patients from sleep more often than "psychogenic" pruritus does.]

VI. Mode of onset and course
    A. Coincident symptoms or events?
    B. Similar episodes in past?
    C. Gradual or sudden?
    D. Total duration?
    E. Getting better or worse?

VII. Specific temporal relationships (e.g., nocturnal, morning, monthly); does it waken the patient from sleep?

    [Comment: Most forms of itching worsen at night, but scabies is particularly notable for this. It is said that itching from scabies is most intense immediately on going to bed; itching from bedbugs occurs later at night. Severe itching that wakens the patient from sleep may be of organic origin. Many patients with severe skin diseases such as psoriasis may also have other sleep disturbances or psychological problems that lead to nocturnal wakening.]

VIII. Past treatment and evaluation
    A. When, where, by whom?
    B. What studies were performed? What were the results?
    C. Previous diagnoses
    D. Past prescribed treatment and home treatment?
    E. Results of past treatment?

IX. Assessment of personality and response to other discomforts; specific emotional stresses.

[a] Modified from Bernhard JD: Clinical aspects of pruritus, in: Fitzpatrick TB, Eisen AZ, Wolff K et al (eds): *Dermatology in General Medicine,* 3d ed, New York, McGraw-Hill, 1987, pp 78–90. And from the Worcester Itch Index (WITCH).

ATOPIC DERMATITIS (ATOPIC ECZEMA, AD)[30–32]

Atopic eczema is a chronic or chronically relapsing disorder in which severe itching is accompanied (or followed) by erythema, scaling, papulovesicles, and excoriations. Pruriginous papules, nodules, and lichenification are often present as well. Exudative, eczematous lesions, characteristically over the head, trunk, and extensor aspects of the extremities predominate in the infantile phase. In childhood and later, the flexural aspects of the elbows, knees, wrists, ankles, and neck are more typically involved, and acute eczematous changes may be replaced by lichenification and scaling. The hands may also be involved. Although IgE serum levels are often increased in AD patients, there is no laboratory marker for the disease, so that the diagnosis is based on several major and minor clinical criteria.[48] These include pruritus, typical distribution and morphology of lesions, chronic relapsing course, and personal or family history of atopic diseases.

"Atopic" is coined from the Greek for "wrongly placed," and refers to a specific group of disorders in which allergy is presumed to play a basic role, namely, atopic eczema, allergic bronchial asthma, and hay fever (allergic rhinitis and conjunctivitis due to pollen). The pathogenesis of atopic eczema is not known, but it is clear that genetic factors, disturbances in humoral and cell mediated immunity, alterations in cutaneous vascular responses, pharmacologic abnormalities, and other functional skin disturbances such as "dryness" of the skin and disturbed sweating, may be involved.[33–35] Cutaneous reactivity to neuropeptides such as Substance P may be altered.[36,37]

Altered immunologic reactivity to pollens,[38] to molds, to house dust mite antigens,[39–42] to certain foods,[43] and to staphylococci[44] each seem to be of importance to variable degrees in different patients. Marked deposition of eosinophil-granule major basic protein has been detected in affected skin of AD patients, indicative of eosinophil involvement in lesion pathogenesis.[45] Atopic dermatitis patients appear to have a lower itch threshold to any one of a number of physical stimuli, and are more likely than controls to experience "pure itching" without any pricking sensation after exposure to wool.[46,47]

Itch is such an important aspect of atopic dermatitis that "the diagnosis of active atopic dermatitis cannot be made if there is no history of itching."[48] Indeed, atopic eczema has been dubbed "the itch that rashes." As a primary cutaneous lesion has not been established, it is widely accepted that itch is the primary event in AD, and that rubbing and scratching are what cause the rash to appear.

The pruritic mediator or mediators of itching in AD have not been identified. Although histamine may play some role in some cases, there is substantial disagreement about just how important it may be, and there is conflicting evidence about how much it may or may not be elevated in the skin and blood of patients with AD. The fact that antihistamines are of only minimal to moderate help in relieving the itch of AD indicates that histamine cannot be the only itch mediator and is probably not the most important one. As the number of mast cells is increased in atopic skin, mast cell mediators other than histamine may be important. Immunologic and non-immunologic mediators of itching in AD must act by directly stimulating the itch receptor (presumably free nerve endings near the dermal–epidermal junction) or indirectly through sequential release of other mediators that act on the receptor.[32] Rajka reported a correlation between experimental trypsin-induced itch duration and high IgE levels, but serum IgE levels are not elevated in all AD patients, so both parameters might simply reflect the severity of the disease rather than primary causal relationships.[49] It is also possible that levels of IgE bound to epidermal cells may have more to do with atopic dermatitis than circulating levels do, and that atopics may have higher levels of high-affinity IgE-receptors on their epidermal Langerhans cells.[50] Other features of atopic skin, such as dryness and "microcracking" may also lead directly to itching—perhaps through direct physical stimulation of the itch receptor—and to enhanced sensitivity to pruritogenic substances such as wool.

Itching in AD can be extremely intense but is usually intermittent. In Wahlgren's study, two-thirds of the patients complained that itching had disturbed their sleep frequently for the preceding 3 months, and two-thirds of the people who shared bedrooms with AD patients complained of the patient's nightly scratching. Patients with AD frequently resort to towels, combs, back-scratchers, brushes, and even scissors to scratch. Paroxysmal itching may occur in the evening and at bedtime, and a number of both immunologic and nonimmunologic stimuli may provoke it (see Table 3-5).

One dramatic feature of itching in many patients with AD is its dramatic precipitation on undressing—the impression (if not the actuality) that itch

Table 3-5 Factors that provoke itch in patients with atopic dermatitis[a]

	Percent
heat and perspiration	96
wool	91
emotional stress	81
certain foods	49
alcohol	44
common colds	36

[a] From C-F Wahlgren. Itch and atopic dermatitis: Clinical and experimental studies. *Acta Derm Venereol* Suppl 165, 1991.

may be provoked by contact with air led to this symptom being called "atmoknesis."[51] Other factors that precipitate or exacerbate itching in AD include sweating, dry skin, contact with wool, erythema, and flushing. Stress may trigger itching in AD through several pathways: one may be through the stimulus of cutaneous flushing.[52,53] An increased sensitivity and decreased threshold to pruritic stimuli such as trypsin, cowhage spicules, and wool, along with prolonged itch duration seem to be important features of itching in AD.[54,55] On the other hand, Heyer and colleagues demonstrated that control subjects perceived a higher itch intensity from a strong histamine stimulus than AD patients did when the stimulus was delivered to their normal-appearing skin.[56] Moreover, atopics were less able to discriminate between strong and weak histamine stiumuli. They conclude that afferent cutaneous nerve fibers in AD patients may be desensitized to histamine and that neurogenic vasodilatation may be involved in the pathophysiology of AD. While these findings might seem contradictory to others in which itch threshold was diminished in atopics, it is important to recognize that different stimuli were used by different investigators. If histamine is only one of any number of possible itch mediators or pruritogens in atopic dermatitis, then some desensitization to it could occur without necessarily altering the itch threshold to other pruritogens such as trypsin.

Treatment of Atopic Dermatitis

General measures are discussed in Chap. 26 and 27, and by Hanifin[57] and Shelley and Shelley.[58] Phototherapy and photochemotherapy, which may be particularly effective in severe cases of AD, are discussed in Chap. 28. Antihistamines are discussed in detail in Chap. 29, but will be discussed briefly here because of their controversial role in AD. The other basic measures include protection from recognized environmental and food allergens, avoidance of excessive heat and sweating, treatment of secondary infection, and reduction of emotional stresses. The list of agents currently under investigation is a testimony to the difficulty of treating AD, and to the urgent necessity to unravel its cause. These include cyclosporin,[59] thymopentin, interferons, evening primrose oil, and a Chinese herb decoction.[60,61]

To some degree, treating the rash and treating the itch of atopic dermatitis amount to nearly the same thing. Agents that help the eczematous rash, such as topical corticosteroids, may have a dual effect in directly decreasing the itch as well, or in decreasing the itch as a consequence of improvement in the rash. In practice it may not be possible to separate these effects, except to note that topical corticosteroids are not particularly effective in reducing itching that is not caused by a rash in other circumstances (such as primary biliary cirrhosis). Given the controversy over the extent and nature of histamine's role in atopic dermatitis, it is not surprising that the use of antihistamines in treating AD is controversial as well. There is no doubt that the sedative effect of many conventional antihistamines can provide some relief because of that effect. When it comes to nonsedating or low-sedative antihistamines in atopic dermatitis, however, the weight of evidence from randomized, placebo-controlled, cross-over clinical trials suggests that they are of no value.[62,63] In a parallel rather than cross-over study, low sedative antihistamines did seem to have a mildly beneficial effect, however, so the possibility that a small subgroup of atopic dermatitis patients may benefit from nonsedative antihistamines because of their antihistamine rather than soporific effect remains a tantalizing possibility.[64] Considering the wide variety of actions other than H1-receptor antagonism that some of the newer antihistamines may have, the final word on antihistamine treatment in AD remains to be heard.

Cyclosporin

Several groups have investigated cyclosporin as a treatment for atopic dermatitis. Wahlgren and colleagues used oral cyclosporin A to treat 10 AD patients and observed an antipruritic effect within 10 days in 9 of the 10.[65] They observed that cyclosporin markedly reduced erythema, which is especially interesting in terms of the frequently noted association between erythema and itching in AD. Sowden and colleagues confirmed the efficacy of oral cyclosporin in an 8-week placebo-controlled trial.[66] Given its well-known side effects and risks, however, cyclosporin must still be considered an investigational treatment for AD.

Papaverine*

Although two double-blind trials have failed to confirm the efficacy of papaverine treatment in AD,[67,68] and the risk of hepatotoxicity has come to light, the possibility that papaverine might help some individuals or subgroups of AD patients has not been excluded.[69] Papaverine is a phosphodiesterase inhibitor. Phosphodiesterase levels may be elevated in leukocytes of AD patients,[70] and it was hoped that phosphodiesterase inhibiton and the consequent elevation of cAMP levels would be helpful, perhaps by decreasing degranuation of mast cells. Alternatively, papaverine might have exerted an antipruritic effect because of its vasodilatory action, as first suggested by Wirth in 1947.[71] Neither of these hypotheses has been proven experimentally, however, and the two negative controlled studies force us to grope for explanations that might account for papaverine's anecdotal effectiveness in the clinic. One possibility is that neither controlled study was actually sensitive

---

* Parts of this section are adapted from Bernhard, JD. Itching XXXIV. Is papaverine effective in atopic dermatitis? *Dermatologic Capsule & Comment* 14:11–12, 1992.

enough to detect differences, especially given how crude our methods for measuring itching and extent of eczema are. Another possibility is that the drug was not given in high enough dosage for a sufficiently long period of time. Another is that patient selection is important and that only certain subgroups of AD patients will respond. Over more than 35 years, Baer chose patients whose AD was moderately severe to severe and whose itching "had not responded to other commonly used forms of treatment, exclusive of systemic corticosteroids," or who had not responded to anything but systemic corticosteroids. Furthermore, he never advocated papaverine as monotherapy for AD, and he noted that even if it were effective against itching, it could not be expected "to reverse the chronic skin changes brought about by months or years of scratching and rubbing." The last possibility is that papaverine is an especially effective placebo. (Can one placebo be stronger than another? The answer may be yes, especially if a minor but tolerable side effect unrelated to the putative therapeutic effect ensures that the patient knows that the "medication" is "working.") Considering how substantial psychological and attention factors can be on itching, and how potent the placebo effect can be in such a subjectively experienced symptom, the placebo effect is one that cannot be ignored, and that we cannot afford to ignore.[72] My own experience with papaverine treatment of AD is rather limited, but one anecdote may be revealing. I treated a 40-year-old woman with steroid-dependent asthma and severe refractory atopic dermatitis whose skin disease was becoming even more severe and unresponsive as her pulmonologist attempted to decrease her systemic corticosteroid dose. Within 5 days of starting papaverine she noted a dramatic decrease in itching and her rash began to improve as well. Over the next few weeks her skin continued to get better but she began to lose her appetite and became disturbingly fatigued. She had developed a chemical hepatitis; it resolved some weeks after the papaverine was discontinued. Conclusion: Papaverine may still be worth considering in the treatment of patients with severe AD, but liver enzymes should be monitored and patients should be warned to discontinue the medication if symptoms of hepatitis develop. The hepatic effects may be dose related. Some of Shupack's patients who developed liver enzyme abnormalities were treated with doses as high as 900 mg; Baer usually used 400 mg per day and did not go above 450 mg.[73]

PSORIASIS[74–77]

"Psoriasis" comes from the Greek word for itch (*psora*). Although some patients with psoriasis do not itch, and many textbooks even say that itching is not a prominent feature of the disease, anyone who treats many patients with psoriasis knows that itching is a frequent, distressing, and often predominant complaint. Psoriasis is the prototypical papulosquamous or erythematosquamous disorder of the skin. It is extremely common and has many clinical varieties, but the most typical lesion is an erythematous plaque with silvery, micaceous scale, preferentially located over extensor aspects of the extremities but often involving the scalp and other areas as well. Psoriasis may be accompanied by a specific arthropathy. It is primarily an inherited disorder but its pathogenesis, and the pathogenesis of itching when it occurs in psoriasis, remain unknown.

Inflammatory, immunologic, regulatory, and proliferative derangements have been detected in both the involved and uninvolved skin of patients with psoriasis, and it is likely that some or all of these may play a role in causing psoriatic itch. Neuropeptides such as Substance P may also be important in psoriasis and its itch. Increased levels of Substance P, vasoactive intestinal peptide, and Substance P-containing nerves have been detected in psoriatic lesions.[78–80] Topical capsaicin depletes Substance P; in several studies it has had a beneficial effect in reducing itch and in improving or clearing psoriatic plaques.[81–83] As early psoriatic papules may have significant numbers of mast cells, histamine and other mast cell mediators could be important in psoriatic itching as well.[84] Psoriatic papules and plaques may also itch because of the actual physical effects of dryness and scales with rough, sharp, or irritating edges—and it is noteworthy that the normal-appearing, uninvolved skin of patients with psoriasis does not itch. Although we have seen many patients whose psoriasis continued to itch even after the lesions had stopped scaling (but still remained as erythematous plaques), the link between itching and scaling seems strong. Although we have not conducted a formal study, some of our most carefully observant patients report that their first noticeable response to PUVA photochemotherapy is disappearance of the itch with nearly simultaneous reduction in scaling. One must wonder if itching is directly related to the developmental pathophysiology of psoriasis, or if it is a secondary, epiphenomenon. (Should it be, "I itch, therefore I scale," or "I scale, therefore I itch"?) In any event, there can be no doubt that the injury caused by scratching provides an important pathway for the Koebner reaction (isomorphic response)[85] and exacerbation of psoriasis.

Newbold studied itching in 200 consecutive hospitalized psoriasis patients:[86] 92 percent had had pruritus at some time and in 89 percent it was the main complaint; 80 percent had never had a total remission. The scalp was the most frequently involved site, followed by shins, elbows, back, flexures, and face. Newbold concluded that psoriatic itching was often paroxysmal and severe, especially at night; that it was worse when lesions were dry and when the disease was active, and that provocative factors included heat, scratching, and stress. Atmoknesis, itching provoked by open exposure of the skin to air upon undressing, is also a common feature.[51] Newbold also observed that small lesions were more likely to itch than large ones, that the edges of lesions, especially in flexural areas, were often very irritable, that itching could be a particular feature of "unstable" psoriasis, and that there was no link between the extent of the disease and severity of itching. Other authors have also noted an association between itching and eruptive psoriasis. Itching is a prominent feature of psoriasis in children and in eruptive guttate psoriasis.

In Gupta and colleague's study of 82 inpatients with psoriasis, 67 percent reported moderate or severe itching.[87] They also found that the severity of itching was directly related to the severity of scaling at the time of admission. Intrapsychic factors, particularly depression, also correlated significantly with the degree of itching. Gupta and colleagues also found that nocturnal wakening is an important problem for many patients with psoriasis, and that psychiatric and sleep pathologic factors seemed to contribute to this phenomenon.[88] It is likely that the complex interaction between psychogenic factors and the "organic" itch triggered by the skin disease itself leads to many nights of misery for patients with psoriasis.[89]

Allergic contact reactions, sometimes to components of medications used to treat the disease, may also contribute to itching in psoriasis. Rebora found that more than half of a group of 31 patients with itchy psoriasis had positive patch test reactions to cutaneous allergens including potassium dichromate, nickel, triethylenetetraamine, and neomycin.[90]

Aside from Newbold's observation that the scalp is one of the sites most frequently affected by itching in psoriasis, there is something special about psoriatic scalp itch. Based on observations of my patients and discussions with my colleague, Dr. Karen Rothman, the following postulates seem to hold: (1) When psoriasis on the scalp itches, psoriasis on the body often, but not always, itches as well; (2) When psoriasis on the scalp does not itch, psoriasis on the body usually does not itch, either; (3) If only one spot of psoriasis itches, it will usually be on the scalp.

PUVA Itch

Psoriasis patients who undergo PUVA photochemotherapy may develop localized or generalized itching related to the treatment.[91,92] Some develop skin pain, which may be localized to the interscapular area and often has an itching, prickling, or smarting character.[93,94] PUVA itch could be related to low-grade phototoxicity, to the production of a new pruritogen, to a lowering of the itch threshold, or, as Roelandts and Stevens[94] suggest, to stimulation of cutaneous or joint—capsule nerve receptors. PUVA itch or pain can require discontinuation of the treatment, and in some patients may persist for weeks or months. In some patients, it may be possible to "treat through" the problem, in others, there are anecdotal reports of dilantin, transcutaneous nerve stimulation, and the administration of a few ultraviolet B treatments being helpful.

Treatment of Itching in Psoriasis

The best treatment for psoriatic itching is to treat the underlying psoriasis itself. A large number of modalities, ranging from topical corticosteroids to PUVA photochemotherapy to oral methotrexate treatment are available and reviewed in standard tests. The basic principles of symptomatic treatment of psoriatic itching, aside from treating the psoriasis itself, are discussed in Section V, of this book. It is fair to say that, aside from their soporific effect, antihistamines are not particularly helpful, and that measures designed to hydrate or moisturize the skin and to nontraumatically reduce scaling generally are. Stress-reduction and relaxation measures may also be helpful.[95]

SPECIAL PROBLEMS

Many disorders and special problems defy categorization as dermatologic or nondermatologic. Some are born on the skin, some achieve their recognition only because of their presentation on the skin, and some have the label "dermatologic" thrust on them for lack of a better category or because their deeper cause is unknown. For example, aquagenic pruritus could be considered a "dermatologic" disorder and appropriately discussed in this chapter (as it will be), but must be mentioned in the chapters on hematologic causes of itching (Chap. 17), strange skin sensations (Chap. 12), and pruritic curiosities (Chap. 13) as well. Notalgia paresthetica is usually considered a dermatologic problem but is probably an isolated sensory neuropathy that can also lead to secondary macular amyloidosis; it will be considered in Chap. 12. Given overlapping categories, it is hoped that the index and the tables throughout the book will enable readers to find their way to what they need. Several selected special problems are discussed in the following sections.

The Itchy Scalp

Any pruritic skin disorder that can involve the scalp can present with itching localized to the scalp. Psoriasis is probably the most frequent cause. Other causes are listed in Table 3-6.

Diagnosis can be very challenging because the scalp presents a limited number of reaction patterns—redness, scaling, papules, pustules, infiltration, and scars. Samuel Moschella has commented on the difficult problem of "diffuse red scalp disease which can also be itchy and burning. There is no scaling, no hair loss, and no scarring. It is non-responsive to any therapy including potent topical steroids or anti-seborrheic therapy."[112] The burning component raises the question of dermatitis herpetiformis or of psychogenic

Table 3-6 Differential diagnosis of the itchy scalp

With identifiable (but not necessarily diagnostic) skin lesions on clinical examination or on histopathologic examination
  seborrheic dermatitis
  psoriasis[96]
  lichen simplex chronicus
  seborrhea nuchae
  atopic dermatitis
  contact dermatitis (irritant and allergic)
  pyogenic infection
  dermatitis herpetiformis (often "burning," sometimes without lesions)
  folliculitis
  acne necrotica
  acne keloidalis
  dissecting folliculitis
  folliculitis decalvans
  perifolliculitis abscendens et suffodiens
  eosinophilic pustular folliculitis[97]
  eosinophilic pustulosis of the scalp in childhood[98]
  lichen planopilaris (often a "burning" or "tingling" itch)
  lichen planus
  active discoid lupus erythematosus (occasionally)
  xerosis
  neurotic excoriation
  active alopecia areata (unusual)
  prurigo simplex subacuta
  angiosarcoma
Without specific skin lesions
  generalized pruritus (any cause)
  pediculosis (nits, secondary pyoderma may be present)
  scabies in children or immunocompromised host[99]
  external agents (e.g., fiberglass)
  drug reactions[100,101]
  iron deficiency[102]
  diabetes mellitus (?)
  book lice infestation[103]
  thinker's itch[104]
Psychogenic or psychiatric causes[a]
  psychogenic (stress) pruritus[105]
  dermatologic nondisease[106]
  coenestopathic states[107] (itching; other strange sensations)
  early schizophrenia[108]
The burning, painful, or tender scalp
  infections of the scalp
  psychogenic or psychiatric states listed earlier
  temporal arteritis
  eosinophilia-myalgia syndrome[109]
  cranial myositis
  mononeuritis multiplex
  post-herpetic neuralgia
  trigeminal neuralgia, occipital neuralgia
  atypical facial neuralgia[100]
  tension, cluster, or migraine headache[111]

  [a] Several of these may be different names for the same thing.

pruritus. Psychogenic and stress-related causes are probably not uncommon, but the diagnosis should be made after careful examination and care. Follow-up physical examination may be required, as demonstrated in the case of a 76-year-old man who presented with a 2-month history of scalp pruritus who developed an area that would bleed after scratching 1 month after onset of the symptom. Biopsy of a plaque revealed angiosarcoma.[113]

THE ITCHY FACE

Itching with a rash can occur in any of the classic causes of dermatitis of the face, (see Table 3-7). One cause of increasing importance in the age of electronics is excessive dryness as a manifestation of low-humidity micro-trauma,[114] an occupational dermatosis from work in so-called "clean rooms."[115,116] Some cases may be localized to the eyelids, but contactants are the more frequent cause of eyelid dermatitis.[117]

Seborrheic dermatitis and allergic contact dermatitis, especially from cosmetics, must be among the most important and frequent causes. Sometimes very little if any dermatitis can be detected, so the absence of erythema and scaling should not be taken to exclude the possibility of a contact dermatitis. Cosmetics must often be interdicted despite protestation, and it is often necessary to take and retake a painstaking history before the cause is finally uncovered. Moisturizers, cold creams, "skin creams," hair and nail formulations, shampoos, and myriad other products containing vitamins, aloe, and a multitude of fragrances and preservatives present a bewildering variety of potential allergens and irritants. Some patients are so "hooked" to

Table 3-7 Differential diagnosis of the itchy face

> seborrheic dermatitis
> atopic dermatitis
> allergic contact dermatitis
> irritant contact dermatitis
> xerosis; low-humidity microtrauma
> flushing syndromes (e.g., carcinoid)
> rosacea (flushing or burning sensations may occur)
> so-called "video display terminal (VDT) dermatitis" (usually
>   related to dryness or some other cause)[118]
> status cosmeticus (from allergenic or irritant contactants)
> post-herpetic pruritus
> other inflammatory dermatoses
> unilateral facial pruritus secondary to brainstem glioma[119]
> dysmorphophobia (dermatologic nondisease)[106]
> facial dysesthesias (can also be caused by contactants such as
>   synthetic pyrethroids)
> photosensitivity[120]
> spinal or epidural opioid injection

cosmetic products that the problem becomes exceedingly difficult to sort out, especially when one or more of the products is being used for symptomatic relief of a reaction that it may itself be exacerbating. Fisher has coined the term "status cosmeticus" to describe the syndrome in which a vicious cycle of cosmetic product usage contributes to perpetual cutaneous reactions.[121] According to Fisher, these patients usually present

> with an unremarkable clinical picture. They may have a mild erythema of the "butterfly" area of the face with slight edema of the eyelids. Occasionally, there is follicular eruption. The signs are, however, not as vivid as the patients' vivid complaints of burning, stinging sensations. These persons usually complain that they have tried at least twenty different cosmetics, all of which "disagree" with them.

Engasser and Maibach have described this phenomenon as "the intolerant skin syndrome."[122] Exactly where "sensitive skin"[123] ends and "intolerant" skin begins may be difficult to say, especially insofar as the definition of "dry skin" is subject to some debate.[124] Fisher listed a number of "stinging agents" that can produce status cosmeticus; these are included in Table 3-8. Certain anti-irritant cosmetic ingredients may neutralize this effect under some circumstances.

Fragrances and sunscreen lotions are among the major causes of itching among cosmetic products.[125,125a] When low-grade allergens are involved, the pathophysiology may also include that of chronic allergic contact dermatitis. When low-grade irritants alone are involved, the picture may be harder to recognize and the diagnosis harder to prove.

Table 3-8 Stinging substances that can produce "status cosmeticus"[a]

benzoic acid
bronopol
cinnamic acid compounds
dowicil 200
formaldehyde
lactic acid
nonionic emulsifiers
propylene glycol
quaternary ammonium compounds
sodium lauryl sulfate
sorbic acid
urea
fragrances
certain sunscreen agents

[a] Modified from Fisher.[121]

Flushing

Flushing of the face, whether caused by emotion, physical agents such as heat, chemicals such as ethanol, drugs such as nicotinic acid, foods such as glutamate, hormones as in menopause or the hyperendorphin syndrome, or mediator release as in mastocytosis or from carcinoid and pancreatic tumors, can be associated with itching of the face. Other symptoms, such as weakness, sweating, headache, and diarrhea, may also occur, depending on the cause.[126]

Demodicidosis

The hair follicle mite, demodex folliculorum, is not ordinarily pathogenic. Under certain circumstances, however, the follicles may become overpopulated and reaction can occur, particularly if the mite escapes into the surrounding dermis.[127] Although this topic has been somewhat controversial, I believe that it is a genuine problem, as first described by Ayres in 1930.[128,129] Patients, usually women, may present with minimal but persistent dry, rough, fine scaling of the cheeks, forehead, and chin. Erythema may be present and the follicles may be prominent. The chief complaint is usually irritation, itching, burning, stinging, or heat. A rosacea-like eruption, in which small pustules may be present as well, can probably also be caused by demodex. In some cases, the exclusive use of oily cleansing or cold creams, combined with an avoidance of soap and water for facial cleansing, seems to be an important contributory factor. Although it is usually a facial eruption, demodicidosis can present with more widespread pruritic, erythematous, scaling eruptions in special circumstances such as Cushing syndrome and deficient body hygiene.[130]

"Exhausted Skin," Chronic Irritant Contact Dermatitis

M.V. Dahl uses the term "exhausted skin" to describe the situation in which a continual dermatitis with itching and scratching results from repetitive exposures to irritants.[131] This can be a particularly insidious and pesky problem because cumulative damage to the skin over time results when weak irritants lead to subclinical damage each time any one of a variety of irritants is encountered. Clinical signs may be subtle or absent, but sooner or later "the skin's repair systems become drained," its ability to recover diminished, the "irritation threshold" is exceeded, and clinical dermatitis appears. To make matters worse, new irritants can perpetuate the problem and new allergens can complicate it. This ties into the "sputnik effect" of irritant dermatitis because, "Like sputnik, once launched, the dermatitis can continue in orbit for a long time without further propulsive power apparently being supplied."[131] Patch testing may be helpful in unravelling irritant and/or allergic contact dermatitis, and a biopsy of the reaction site at 48 hours may yield features that can be helpful in making distinctions. Because certain sites, such as the face and eyelids, are especially sensitive; and others, such as those with thicker skin, may be less so, testing away from the actual site involved may not be truly reflective of the clinical circumstances. Even daily dish washing with commercial dish-washing products can lead to itching, dryness, and smarting of the hands, usually in association with objective signs of erythema, scaling, or fissures.[132]

CONNUBIAL CONTACT DERMATITIS

For general and detailed discussions of contact dermatitis, the reader is referred to general textbooks of dermatology and to several specific comprehensive textbooks of contact dermatitis.[133–137] Because it can be so easy to miss if it is not considered, however, brief mention of "connubial contact dermatitis" will be made here.[138,139] Other terms for this phenomenon include "consort contact dermatitis," "dermatite par procuration," "dermatitis by proxy," and "intercourse related pruritus."[140] A variety of allergenic and/or irritating substances can be transmitted from one person to another via direct skin-to-skin contact, or via clothing, or even via washing machines. One increasingly important cause of such contact sensitivity reactions is latex, which can even cause anaphylactic reactions in highly sensitive individuals exposed via condoms or latex gloves.[141,142] Other sources of reactions include fragrances from cosmetic products and perfumes, lipstick, sunscreens, and fiberglass. The photocontact variety of connubial contact dermatitis may be even harder to recognize, as it requires exposure to the chemical, exposure to sunlight, and usually some latency period before the rash appears.[143]

SENILE PRURITUS

When itching without a rash occurs in elderly people and cannot be explained in any other way, such as xerosis ("winter itch"), an underlying systemic illness, or as a depressive equivalent, the diagnosis of senile pruritus may be made.[144–146] Its cause is not known, but it has been suggested that it may be related to neural phenomena such as those responsible for "phantom itching" in phantom limbs or cases of nerve injury.[147] Alternatively, Long and Marks have suggested that elderly patients with generalized pruritus may have an acquired abnormality of keratinization.[147a] The most common cause of itching in elderly people is probably dry skin (xerosis), and it is known that aged skin has a lower water content than younger skin.[148] Itching because of xerosis ordinarily responds to measures designed to hydrate the skin, such as topical emollients and reduction of exposure to soaps and excessive bathing. When xerosis, or any other of the recognized causes of itching can be diagnosed in an elderly person, the diagnosis of "senile pruritus" no longer applies.

AQUAGENIC PRURITUS

The classic setting for aquagenic pruritus is in polycythemia rubra vera, and it is discussed in Chap. 17. As Table 3-9 shows, however, polycythemia vera is not the only cause of aquagenic pruritus.

Aquagenic pruritus was recognized as a diminutive variant of the more rare aquagenic urticaria[154] and named by Walter B. Shelley in 1970.[155] It was characterized as a clinical entity by Greaves and colleagues in 1979.[156] In classic aquagenic pruritus, itching or a prickling, tingling, burning, or stinging sensation (also described as "irritation") occurs within 30 minutes of water contact—regardless of temperature—and lasts for as long as 2 hours. It often starts on the lower extremities but can begin anywhere and it may generalize. Many patients experience concomitant psychological changes including irritability, emotional lability, aggression, anger and depression.[157,158] Criteria

Table 3-9 Differential diagnosis of pruritus or prickling sensations provoked by water contact

Without visible skin lesions
    polycythemia rubra vera
    Hodgkin's disease (uncommon)
    mastocytosis
    hypereosinophilic syndrome[149]
    myelodysplastic syndrome[150]
    essential thrombocythemia[151]
    idiopathic hemochromatosis (one case)[152]
    cold pruritus
    heat pruritus[a]
    alcohol-induced itching on hot shower in sarcoidosis[153]
    aquagenic pruritus (isolated or idiopathic)

With visible skin lesions
    cold urticaria
    symptomatic dermographism (from impact of shower jet)
    cholinergic urticaria (hot water)
    aquagenic urticaria
    aquagenic pruritus of the elderly (xerosis; may be subtle)
    eczematous dermatoses (incidental exacerbation by water contact)

[a] Presumed to exist as a diminutive variant of heat urticaria provoked by contact with hot water, by analogy with aquagenic urticaria and aquagenic pruritus, but not yet reported.

for the diagnosis of aquagenic pruritus, according to Steinman and Greaves,[157] include the following:

1. Severe pruritus occurs after water contact, regardless of water temperature.
2. Pruritus develops within minutes after water contact.
3. No visible skin changes occur.
4. No chronic skin disease or internal disorder is present that could explain the discomfort, nor can drugs be implicated.
5. Cold, vibratory, pressure, aquagenic, cholinergic, and heat urticaria and symptomatic dermatographism are excluded.
6. Polycythemia rubra vera and other myeloproliferative disorders are excluded.

Although itching after water contact may be common among patients with skin diseases, strict application of these criteria reveal that true idiopathic or "isolated" aquagenic pruritus is not common,[159] although estimates of its prevalence vary.[160]

When old age, seasonal weather variation, and dry skin act in concert, a variation without the associated psychologic symptoms may occur and is called aquagenic pruritus of the elderly.[161] It responds readily to measures addressed toward hydrating the skin, such as emollients.

The pathogenesis of aquagenic pruritus in other cases (i.e., those not associated with mere dryness of the skin) is not known, but there are several clues. Greaves and colleagues observed increased levels of blood histamine, evidence of cutaneous mast cell degranulation, and pharmacological evidence of local release of acetyl choline.[156] There is evidence for water-induced activation of acetylcholinesterase[162] and there is also evidence that the cutaneous fibrinolytic system may be involved.[163,164] Czarnetzki and colleagues have suggested that water acts as a carrier for an epidermal antigen that diffuses into the dermis to cause mediator release from sensitized dermal mast cells.[165] Bath pruritus in polycythemia vera is discussed further in Chap. 17; there is evidence for an increase in cutaneous fibrinolytic activity[166] and for an increase in the number of cutaneous mast cells.[167] Although the final mechanism for water-induced itching in different settings may vary, it is possible to envision a scenario in which water either carries a chemical signal from the epidermis or triggers a structural change in the skin in such a way that mast cells are triggered or cutaneous nerves are fired directly.

Based on the fact that aquagenic pruritus may occur as an idiopathic disorder, as a harbinger or concomitant of serious diseases, as a concomitant of xerosis in the elderly, or as a feature of banal dermatoses, the classification system shown in Table 3-10 has been proposed, partly to ensure that patients are followed appropriately for the potential development of lymphoproliferative disorders.[168]

Table 3-10 Aquagenic pruritus types

Type I. Isolated aquagenic pruritus (IAP): no associated systemic disease and no visible skin lesions.

Type II. Rash aquagenic pruritus (RAP): associated with visible skin disorders such as atopic dermatitis and psoriasis.

Type III. Aquagenic pruritus of the elderly (APE): associated with dry skin in the elderly.

Type IV. Systemic aquagenic pruritus (SAP): associated with or presenting as a harbinger of a systemic disease such as polycythemia vera,[169,170] hypereosinophilic syndrome, or myelodysplastic syndrome.

Symptomatic treatment options for aquagenic pruritus include the addition of baking soda to the bath water,[171,172] ultraviolet B phototherapy,[173] and PUVA photochemotherapy.[174] It may be necessary to raise the pH to 8 and to use as much as 0.5 to 1.0 kg of baking soda to be effective. In polycythemia vera, aspirin (which must be used with caution),[175,176] and antiserotoninergic antihistamines such as cyproheptidine may be helpful.[177] There are also reports of single cases or small series treated with cimetidine,[178] cholestyramine,[179] and other agents.

ITCHY SKIN DISORDERS WITH BLISTERS

Bullous pemphigoid is the classic example of an itchy, vesiculo-bullous skin disorder. As Table 3-11 demonstrates, however, a fairly extensive variety of skin diseases can present with vesicular or bullous lesions, which can be an important clue to the diagnosis. A geometric configuration may point to the diagnosis of allergic contact dermatitis, such as poison ivy. Other aspects of the history and physical examination will point to other diagnoses, but in many cases a skin biopsy with specimens provided for both routine histology and direct immunofluorescence testing will be required to establish the diagnosis.

URTICARIA

Urticaria (hives) are usually intensely itchy. It is said that their "clinical features and natural history are as varied and unpredictable as the aetiology."[186] For the most part, early lesions and small superficial wheals are most itchy. Urticarial wheals occur in myriad sizes and shapes; many have a blanched palpable center and a variable halo of erythema. Others are simply pink or red. The defining feature of classic hives are changing shape over a short period of time and the short life-span (less than 24 hours) of individual lesions. If this single feature (evanescence), along with the characteristic absence of

Table 3-11 Pruritic skin disorders with blisters (vesicles or bullae)

dermatitis herpetiformis[a]
miliaria crystallina
pemphigoid—often/usual[b]
pemphigoid nodularis[180]
pemphigus—inconstant[b]
Hailey–Hailey disease (benign familial chronic pemphigus)
herpes gestationis (pemphigoid gestationis)
linear IgA disease[a]
bullous lupus erythematosus
bullous lichen planus[181]
epidermolysis bullosa[a]—some types
vesicular pityriasis rosea[182]
varicella
scabies[21]
insect bite reactions (at site of bites and secondary
    hypersensitivity reactions at other or prior sites)
bullous impetigo (inconstant)
acute eczematous dermatitis
eczema: pompholyx on hands and feet
allergic contact dermatitis (e.g., poison ivy)
phytophotodermatitis
id reactions/autoeczematization
bullous tinea infection[183]
Darier–White disease (uncommon)[184,185]

[a] Itch may have burning character.
[b] Erosions often painful.

epidermal changes such as scaling were more often borne in mind, far fewer diagnoses of urticaria would be missed. Treatment of urticaria depends on elimination of identifiable causes and judicious use of oral antihistamines. For full discussions of urticaria, the reader is referred to standard textbooks of dermatology, medicine, allergy, and pediatrics, as well as to several monographic sources (references 4 and 5).

REFERENCES

1. Katz SI, moderator: Dermatitis herpetiformis: The skin and the gut. *Ann Intern Med* 93:857–874, 1980.
2. Alexander JO'D: *Dermatitis Herpetiformis.* London, Saunders. 1975.
3. Fitzpatrick TB, Johnson RA, Polano MK, et al: *Color Atlas and Synopsis of Clinical Dermatology: Common and Serious Diseases,* 2d ed. New York, McGraw-Hill, 1992, pp 28–29.

4. Warin RP, Champion RH: *Urticaria.* London, Saunders, 1974.
5. Czarnetzki BM: *Urticaria.* Berlin, Springer-Verlag. 1986.
6. Heenan PJ, Quirk CJ: Transient acantholytic dermatosis. *Br J Dermatol* 102:515–520, 1980.
7. Herman LE, Harawi SJ, Ghossein RA, et al: Folliculitis: A clinicopathological review. *Pathology Annual* 26:210–246, 1991.
8. Patterson JW, Brown PC: Ultrastructural changes in acquired perforating dermatosis. *Int J Dermatol* 31:201–205, 1992.
9. Zelger B, Hintner H, Aubock J, et al: Acquired perforating dermatosis. Transepidermal elimination of DNA material and possible role of leukocytes in pathogenesis. *Arch Dermatol* 127:695–700, 1991.
10. Giard F, Marcoux D, McCuaig C, et al: Eosinophilic pustular folliculitis in childhood: A review of four cases. *Pediatr Dermatol* 8:189–193, 1991.
11. Hitch JM, Lund HZ: Disseminate and recurrent infundibulofolliculitis: Report of a case. *Arch Dermatol* 97:432, 1968.
12. Ross V, Baxter DL: Widespread candida folliculitis in a nontoxic patient. *Cutis* 49:241–243, 1992.
13. Helm KF, Lookingbill DP: Pityropsorum folliculitis and severe pruritus in two patients with Hodgkin's disease. *Arch Dermatol* 129:380–381, 1993.
14. Burge SM, Wilkinson JD: Darier-White disease: A review of the clinical features in 163 patients. *J Am Acad Dermatol* 27:40–50, 1992.
15. Bernhard JD, Owen WR, Steinman HK, et al: Inflammatory linear verucous epidermal nevus. Epidermal protein analysis in four patients. *Arch Dermatol* 120:214–215, 1984.
16. Editorial: Winter's skin. *Lancet* 335:266, 1990.
17. Kligman AM: The spectrum of contact urticaria: Wheals, erythema, and pruritus. *Dermatol Clin* 8:57–60, 1990.
18. Barker DJ: Generalised pruritus as a presenting feature of bullous pemphigoid. *Br J Dermatol* 109:237–238, 1983.
19. Bingham EA, Burrows D, Sandford JC: Prolonged pruritus and bullous pemphigoid. *Clin Exp Dermatol* 9:564–570, 1984.
20. Ross JS, McKee PH, Smith NP, et al: Unusual variants of pemphigoid: From pruritus to pemphigoid nodularis. *J Cutan Pathol* 19:212–216, 1992.
21. Bhawan J, Milstone E, Malhotra R, et al: Scabies presenting as bullous pemphigoid-like eruption. *J Am Acad Dermatol* 24:179–181, 1991.
22. Kendall ME, Fields JP, King LE: Cutaneous mastocytosis without clinically obvious skin lesions. *J Am Acad Dermatol* 10:903–905, 1984.
23. Bjornberg A: Glass fiber dermatitis. *Am J Ind Med* 8:305–400, 1985.
24. Chernosky ME: Pruritic skin disease and summer air conditioning. *JAMA* 179:1005–1010, 1962.
25. Silverman AR, Nieland ML: Clinical and laboratory studies in hot tub dermatitis: A familial outbreak of Pseudomonas folliculitis. *J Am Acad Dermatol* 8:153–156, 1983.
25a. Slaba R: *The Illustrated Guide to Cacti.* New York, Sterling Publication, 1992, p 98.
26. Hippocrates: The genuine works of Hippocrates. Translated from the Greek with a preliminary discourse and annotations, by F. Adams. Vol I. London, The New Sydenham Society. 1849, p 753.
27. Sober AJ: The changing mole. *JAMA* 253:1612–1613, 1985.
28. Carmichael AJ, McHugh MI, Martin AM: Renal itch as an indicator of poor outcome. *Lancet* 337:1225–1226, 1991.
29. Austen KF: Quoted in Macklis RM, Mendelsohn ME, Mudge GH: *Manual of Introductory Clinical Medicine. A Student-to-Student Guide.* Boston, Little, Brown and Co. 1984, p 20.
30. Rajka G: *Atopic Dermatitis.* London, Saunders, 1975.

31. Hanifin JM: Atopic dermatitis. *J Am Acad Dermatol* 6:1–13, 1982.

32. Wahlgren C-F: Itch and atopic dermatitis: Clinical and experimental studies. *Acta Dermatovener* (Stockh) Suppl 165, 1991.

33. Hanifin JM: Pharmacological abnormalities in atopic dermatitis. *Allergy* 44, Suppl 9:41–46, 1989.

34. Hanifin JM: Immunobiochemical aspects of atopic dermatitis. *Acta Derm Venereol* (Stockh) Suppl 144:45–47, 1989.

35. Trask DM, Chan SC, Sherman SE, et al: Altered leukocyte protein kinase activity in atopic dermatitis. *J Invest Dermatol* 90:526–531, 1988.

36. Giannetti A, Girolomoni G: Skin reactivity to neuropeptides in atopic dermatitis. *Br J Dermatol* 121:681–688, 1989.

37. Coulson IH, Holden CA: Cutaneous reactions to substance P and histamine in atopic dermatitis. *Br J Dermatol* 122:343–349, 1990.

38. Tuft L: Importance of inhalant allergens in atopic dermatitis. *J Invest Dermatol* 12:211–219, 1949.

39. Platts-Mills TAE, Mitchell EB, Rowntree S, et al: The role of dust mite allergens in atopic dermatitis. *Clin Exp Dermatol* 8:233–247, 1983.

40. Norris PG, Schofield O, Camp RDR: A study of the role of house dust mite in atopic dermatitis. *Br J Dermatol* 118:435–440, 1988.

41. Beck HI, Korsgaard J: Atopic dermatitis and house dust mites. *Br J Dermatol* 120:245–251, 1989.

42. Roberts DLL: House dust mite avoidance and atopic dermatitis. *Br J Dermatol* 110:735–739, 1984.

43. Sampson HA, Jolie PL: Increased plasma histamine concentrations after food challenges in children with atopic dermatitis. *N Engl J Med* 311:372–376, 1984.

44. Dahl MV. Staphylococcus aureus and atopic dermatitis. *Arch Dermatol* 119:840–846, 1983.

45. Leiferman KM, Ackerman SJ, Sampson HA, et al: Dermal deposition of eosinophil-granule major basic protein in atopic dermatitis. Comparison with onchocerciasis. *N Engl J Med* 313:282–285, 1985.

46. Wahlgren CF, Hagermark O, Bergstrom R: Patients' perception of itch induced by histamine, compound 48/80 and wool fibres in atopic dermatitis. *Acta Derm Venereol* (Stockh) 71:488–494, 1990.

47. Wahlgren CF: Pathophysiology of itching in urticaria and atopic dermatitis. *Allergy* 47:65–75, 1992.

48. Hanifin JM, Rajka G: Diagnostic features of atopic dermatitis. *Acta Dermatovener* Suppl 92:44, 1980.

49. Rajka G: Itch and IgE in atopic dermatitis. *Acta Derm Venereol* (Stockh) Suppl 92:38–39, 1980.

50. Haas N, Hamann K, Grabbe J, et al: Expression of the high affinity IgE-receptor on human Langerhans' cells. Elucidating the role of epidermal IgE in atopic eczema. *Acta Derm Venereol* (Stockh) 72:271–272, 1992.

51. Bernhard JD: Nonrashes 5. Atmoknesis: pruritus provoked by contact with air. *Cutis* 44:143–144, 1989.

52. Graham DT, Wolf S: The relation of eczema to attitude and to vascular reactions of the human skin. *J Lab Clin Med* 42:238–254, 1953.

53. Edwards AE, Shellow WVR, Wright ET, et al: Pruritic skin disease, psychological stress, and the itch sensation. *Arch Dermatol* 112:339–343, 1976.

54. Arthur RP, Shelley WB: The nature of itching in dermatitic skin. *Ann Intern Med* 49:900–908, 1958.

55. Rajka G: Itch duration in the involved skin of atopic dermatitis (prurigo Besnier). *Acta Derm Venereol* (Stockh) 47:320–321, 1968.

56. Heyer G, Hornstein OP, Handwerker HO: Skin reactions and itch sensation induced by epicutaneous histamine application in atopic dermatitis and controls. *J Invest Dermatol* 93:492–494, 1989.
57. Hanifin JM: Basic and clinical aspects of atopic dermatitis: A review. *Ann Allergy* 52:386–395, 1984.
58. Shelley WB, Shelley ED: Atopic dermatitis, in Shelley WB, Shelley ED: *Advanced Dermatologic Treatment*. Philadelphia, Saunders. 1987, pp 78–87.
59. Camp RDR, Reitamo S, Friedmann PS, et al: Cyclosporin A in severe, therapy-resistant atopic dermatitis: Report of an international workshop, April 1993. *Br J Dermatol* 129:217–220, 1993.
60. Galloway JH, Marsh ID, Bittiner SB, et al: Chinese herbs for eczema, the active compound? *Lancet* 337:566, 1991.
61. Sheehan MP, Rustin MHA, Atherton DJ, et al: Efficacy of traditional Chinese herbal therapy in adult atopic dermatitis. *Lancet* 340:13–17, 1992.
62. Wahlgren CF, Hagermark O, Bergstrom R: The antipruritic effect of a sedative and a non-sedative antihistamine in atopic dermatitis. *Br J Dermatol* 122:545–551, 1990.
63. Berth-Jones J, Graham-Brown RAC: Failure of terfenadine in relieving the pruritus of atopic dermatitis. *Br J Dermatol* 121:635–637, 1989.
64. Doherty V, Sylvester DGH, Kennedy CTC, et al: Treatment of itching in atopic eczema with antihistamines with a low sedative profile. *BMJ* 298:96, 1989.
65. Wahlgren CF, Scheynius A, Hagermark O: Antipruritic effect of oral cyclosporin A in atopic dermatitis. *Acta Derm Venereol* (Stockh) 70:322–329, 1990.
66. Sowden JM, Berth-Jones J, Ross JS, et al: Double-blind, controlled, cross-over study of cyclosporin in adults with severe refractory atopic dermatitis. *Lancet* 338:137–140, 1991.
67. Berth-Jones J, Graham-Brown RAC: Failure of papaverine to reduce pruritus in atopic dermatitis: A double-blind, placebo-controlled cross-over study. *Br J Dermatol* 122:553–557, 1990.
68. Shupack J, Stiller M, Meola T, et al: Papaverine hydrochloride in the treatment of atopic dermatitis: A double-blind, placebo-controlled crossover clinical trial to reassess safety and efficacy. *Dermatologica* 183:21–24, 1991.
69. Baer RL: Papaverine therapy in atopic dermatitis. *J Am Acad Dermatol* 13:806–808, 1985.
70. Grewe SR, Chan SC, Hanifin JM: Elevated leukocyte cyclic AMP-phosphodiesterase in atopic disease: A possible mechanism for cyclic AMP-agonist hyporesponsiveness. *J Allergy Clin Immunol* 70:452–457, 1982.
71. Wirth L: Antipruritic qualities of papaverine hydrochloride. *J Invest Dermatol* 8:63–64, 1947.
72. Epstein E, Pinski JB: A blind study. *Arch Dermatol* 89:548–549, 1964.
73. Baer RL: Personal communication. May 20, 1992.
74. Mier PD, van de Kerkhof PCM: *Textbook of Psoriasis*. Edinburgh, Churchill Livingstone, 1986.
75. Camp RDR: Psoriasis, in Champion RH, Burton JL, Ebling FJG (eds): *Textbook of Dermatology*, 5th ed. Oxford, Blackwell Scientific Publications. 1992, pp 1391–1457.
76. Christophers E, Krueger GC: Psoriasis, in Fitzpatrick TB, Eisen AZ, Wolff K, et al (eds): *Dermatology in General Medicine*, 3d ed. New York, McGraw Hill. 1987, pp 461–491.
77. Roenigk HH, Maibach HI: *Psoriasis*, 2d ed. New York, Marcel Dekker, 1991.
78. Naukkarinen A, Nickoloff BJ, Farber EM: Quantification of cutaneous sensory nerves and their substance P content in psoriasis. *J Invest Dermatol* 92:126–129, 1989.
79. Kurkcuoglu N, Cakar N: Substance-P immunoreactivity in active edges of psoriatic plaques. *Clin Exp Dermatol* 15:467, 1990.
80. Eedy DJ, Johnston CF, Shaw C, et al: Neuropeptides in psoriasis: An immunocytochemical and radioimmunoassay study. *J Invest Dermatol* 96:434–438, 1991.

81. Bernstein JE, Parish LC, Rappaport M, et al: Effects of topically applied capsaicin on moderate and severe psoriasis vulgaris. *J Am Acad Dermatol* 15:504–507, 1986.
82. Berberian B, Bernstein JE, Dodd WA, et al: Double-blind evaluation of capsaicin cream in pruritic psoriasis. Abstract. *J Invest Dermatol* 94:506, 1990.
83. Kurkcuoglu N, Alaybeyi F: Topical capsaicin for psoriasis, (letter). *Br J Dermatol* 123:549–550, 1990.
84. Toruniowa B, Jablonska S: Mast cells in the initial stages of psoriasis. *Arch Dermatol Res* 280:189–193, 1988.
85. Melski JW, Bernhard JD, Stern RS: The Koebner (isomorphic) response in psoriasis. Associations with early age-at-onset and multiple previous therapies. *Arch Dermatol* 119:655–659, 1983.
86. Newbold PCH. Pruritus in psoriasis, in Farber EM, Cox AJ (eds): *Psoriasis: Proceedings of the Second International Symposium.* New York, Yorke Medical Books. 1977, pp 334–336.
87. Gupta MA, Gupta AK, Kirkby S, et al: Pruritus in psoriasis. A prospective study of some psychiatric and dermatologic correlates. *Arch Dermatol* 124:1052–1057, 1988.
88. Gupta MA, Gupta AK, Kirkby S, et al: Pruritus associated with nocturnal wakenings: Organic or psychogenic? *J Am Acad Dermatol* 21:479–484, 1989.
89. Bernhard JD: Nocturnal wakening caused by pruritus: Organic or psychogenic? *J Am Acad Dermatol* 23:767, 1990.
90. Rebora A, Aratari E, Bertamino R, et al: The itching psoriasis. *Acta Derm Venereol* (Stockh) Suppl 113:118–120, 1984.
91. Jordan WP: PUVA, pruritus and the loss of the axon flare. *Arch Dermatol* 115:636, 1979.
92. Rogers S, Marks J, Shuster S: Itch following photochemotherapy for psoriasis. *Acta Derm Venereol* (Stockh) 61:178–180, 1981.
93. Tegner E: Severe skin pain after PUVA treatment. *Acta Derm Venereol* (Stockh) 59:467–470, 1979.
94. Roelandts R, Stevens A: PUVA-induced itching and skin pain. *Photodermatol Photoimmunol Photomed* 7:141–142, 1990.
95. Bernhard JD, Kabat-Zinn J, Kristeller J: Effectiveness of relaxation and visualization techniques as an adjunct to phototherapy and photochemotherapy of psoriasis. *J Am Acad Dermatol.* 19:572–573, 1988.
96. Farber EM, Nall L: Natural history and treatment of scalp psoriasis. *Cutis* 49:396–400, 1992.
97. Giard F, Marcoux D, McCuaig C, et al: Eosinophilic pustular folliculitis (Ofjui disease) in childhood, a review of four cases. *Pediatr Dermatol* 8:189–193, 1991.
98. Taieb A, Bassan-Andrieu LB, Maleville J: Eosinophilic pustulosis of the scalp in childhood. *J Am Acad Dermatol* 27:55–60, 1992.
99. Venning VA, Millard PR: Recurrent scabies with unusual clinical features in a renal transplant recipient. *Br J Dermatol* 126:204–205, 1992.
100. McCauley CS, Blumenthal MS: Dobutamine and pruritus of the scalp. *Ann Intern Med* 105:966, 1986.
101. Sowunmi A, Walker O, Salako LA: Pruritus and antimalarial drugs in Africans. *Lancet* 2:213, 1989.
102. Tucker WFG, Briggs C, Challoner T: Absence of pruritus in iron deficiency following venesection. *Clin Exp Dermatol* 9:186–189, 1984.
103. Burgess I, Coulthard M, Heaney J: Scalp infestation by Liposcelis mendax. *Br J Dermatol* 125:400–401, 1991.
104. Bernhard JD: Does thinking itch? *Lancet* i:589, 1985.
105. Calnan CD, O'Neill D: Itching in tension states. *Br J Dermatol* 64:274–280, 1952.
106. Cotterill JA: Dermatological nondisease: A common and potentially fatal disturbance of cutaneous body image. *Br J Dermatol* 104:611–618, 1981.
107. Dupre E. Coenestopathic states, in Hirsch SR, Shepherd M (eds): *Themes and Variations*

in European Psychiatry. An anthology. Charlottesville, University Press of Virginia. 1974, pp 385–394.

108. Rook A, Wilkinson DS: Psychocutaneous disorders, in Rook A, Wilkinson DS, Ebling FJG (eds): *Textbook of Dermatology,* 3d ed. Oxford, Blackwell. 1979, p 2029.

109. Scheff RJ, Rolla AR: The eosinophilia-myalgia syndrome. *Ann Intern Med* 112:964–965, 1990.

110. Cooper BC, Lucente FE: Management of facial, head and neck pain. Philadelphia, Saunders. 1989, pp 44–46.

111. Drummond PD: Scalp tenderness and sensitivity to pain in migraine and tension headache. *Headache* 27:45–50, 1987.

112. Moschella SL: Written personal communication. August 14, 1992.

113. Schmidt K, Medenica M: Pruritic ulcerating bruise in an elderly Hispanic man. *Arch Dermatol* 128:1115–1120, 1992.

114. Rycroft FJG: Low humidity and microtrauma. *Am J Ind Med* 8:371, 1985.

115. White IR, Rycroft RJG: Low humidity occupational dermatoses—an epidemic. *Contact Dermatitis* 8:287, 1982.

116. Guest R: Clean rooms and itchy faces. *J Soc Occup Med* 41:37, 1991.

117. Nethercott JR, Nield G, Holness DL: A review of 79 cases of eyelid dermatitis. *J Am Acad Dermatol* 21:223–230, 1989.

118. Berg M: Facial skin complaints and work at visual display units. Epidemiological, clinical and histopathological studies. *Acta Derm Venereol* (Stockh) Suppl 150, 1989.

119. Summers CG, MacDonald JT: Paroxysmal facial itch: A presenting sign of childhood brainstem glioma. *J Child Neurol* 3:189–192, 1988.

120. Bernhard JD: Photosensitivity, in Lebwohl M (ed): *Difficult Diagnoses in Dermatology.* Edinburgh, Churchill-Livingstone. 1988, pp 405–417.

121. Fisher AA: Status cosmeticus: A cosmetic intolerance syndrome. *Cutis* 46:109–110, 1990.

122. Engasser PG, Maibach HI: Dermatitis due to cosmetics, in Fisher AA (ed): *Contact Dermatitis.* Philadelphia, Lea & Febiger, 1986.

123. Maibach HI, Lammintausta K, Berardesca E, et al: Tendency to irritation: sensitive skin. *J Am Acad Dermatol* 21:833–835, 1989.

124. Pierard GE: What do you mean by dry skin? *Dermatologica* 179:1, 1989.

125. Frosch P, Kligman AM: A method for appraising the stinging capacity of topically applied substances. *J Soc Cosmet Chem* 28:197, 1981.

125a. Foley P, Nixon R, Marks R, et al: The frequency of reactions to sunscreens: Results of a longitudinal population-based study on the regular use of sunscreens in Australia. *Br J Dermatol* 128:512–518, 1993.

126. Braun-Falco O, Plewig G, Wolff HH, et al: *Dermatology.* Chapter 14. Erythematous and erythematosquamous skin diseases. Berlin, Springer-Verlag. 1991, pp 403–466.

127. Alexander JO'D: *Arthropods and Human Skin.* Berlin, Springer-Verlag. 1984, pp 293–302.

128. Ayres S: Pityriasis folliculorum (Demodex). *Arch Dermatol Syphilol* 21:19–24, 1930.

129. Ayres S Jr, Ayres S III: Demodectic eruption (demodicidosis) in the human. *Arch Dermatol* 83:816–827, 1961.

130. Sevinsky L, Hoyo OE, Santos P, et al: Demodicidosis: A case report. *Eur J Dermatol* 2:246–248, 1992.

131. Dahl MV: Chronic, irritant contact dermatitis: Mechanisms, variables, and differentiation from other forms of contact dermatitis. *Adv Dermatol* 3:261–276, 1988.

132. Klein G, Grubauer G, Fritsch P: The influence of daily dish-washing with synthetic detergent on human skin. *Br J Dermatol* 127:131–137, 1992.

133. Fisher AA: *Contact Dermatitis,* 3d ed. Philadelphia, Lea & Febiger, 1986.

134. Cronin E: *Contact Dermatitis.* London, Churchill Livingstone, 1980.

135. Jackson EM, Goldner R (eds): *Irritant Contact Dermatitis.* New York, Marcel Dekker, 1989.
136. Nater JP, de Groot AC: *Unwanted Effects of Cosmetics and Drugs Used in Dermatology,* 2d ed. New York, Elsevier, 1985.
137. Adams RM (ed): *Occupational Skin Disease,* 2d ed. Philadelphia, Saunders, 1990.
138. Morren M, Rodrigues R, Dooms-Goossens A, et al: Connubial contact dermatitis: A review. *Eur J Dermatol* 2:219–223, 1992.
139. Cochfeld M, Burger J: Sexual transmission of nickel and poison oak contact dermatitis. *Lancet* 1:589, 1983.
140. Bernhard JD. Editorial comment, in Sober AJ, Fitzpatrick TB (eds): *Year Book of Dermatology 1990.* St. Louis, Mosby Year Book. 1990. p 86.
141. Morales C, Basomba J, Carreira J: Anaphylaxis produced by rubber glove contact: Case reports and immunological identification of the antigens involved. *Clin Exp Allergy* 19:425–430, 1989.
142. Turjanmaa K, Reunala T: Condoms as a source of latex allergen and cause of contact dermatitis. *Contact Dermatitis* 20:360–364, 1989.
143. Leroy D, Dompmartin A: Connubial photosensitivity to musk ambrette. *Photodermatol* 6:137, 1989.
144. Hunter JAA: Seventh age itch. *BMJ* 291:842, 1985.
145. Young AW: The diagnosis of pruritus in the elderly. *J Am Geriatr Soc* 15:750–758, 1967.
146. Graham-Brown RAC, Monk BE: Pruritus and xerosis, in Monk BE, Graham-Brown RAC, (eds): *Skin Disorders in the Elderly.* Oxford, Blackwell, 1988, pp 133–146.
147. Bernhard JD: Phantom itch, pseudophantom itch, and senile pruritus. *Int J Dermatol,* 31:856–857, 1992.
147a. Long CC, Marks R: Stratum corneum changes in patients with senile pruritus. *J Am Acad Dermatol* 27:560–564, 1992.
148. Potts RO, Buras EM, Chrisman DA: Changes with age in the moisture content of human skin. *J Invest Dermatol* 82:97–100, 1984.
149. Newton JA, Singh AK, Greaves MW, et al: Aquagenic pruritus associated with the idiopathic hypereosinophilic syndrome. *Br J Dermatol* 122:103–106, 1990.
150. McGrath JA, Greaves MW: Aquagenic pruritus and the myelodysplastic syndrome. *Br J Dermatol* 123:414–415, 1990.
151. Itin PH, Winkelmann RK: Cutaneous manifestations in patients with thrombocythemia. *J Am Acad Dermatol* 24:59–63, 1991.
152. Nestler JE: Hemochromatosis and pruritus. *Ann Intern Med* 98:1026, 1983.
153. Sharma OP, Balchum OJ: Alcohol-induced pain and itching on hot shower in sarcoidosis. An unusual association. *Am Rev Respir Dis* 106:763–766, 1972.
154. Shelley WB, Rawnsley HM: Aquagenic urticaria: Contact sensitivity reaction to water. *JAMA* 189:895–898, 1964.
155. Shelley WB: Questions and answers. *JAMA* 212:1385, 1970.
156. Greaves MW, Black AK, Eady RAJ, et al: Aquagenic pruritus. *BMJ* 282:2008–2010, 1981.
157. Steinman HK, Greaves MW: Aquagenic pruritus. *J Am Acad Dermatol* 13:91–96, 1985.
158. Bircher AJ: Water-induced itching. *Dermatologica* 181:83–87, 1990.
159. Logan RA, Fehrer MD, Steinman HK: The prevalence of water-induced itching. *Br J Dermatol* 111:734–736, 1984.
160. Potasman I, Heinrich I, Bassan HM: Aquagenic pruritus: Prevalence and clinical characteristics. *Isr J Med Sci* 26:499–503, 1990.
161. Kligman AM, Greaves MW, Steinman H: Water-induced itching without cutaneous signs. Aquagenic pruritus. *Arch Dermatol* 122:183–186, 1986.
162. Bircher AJ, Meier-Ruge W: Aquagenic pruritus. Water-induced activation of acetylcholinesterase. *Arch Dermatol* 124:84–89, 1988.
163. Lotti T, Steinman HK, Greaves MW, et al: Increased cutaneous fibrinolytic activity in aquagenic pruritus. *Int J Dermatol* 25:508–510, 1986.

164. Lotti T, Casigliani R, Panconesi E: Plasminogen activation in pruritus aquagenicus and aquagenic urticaria. *Ital Gen Rev Dermatol* 24:159–162, 1987.
165. Czarnetzki BM, Breetholt KH, Traupe H: Evidence that water acts as a carrier for an epidermal antigen in aquagenic urticaria. *J Am Acad Dermatol* 15:623–627, 1986.
166. Steinman HK, Kobza-Black A, Lotti TM, et al. Polycythaemia rubra vera and water-induced pruritus: Blood histamine levels and cutaneous fibrinolytic activity before and after water challenge. *Br J Dermatol* 116:329–333, 1987.
167. Jackson N, Burt D, Croker J, et al: Skin mast cells in polycythaemia vera: Relationship to the pathogenesis and treatment of pruritus. *Br J Dermatol* 116:21–29, 1987.
168. Bernhard JD: Editorial comment, in Sober AJ, Fitzpatrick TB, (eds): *1992 Year Book of Dermatology.* St Louis, Mosby Year Book. 1992, 402–403.
169. Archer CB, Camp RDR, Greaves MW: Polycythaemia vera can present with aquagenic pruritus. *Lancet* 1:1451, 1988.
170. Reid CDL: Pruritus preceding the development of polycythaemia vera. *Lancet* 2:964, 1988.
171. Bayoumi AHM, Highet AS: Baking soda baths for aquagenic pruritus. *Lancet* 2:464, 1986.
172. Wolf R, Krakowski A: Variations in aquagenic pruritus and treatment alternatives. *J Am Acad Dermatol* 18:1081–1083, 1988.
173. Handfield-Jones SE, Greaves MW: Aquagenic pruritus: Update on diagnosis and treatment. *Br J Dermatol* 125, Suppl 38:13, 1991.
174. Swerlick RA: Photochemotherapy treatment of pruritus associated with polycythemia vera. *J Am Acad Dermatol* 13:675–677, 1985.
175. Fjellner B, Hagermark O: Pruritus in polycythaemia vera: Treatment with aspirin and possibility of platelet involvement. *Acta Derm Venereol* (Stockh) 59:505–512, 1979.
176. Jackson N, Burt D, Crocker J, et al: Skin mast cells in polycythaemia vera: Relationship to the pathogenesis and treatment of pruritus. *Br J Dermatol* 116:21–29, 1987.
177. Gilbert HS, Warner RRP, Wasserman LR: A study of histamine in myeloproliferative disease. *Blood* 28:795–806, 1966.
178. Weick JK, Donovan PB, Najean Y, et al: The use of cimetidine for the treatment of pruritus in polycythemia vera. *Arch Intern Med* 142:242–243, 1981.
179. Chanarin I, Szur L: Relief of intractable pruritus in polychthaemia rubra vera with cholestyramine. *Br J Hematol* 29:669–670, 1975.
180. Ross JS, McKee PH, Smith NP, et al: Unusual variants of pemphigoid: From pruritus to pemphigoid nodularis. *J Cutan Pathol* 19:212–216, 1992.
181. Camisa C, Neff JC, Rossana C, et al: Bullous lichen planus: Diagnosis by indirect immunofluorescence and treatment with dapsone. *J Am Acad Dermatol* 14:464–469, 1986.
182. Crosby DL, Feldman SD: A pruritic vesicular eruption. *Arch Dermatol* 126:1497–1502, 1990.
183. Bennion SD. Annular vesiculation. *Arch Dermatol* 125:1569–1574, 1989.
184. Hori Y, Tsuru N, Niimura M: Bullous Darier's disease. *Arch Dermatol* 118:278–279, 1982.
185. Telfer NR, Burge SM, Ryan TJ: Vesiculo-bullous Darier's disease. *Br J Dermatol* 122:831–834, 1990.
186. Champion RH. Urticaria, in: Champion RH, Burton JL, Ebling FJG, (eds): *Textbook of Dermatology,* 5th ed. Oxford, Blackwell, 1992, pp 1865–1880.

FOUR

ITCHY PAPULAR ERUPTIONS

Jeffrey D. Bernhard

The differential diagnosis of itchy papular eruptions is broad (Tables 4-1, 4-2, 4-3, and 4-4). One of the most common causes, insect bites, is often difficult to prove or, when suspected as a diagnosis, is met with resounding incredulity by the patient. The diagnostic challenge and frustration is epitomized by the diagnosis rashly dubbed "itchy red bump disease." We shall return to itchy red bump disease and its relatives (or twins) at the end of this chapter.

PAPULAR URTICARIA FROM INSECT BITES, AND ITS RELATIONSHIP TO PRURITIC PAPULAR ERUPTIONS AND THE VARIOUS "PRURIGOS"*

The smaller the bite, the bigger the diagnostic problem.
W.B. Shelley and E.D. Shelley[40]

This is one of the most challenging problems in all of clinical dermatology. The history, laboratory examination, and a skin biopsy may be extremely helpful, but even then, the clinician is often faced with a bewildering variety of diagnostic and synonymous labels of the type for which dermatologists are justly famous, and, with label in hand or not, a therapeutic challenge.

---

* Small parts of this section are adapted from reference 46. Some passages have been reproduced unchanged. Some material has been updated, expanded, and partially rearranged.

Table 4-1 Differential diagnosis of itchy papular eruptions

Infestations and infections
    scabies (see Chap. 9)
    other mites
    pediculosis
    other arthropod bites (especially fleas, bedbugs; papular urticaria)
    swimmer's itch (schistosomal cercarial dermatitis; clam-digger's itch)
    sea bather's eruption (see Chap. 9)
    strongyloidiasis ("ground itch")
    hookworm ("ground itch" at portal of entry; secondary urticaria)
    ascariasis
    other intestinal nematodes (may cause, e.g., urticaria)
    other helminth; filaria, e.g., onchocerciasis[1,2]
    certain protozoan infections (e.g., acute phase of African trypanosomiasis)[2]

Contactants
    sponge dermatitis (e.g., *Tedania ignis*—fire sponge)
    bristle worm (fireworm)
    papular contact dermatitis (irritant or allergic)
    certain plants (e.g., nettle)
    caterpillar hairs

Inflammatory dermatoses
    dermatitis herpetiformis
    pityriasis rosea
    eczematous dermatitis, especially follicular eczema[3]
    atopic prurigo reaction[4]
    psoriasis
    folliculitis (infectious and noninfectious) see Table 4-2
    perifolliculitis
    Fox-Fordyce disease
    miliaria
    other sweat retention syndromes[4]
    autoeczematization reaction
    id reaction (may be papulovesicular)[6,7]
    Darier–White disease (keratosis follicularis)[8]
    Grover's disease (transient acantholytic dermatosis;[9] papules, papulovesicles, and
        excoriated papules)
    persistent acantholytic dermatosis[10]
    other/related papular acantholytic & dyskeratotic eruptions[11]
    infantile acrolocalized papulovesicular syndrome[12]
    papular acrodermatitis (Gianotti-Crosti syndrome)[13]
    follicular and papular forms of urticaria and dermographism (see Tables 4-2 and 4-3)
    lichen planus
    disseminated granuloma annulare

Miscellaneous
    pruritic urticarial papules and plaques of pregnancy (see Chap. 19).
    eruptive syringomas[14] (usually asymptomatic)
    papular mucinosis (lichen myxedematosus)[15]
    Waldenstrom's macroglobulinemia[16]
    hypereosinophilic syndrome[17]
    eosinophilia-myalgia syndrome[18]

Table 4-1 Continued

Miscellaneous (continued)
    adult T-cell leukemia/lymphoma[19]
    pruritic papular eruption of HIV infection (see Chap. 20)
    papuloerythroderma[20]
    papular eruption of black men[21]
    hamartoma moniliformis[22]
    prurigo simplex subacuta/subacute prurigo/papular dermatitis (see text)
    prurigo nodularis (see Chap. 7)
    prurigo pigmentosa[23]
    actinic prurigo[24,25]
    perforating disorders (e.g., Kyrle's disease; see Table 4-4)
    "scratch papules" secondary to rubbing and excoriation when an underlying systemic
      cause of pruritus is present

Table 4-2 Folliculitis

Infectious folliculitis
    gram-positive
    gram-negative[26]
    pseudomonas[27]
    pityrosporum[28]
    Demodex[29]

Drug-induced folliculitis and acneiform eruptions
    actinomycin D
    granulocyte-colony-stimulating factor[30]
    tetracycline
    rifampin
    diphenylhydantoin
    halogens[31]

Eosinophilic pustular folliculitis[32]
Actinic folliculitis[33]
Pseudofolliculitis[34]
Perforating folliculitis

Table 4-3 Pruritic conditions with urticarial papules or plaques

ordinary urticaria (hives)
arthropod reactions
papular urticaria (insect bite reactions: especially mosquitoes, fleas, bedbugs)
reactions to urticating spicules or nettling hairs of caterpillars
dermatitis herpetiformis
pemphigoid
herpes gestationis
allergic contact dermatitis
leukocytoclastic vasculitis (urticarial vasculitis)
hypersensitivity reactions (drug eruptions, infections, infestations)
pruritic urticarial papules and plaques of pregnancy

This problem is embodied in the diagnoses of prurigo simplex subacuta, lichen Vidal urticatus, subacute prurigo, papular dermatitis of adults, itchy red bump disease, lichen urticatus, strophulus, and papular urticaria. Papular urticaria (PU) probably subsumes most of the above when an arthropod-related cause can be determined.[41] According to Lever,

> Papular urticaria, also known as lichen urticatus, is the result of hypersensitivity to bites from certain insects, especially mosquitoes, fleas, and bedbugs. One observes edematous papules and papulovesicles, which, because of severe itching, usually are excoriated. The eruption is more commonly found in children than adults, and, if caused by mosquitoes, is limited to the summer months. The lesions of papular urticaria are clinically and often histologically indistinguishable from those of prurigo simplex.[42]

In his magisterial text, *Arthropods and Human Skin*, J. O'Donel Alexander defines papular urticaria a shade more restrictedly:

> Chronic re-infestation in persons constantly exposed to fleas produces the condition known as papular urticaria (PU), commonly known as "hives," "heat spots," lichen urticatus or strophulus.[43]

In the foreward to O'Donel's book, Arthur Rook makes a particularly telling comment:

> Every dermatologist of experience will admit that he sees many patients in whom he makes a diagnosis of "insect bites", if he has the confidence to do so, or of "papular urticaria" or "prurigo" when he lacks such confidence, mainly because he is at a loss to know which arthropod is likely to be implicated.[44]

Rook describes papular urticaria (syn. strophulus) as "an historic source of terminologic and diagnostic confusion."[45] According to Rook:

> The very large number of synonyms and the frequent confusion with other prurigos largely explain the acrimonious and protracted disputes on etiology. Papular urticaria is a chronic or recurrent eruption of irritable papules often grouped in irregular clusters, frequently seasonal in incidence, and afflicting predominantly children between the ages of 2 and 7 ... produced by fleas, bedbugs, some other insects, and certain mites, notably *Cheyletiella*.[45]

If there is a classic lesion of papular urticaria, it is a small, extremely itchy, erythematous wheal or papule, with or without an urticarial flare, usually arranged in clusters over the shoulders, upper arms, and buttocks, in a child between the ages of 18 months and 17 years. [13] [p71] Vesicles and bullae may be seen when intense hypersensitivity is present. A central hemmorhagic punctum or tiny vesicle may be seen if the lesion has not been excoriated; when present, these findings are an important aid to diagnosis. Although the initial lesion may be an urticarial wheal, firm pruritic papules may develop and persist for days: in that case, the use of the term "urticaria," which more typically describes an *evanescent* wheal, is slightly misleading. Unfortunately,

Table 4-4 Perforating disorders

Disorder	Associations and references
Kyrle's disease	renal failure
reactive perforating collagenosis (RPC)	renal failure/diabetes[35] Hodgkin's disease[36]
perforating folliculitis	idiopathic vs. secondary to scratching in any case of generalized pruritus
perforating granuloma annulare[37,38]	
perforating lichen nitidus[39]	
elastosis perforans sepiginosa	connective tissue disorders
calcinosis cutis	

the term "urticarial" is sometimes used to describe lesions that are "like urticaria," but which are not strictly urticaria themselves.

Unrecognized assaults from insects can produce a variety of problems.[46] The patient may present with papular urticaria, papules alone, excoriated papules, papulovesicles, persistent bite reactions (including granulomas and pseudolymphomatous reactions), secondary urticarial eruptions, excoriations alone, secondary eczematization, secondary infection, or any combination of the above. Patients must be questioned, requestioned, and questioned again about their exposure to animals, pets, and other people's pets. Pets and the home may need to be investigated.[47] Shelley and Shelley have drawn particular attention to the diagnostic challenge presented by nonburrowing mites.[48,49] A skin biopsy is often helpful. According to Lever, the presence of large numbers of eosinophils in the biopsy specimen favor the diagnosis of papular urticaria (insect bite reaction).[45]

Although, bites and infestations will be considered in detail in Chap. 9, they must be touched on here because they are still a leading cause of itchy papular eruptions or P.U.O. (pruritus of undetermined origin) even when doctor and patient alike are convinced that bugs or pets are out of the question. It must be stressed that infestations (e.g., by fleas from pets or scabies mites from human or other animal contacts) can occur even in people and homes with the highest hygienic standards.[50] A physician whose bed was positioned directly under an attic vent was plagued by an itchy papular eruption for 3 months before a sparrow's nest above the vent was removed, along with the avian mites (Northern fowl mites) it contained.[51]

Cats and dogs may show complete tolerance to heavy flea infestations, but their owners may not![52] In one study, 57 of 101 patients with unexplained itching were shown, after veterinary examination of their pets, to have been exposed to ectoparasites from animals.[53] Of these patients, 50 were cured within 1 month by ridding their animals of mites and fleas. Cats and dogs can harbor mite species that cannot establish residence or burrow in human skin but that can nonetheless cause transient, repetitive pruritic reactions. Sarcoptes scabiei from dogs and Cheyletiella parasitovorax[54] from dogs or cats can cause a "hit and run" itch in which burrows do not occur. The arms, torso, and legs may be sites of predilection. Another striking feature of pet- or insect-related itching and rashes is that not all members of a given household are necessarily affected. Some people have respiratory as well as cutaneous allergies to animal hair and dander.

Specific arthropods associated with papular urticaria will be addressed in Chap. 9.

SCRATCH PAPULES, FOLLICULAR DERMOGRAPHISM, DERMOGRAPHIC PRURIGO

The problem of itchy papules is made all the more challenging and complex because scratching an itch of any cause can lead to papular or follicular dermographism or to the formation of more persistent, so-called "prurigo papules" or "scratch papules."[55] This term may have been coined by Irwin Braverman, although he thinks he may have absorbed it from other teachers and colleagues over the years.[56]

Dermographism—also known as dermatographia or skin writing—is a form of physical urticaria that develops on scratching or stroking the skin. It occurs in at least 10 varieties,[57] one of which is a papular variant that may be a sign of urticaria pigmentosa.[58,59] Another variety is called follicular dermographism. It appears as "transitory, discrete, follicular urticarial papules" at recently scratched sites, and may occur during periods of transient antigenemia.[60] Dermatographic prurigo may be papular or follicular dermographism by another name, or a simple variant of constitutional dermographism.[61] Marcussen felt that it occurred "in patients with constitutional dermographism when a neurosis brings the weak itching, which in these patients is normally excited by friction, within the focus of consciousness," and that the clinical picture could "thus be explained by the scratching of the places where dermographism is excited by the friction and pressure of garments."[61] Marcussen also found that symptomatic (i.e., itching) dermographism occurred frequently among patients with scabies.

Scratching a systemic itch, as in Hodgkin's disease, may also lead to follicular or papular dermographism, especially (and obviously) in patients who are incidentally dermographic. Similarly, it may lead to the formation of scratch papules, to bacterial or nonbacterial folliculitis, and even to prurigo nodularis.[62] Scratching in systemic illnesses may also be associated with a group of perforating disorders, such as perforating folliculitis. The perforating disorders are listed in Table 4-4. The occurrence of these phenomena means that the entire differential diagnosis of underlying systemic causes of generalized pruritus must be considered in the differential diagnosis of itchy papular eruptions when a primary dermatologic diagnosis cannot be established.

PRURIGO NODULARIS

Prurigo nodularis is easily diagnosed but difficult to treat. Papular rather than nodular lesions may occur. It may arise *ex novo*,[63] in the settings of atopic dermatitis and contact dermatitis, or in the setting of itching related to an underlying systemic illness.[64-66] Chapter 7 is devoted to prurigo nodularis. Greither reviewed the concept of prurigo and its relationship to pruritus in a comprehensive review in 1970, and concluded that prurigo could be rationalized into three groups: an acute form identical to papular urticaria, a subacute form (which has many synonyms and probably many causes), and Hyde's prurigo (prurigo nodularis, nodular prurigo).[67]

Pemphigoid nodularis is a variant of pemphigoid that presents with a pruritic, papular, or nodular eruption, together with clinical, histologic, and immunologic features of bullous pemphigoid. The nodules may be identical to those seen in prurigo nodularis; blisters may be absent. Itching with or without nonspecific skin lesions may be seen before prurigo papules or blisters appear; this confirms the importance of thinking about pemphigoid in the evaluation of an elderly patient with generalized pruritus or a clinically nonspecific persistent pruritic papular eruption. Provost and colleagues described patients with this condition in 1979.[68] Yung and colleagues named it in 1981.[69] At least nine cases have been reported.[70]

Additional Causes of Itchy Papular Eruptions

In recent years itchy papules have also been recognized as a presenting feature in the prodrome of adult T-cell leukemia,[71] in hypereosinophilic syndrome, and in the so-called papuloerythroderma syndrome (references in Table 4-1). Table 4-1 provides a staggering indication of the variety of conditions that may be present with itchy papules, as well as references and citations of other chapters in this book where the topics may be discussed in additional detail. Table 4-2 provides a further indication of the variety of folliculitides and perifolliculitides, many of which are accompanied by pruritus. One of the most frequently overlooked but now increasingly recognized is pityrosporum folliculitis.[72] Another increasingly recognized disorder is eosinophilic pustular folliculitis, which may be related to fungi in some cases,[73] and which is also seen in the setting of HIV infection. This and the so-called pruritic papular eruption of AIDS[74] will be discussed in Chap. 20.

ITCHY RED BUMP DISEASE AND PRURIGO SIMPLEX SUBACUTA

Lastly, the issue of so-called itchy red bump disease must be addressed. Unfortunately, like the itchy bumps themselves sometimes, this is a diagnostic category that will never go away, because it is defined as a pruritic papular eruption that can't be diagnosed as something else! A case that turns out to have been caused by insect bites all along gets relabeled (diagnosed) as "insect bites," "acute prurigo," or "papular urticaria." Some victims turn out to be atopics with papular variants of atopic eczema. As other cases drag on, resistant to further elucidation and often recalcitrant to treatment, they develop Latin names such as "prurigo simplex subacuta," or Latin–English ones such as "subacute prurigo," and "papular dermatitis of adults." Patients who fall into these diagnostic niches (holes?) should be re-examined and carefully re-evaluated over time, with the full range of differential diagnoses, including systemic diseases, in mind (see Chap. 24).[75] Sherertz and colleagues at Bowman Gray recently studied 12 such patients who "had some atopic features" but not enough to meet Hanifin's criteria for atopic dermatitis and in whom no other cause could be determined.[76] Histologic features from skin biopsy specimens "resembled papular urticaria," but there was no "history to suggest arthropod bites" or any other exogenous cause. The patients had multiple flesh-colored to erythematous nonfollicular papules with evidence of excoriation and/or lichenification. Two had vesicles. As in other reports of what must be the same or nearly the same disorder, the lesions were often symmetrically distributed, affected primarily the trunk, extensor aspects of the extremities, and "cape area" of the face, scalp, neck, lower trunk, and buttocks, but spared the palms and soles. The initial lesion is probably a papule, although a short-lived vesicle may exist before the patient scratches it away. The eruptions were chronic, at least 4 months, and 10 of the 12 had been referred by other dermatologists. The most common preceding diagnosis was atopic dermatitis. The common histologic features included a mixed superficial and deep perivascular infiltrate with scattered interstitial eosinophils and spongiosis in most cases. Most of the patients were refractory to simple measures but responded at least partially to treatment with one or more of the following interventions: superpotent topical corticosteroids, tapering doses of systemic corticosteroids, ultraviolet B phototherapy, PUVA photochemotherapy. Uehara and Ofuji studied 28 patients with the "typical picture of prurigo simplex subacuta," but found that the first visible lesion was always a papule and never a vesicle.[77] The striking features in their series were symmetrical distribution, characteristic involvement of the trunk and extensor surfaces of the extremities, sparing of the palms and soles, and occasional involvement of the face and scalp. Differences from one author's experience to the next are to be expected, partly because populations may differ, and partly because it may be difficult to achieve a uniform population of a disorder that is difficult to define and partly diagnosed by the process of exclusion.

Richard Dobson's theory is that itchy red bump disease is a variety of papular urticaria caused by insects. He has observed that it often occurs in retirees who move from the Northeast to the Charleston, South Carolina, area, and who are therefore exposed to a new variety of insects. They develop papular urticaria when bitten the way children do, and after months or years of exposure "the hypersensitivity vanishes (blocking antibody) and the condition clears."[78] Alfred Kopf, who suggested the name prurigo papularis for this disease, also feels that "it may yet prove to be some sort of arthropod assault."[79]

What is itchy red bump disease? Is it the same as prurigo simplex subacuta? Patients whose provisional diagnosis is one or the other but whose rash finally turns out to be caused by insect bites or scratch papules because of an underlying systemic cause of itching turn out to have had something else by definition. Perhaps the safest clinical practice is to assume that itchy red bump disease and/or prurigo simplex subacuta must be considered perpetually provisional diagnoses. Another safe approach would be to view them as other reaction patterns of the skin are viewed. Just as one does not settle for a diagnosis of anemia without pursuing a causal explanation, one should not accept a diagnosis of erythema multiforme, erythema nodosum, or prurigo simplex subacuta without trying to uncover an underlying cause. The last word must be given to Ackerman[80]:

> I believe that itchy red bump disease is a variation on the theme of papular urticaria. There are colleagues, however, . . . who insist that it is a disease sui generis. Some years ago Charlie DeFeo averred that itchy red bump disease is a manifestation of infestation by the mite Cheyletiella parasitovorax. Everyone has a point of view, but nobody knows! . . . [81]

MAKING A DIAGNOSIS

Although one papule may not look that different from another, the trained and careful eye can often discern important features of a papular eruption. Scaling may point to psoriasis or pityriasis rosea. Gentle scraping may reveal the presence of otherwise inapparent scaling, particularly in guttate psoriasis (the candle phenomenon, in which silvery flakes detach from the lesion and look like wax scraped from a candle). Close inspection may reveal that all of the papules are follicular (see Table 4-2). Careful examination of the rest of the body may reveal diagnostic lesions elsewhere, such as burrows on the hands in scabies, the herald patch in pityriasis rosea, or typical psoriasis on the knees, scalp, or anogenital region. Papulovesicles may be detected, so that the differential diagnosis listed in Table 3-11 may be considered.

The importance of the history, bedside scrapings for scabies, bedside

Gram's stain for bacteria, the skin biopsy, appropriate special histologic stains, cultures, and, where indicated, laboratory and radiologic examinations in establishing a diagnosis cannot be overstated. Peripheral blood eosinophilia may point to parasitic infestation but is not always present when infestation is. The exposure, social, and travel history may be especially important as well. For example, tungiasis, an infestation caused by the small sand flea, *Tunga penetrans,* will not be suspected in the patient with a few itchy red papules of the feet unless the history of recent travel to an equatorial or subtropical zone is obtained.[82,83]

REFERENCES

1. Buslau M, Marsch WC: Papular eruption in helminth infestation—a hypersensitivity phenomenon? Report of four cases. *Acta Derm Venereol* (Stockh) 70:526–529, 1990.
2. Canizares O, Harman R: *Clinical Tropical Dermatology,* 2nd ed. Boston: Blackwell Scientific Publications, 1992.
3. Ofuji S, Uehara M: Follecular eruptions of atopic dermatitis. *Arch Dermatol* 107:54–55, 1973.
4. Uehara M: Prurigo reaction in atopic dermatitis. *Acta Derm Venereol* (Stockh) Suppl 92:109–110, 1980.
5. Hu C-H: Sweat-related dermatoses: Old concept and new scenario. *Dermatologica* 182:73–76, 1991.
6. Kaaman T, Torssander J: Dermatophytid—a misdiagnosed entity? *Acta Derm Venereol* (Stockh) 63:404–408, 1983.
7. Brenner S: Pediculid: An unusual id reaction to pediculosis capitis. *J Am Acad Dermatol* 12:125–126, 1985.
8. Burge SM, Wilkinson JD: Darier-White disease: A review of the clinical features in 63 patients. *J Am Acad Dermatol* 27:40–50, 1992.
9. Chalet M, Grover R, Ackerman AB: Transient acantholytic dermatosis. A re-evaluation. *Arch Dermatol* 113:431–435, 1977.
10. Fawcett HA, Miller JA: Persistent acantholytic dermatosis related to actinic damage. *Br J Dermatol* 109:349–354, 1983.
11. Van Joost T, Vuzevski VD, Tank B, et al: Benign persistent papular acantholytic and dyskeratotic eruption: A case report and review of the literature. *Br J Dermatol* 124:92–95, 1991.
12. Crosti A, Gianotti F: Ulteriore contributo alla conoscenza dell'acrodermatite papulosa infantile. *G Ital Derm* 105:477–504, 1964.
13. Weston WL, Lane AT: *Color Textbook of Pediatric Dermatology.* St. Louis, Mosby Year Book. 1991, p 91.
14. Kuttner BJ, Kaplan DL, Rothstein MS: Eruptive pruritic papules. *Arch Dermatol* 125:985–986, 1989.
15. Picascia DD, Magid ML, Minkin RB: Pruritic papular eruption. *Arch Dermatol* 125:989–990, 1989.
16. Green T, Roberts SOB: Waldenstrom's macroglobulinaemia with pruritic papules. *Br J Dermatol* 121 (Suppl 34):115, 1989.
17. Kazmierowski JA, Chusid MJ, Parrillo JE, et al: Dermatologic manifestations of the hypereosinophilic syndrome. *Arch Dermatol* 114:531–535, 1978.
18. Oursler JR, Farmer ER, Roubenoff, et al: Cutaneous manifestations of the eosinophilia-myalgia syndrome. *Br J Dermatol* 127:138–146, 1992.

19. Wright SA, Rothe MJ, Sporn J, et al: Acute adult T-cell leukemia/lymphoma presenting with florid cutaneous disease. *Int J Dermatol* 31:582–587, 1992.
20. Wakeel RA, Keefe M, Chapman RS: Papuloerythroderma. Another case of a new disease. *Arch Dermatol* 127:96–98, 1991.
21. Rosen T, Algra RJ: Papular eruption of black men. *Arch Dermatol* 116:416–418, 1980.
22. Barker JNWN, MacDonald DM: Hamartoma moniliformis: A case report. *Clin Exp Dermatol* 13:34–35, 1988.
23. Teraki Y, Shiohara T, Nagashima M, et al: Prurigo pigmentosa: Role of ICAM-1 in the localization of the eruption. *Br J Dermatol* 125:360–363, 1991.
24. Bernal JE, de Rueda MMD, Oroonez CP, et al: Actinic prurigo among Chimila Indians in Columbia: HLA studies. *J Am Acad Dermatol* 22:1049–1051, 1990.
25. Lane PR, Hogan DJ, Martel MJ, et al: Actinic prurigo: Clinical features and prognosis. *J Am Acad Dermatol* 26:683–692, 1992.
26. Blankenship ML. Gram-negative folliculitis: Follow-up observations in 20 patients. *Arch Dermatol* 120:1301–1303, 1984.
27. Alomar A, Ausina V, Vernis J, et al: Pseudomonas folliculitis. *Cutis* 30:405–409, 1982.
28. Back O, Faergemann J, Hornqvist R: Pityrosporum folliculitis: A common disease of the young and middle aged. *J Am Acad Dermatol* 12:56–61, 1985.
29. Purcell SM, Hayes TJ, Dixon SL: Pustular folliculitis associated with Demodex folliculorum. *J Am Acad Dermatol* 15:1159–1162, 1986.
30. Ostlere LS, Harris D, Prentice HG, et al: Widespread folliculitis induced by human granulocyte-colony-stimulating factor therapy. *Br J Dermatol* 127:193–194, 1992.
31. Hitch JM: Acneform eruptions induced by drugs and chemicals. *JAMA* 200:879–880, 1967.
32. Ofuji S: Eosinophilic pustular folliculitis. *Dermatologica* 174:53–56, 1987.
33. Norris PG, Hawk JLM: Actinic folliculitis—response to isotretinoin. *Clin Exp Dermatol* 14:69–71, 1989.
34. Strauss JS, Kligman AM: Pseudofolliculitis of the beard. *Arch Dermatol* 74:533–542, 1956.
35. Poliak SC, Lebwohl MG, Parris A, et al: Reactive perforating collagenosis associated with diabetes mellitus. *N Engl J Med* 306:81–84, 1982.
36. Pedragosa R, Knobel HJ, Huguet P, et al: Reactive perforating collagenosis in Hodgkin's disease. *Am J Dermatopathol* 9:41–44, 1987.
37. Dabski K, Winkelmann RK: Generalized granuloma annulare: Clinical and laboratory findings in 100 patients. *J Am Acad Dermatol* 20:39–47, 1989.
38. Samlaska CP, Sandberg GD, Maggio KL, et al: Generalized perforating granuloma annulare. *J Am Acad Dermatol* 27:319–322, 1992.
39. Banse-Kupin L, Morales A, Kleinsmith D'A: Perforating lichen nitidus. *J Am Acad Dermatol* 9:452–456, 1983.
40. Shelley WB, Shelley ED: *Advanced Dermatologic Diagnosis.* Philadelphia, Saunders. 1992, p 330.
41. Heng MCY, Kloss SG, Haberfelde GC: Pathogenesis of papular urticaria. *J Am Acad Dermatol* 10:1030–1034, 1984.
42. Lever WF, Schaumberg-Lever G: *Histopathology of the Skin,* 7th ed. Philadelphia, Lippincott. 1990, p 242.
43. Alexander JO'D: *Arthropods and Human Skin.* Berlin, Springer-Verlag. 1984, p 186.
44. Rook A: Foreword, in Alexander JO'D: *Arthropods and Human Skin.* Berlin, Springer-Verlag. 1984, p v.
45. Rook A: Arthropod bites, in M Orkin, HI Maibach (eds): *Cutaneous Infestations and Insect Bites.* New York, Marcel Dekker. 1985, pp 241–315.
46. Bernhard JD: Clinical aspects of pruritus, in Fitzpatrick TB et al (eds): *Dermatology in General Medicine,* 3d ed New York, McGraw-Hill. 1987, pp 78–90.
47. Burns DA: The investigation and management of arthropod bite reactions acquired in the home. *Clin Exp Dermatol* 12:114–120, 1987.

48. Shelley ED, Shelley WB, Pula JF, et al: The diagnostic challenge of non-burrowing mite bites. Cheyletiella yasguri. *JAMA* 251:2690–2691, 1984.
49. Shelley WB, Shelley ED, Welbourn WC: Polypodium fern wreaths (Hagnaya)—a new source of occupational mite dermatitis. *JAMA* 253:3137–3138, 1985.
50. Hewitt M, Walton GS, Waterhouse M: Pet animal infestations and human skin lesions. *Br J Dermatol* 85:215–225, 1971.
51. Gupta AK, Billings JK, Ellis CN: Chronic pruritus: An uncommon cause. *Arch Dermatol* 124:1102–1106, 1988.
52. Thomsett LR: Some manifestations of animal disease transmissible to man: Pruritus. *Proc R Soc Med* 62:1049–1050, 1969.
53. Kieffer M, Kristensen S, Hallas TE: Prurigo and pets: The benefit from vets. *BMJ* 1:1539–1540, 1979.
54. Lee BW: Cheyletiella dermatitis: A report of fourteen cases. *Cutis* 47:111–114, 1991.
55. Braverman IM: *Skin Signs of Systemic Disease,* 2d ed Philadelphia, Saunders, 1981.
56. Braverman IM: Personal communication. August 28, 1989.
57. Wong RC, Fairley JA, Ellis CN: Dermographism: A review. *J Am Acad Dermatol* 11:643–652, 1984.
58. Burkhart CF: Papular dermatographia. *Int J Dermatol* 19:562–563, 1980.
59. Witkowski JA, Parish LC: Papular dermographism: A sign of urticaria pigmentosa. *Int J Dermatol* 22:529, 1983.
60. Shelley WB, Shelley ED: Follicular dermographism. *Cutis* 32:244–260, 1983.
61. Marcussen PV: Dermatographic prurigo. *Acta Derm Venereol* (Stockh) 30:94–113, 1950.
62. Shelnitz LS, Paller AS: Hodgkin's disease manifesting as prurigo nodularis. *Pediatr Dermatol* 7:136–139, 1990.
63. Franciotta D: On the shoulders of giants. *Lancet* 340:64, 1992.
64. Rowland Payne CME, Wilkinson JD, McKee PH, et al: Nodular prurigo—a clinicopathological study of 46 patients. *Br J Dermatol* 113:431–439, 1985.
65. Shelley WB: Prurigo, in *Consultations in Dermatology,* II. Philadelphia, Saunders. 1974, pp 44–49.
66. Brown MA, George CRP, Dunstan CR, et al: Prurigo nodularis and aluminum overload in maintenance haemodialysis. *Lancet* 340:48, 1992.
67. Greither A: On the different forms of prurigo pruritus—prurigo. *Curr Probl Dermatol* 3:1–30, 1970.
68. Provost TT, Maize JC, Ahmed AR, et al: Unusual bullous diseases with immunologic features of bullous pemphigoid. *Arch Dermatol* 115:156–160, 1979.
69. Yung CW, Soltani K, Lorincz AL: Pemphigoid nodularis. *J Am Acad Dermatol* 5:54–60, 1981.
70. Ross JS, McKee PH, Smith NP, et al: Unusual variants of pemphigoid: From pruritus to pemphigoid nodularis. *J Cutan Pathol* 19:212–216, 1992.
71. Pagliuca A, Williams H, Salisbury J, et al: Prodromal cutaneous lesions in adult T-cell leukaemia/lymphoma. *Lancet* 335:733–734, 1990.
72. Potter BS, Burgoon CF, Johnson WC: Pityrosporum folliculitis. *Arch Dermatol* 107:388–391, 1973.
73. Haupt HM, Stern JB, Weber CB: Eosinophilic pustular folliculitis: Fungal folliculitis? *J Am Acad Dermatol* 23:1012–1014, 1990.
74. Hevia O, Jimenez-Acosta F, Ceballos PI, et al: Pruritic papular eruption of the acquired immunodeficiency syndrome: A clinicopathologic study. *J Am Acad Dermatol* 24:231–235, 1991.
75. Jorizzo JL, Gatti S, Smith EB: Prurigo: A clinical review. *J Am Acad Dermatol* 4:723–728, 1981.
76. Sherertz EF, Jorizzo JL, White WL, et al: Papular dermatitis in adults: Subacute prurigo, American style? *J Am Acad Dermatol* 24:697–702, 1991.

77. Uchara M, Ofuji S: Primary eruption of prurIgo simplex subacuta. *Dermatologica* 153:49–56, 1976.
78. Dobson RL: Personal communication. September 2, 1992.
79. Kopf AW: Personal communication. August 26, 1992.
80. Ackerman AB: Histologic diagnosis of inflammatory skin diseases. A method by pattern analysis. Philadelphia, Lea & Febiger. 1978, p 184.
81. Ackerman AB: Personal communication. August 7, 1989.
82. Sanusi DI, Brown EB, Shepard GT, et al: Tungiasis: Report of one case and review of the 14 reported cases in the United States. *J Am Acad Dermatol* 20:941–944, 1989.
83. Trevisan G, Pauluzzi P, Kokelj F: Tungiasis: Report of a case. *J Eur Acad Derm Venereol* 1:73–75, 1992.

HISTOLOGIC CLUES TO THE DIFFERENTIAL DIAGNOSIS OF PRURITIC SKIN DISEASES

Gary R. Kantor

TO BIOPSY OR NOT TO BIOPSY,
THAT IS THE QUESTION.

Anonymous, 1993

When will a skin biopsy help in the diagnostic evaluation of a patient who has itchy skin without rash? What are the appropriate lesions to select for biopsy? What are the findings in the biopsy of itchy skin? Are adjunctive studies, such as immunofluorescence, helpful in the evaluation?

The following discussion will address these queries so that the physician can make an informed judgment when presented with an itchy patient who has either no rash or a nonspecific, inscrutable one.

LESIONS TO BIOPSY IN THE ITCHY PATIENT WITHOUT SPECIFIC RASH

Patients who complain of generalized itch may present with entirely normal looking skin or may present with a host of secondary skin and nail changes, but no primary skin lesions.[1-3] Secondary lesions include excoriations (punctate or linear), lichenification, prurigo (papules or nodules), post-inflammatory pigmentary alteration, and burnished nails, among others. Biopsy of secondary lesions is likely to yield nonspecific findings. For example, biopsy of a superficial ulcer in an excoriated skin eruption may not reveal the characteristic changes of a dermatosis because ulcers are associated with massive recruitment of neutrophils.

As in the evaluation of patients with primary skin disease, biopsy of an early and/or developed lesion will be most helpful for diagnosis if one is present. In many instances, the patient will help in the decision process if he or she can identify an early "lesion." This is especially true in a disease such as dermatitis herpetiformis in which rapid excoriation produces a nondiagnostic clinical lesion. However, a minute papulovesicle may still be present and a biopsy may yield diagnostic information.

In other instances when a biopsy may be desirable, but there are no pristine lesions, biopsy of perilesional normal skin may yield the most information. It must be emphasized that it is critical for the clinician to inform the dermatopathologist interpreting the biopsy of the clinical history and differential diagnosis in order to receive a clinically relevant pathology report. The adage "garbage in, garbage out" pertains very aptly in the biopsy of clinically normal skin.

SKIN BIOPSY IN THE DIAGNOSTIC EVALUATION

Skin biopsy is likely to help after, but not before, the formulation of a clinical differential diagnosis of itch. Histopathology will exclude (and possibly include) differential diagnoses on the list and may yield a specific diagnosis in some instances. However, indiscriminant use of the biopsy will probably produce disappointing results and frustration for both the clinician and dermatopathologist.

Diagnoses that may be uncovered on a biopsy of clinically normal skin are listed in Table 5-1. The presence of eosinophils in an edematous dermis with or without epidermal changes suggests an allergic hypersensitivity reaction so that exclusion of a drug (most common) or arthropod reaction needs to be made. Eosinophils that align along the dermal–epidermal junction with or without spongiosis may be a sign of the urticarial stage of pemphigoid. Because the lesions of dermatitis herpetiformis are so rapidly excoriated from the severe associated itch, this diagnosis may often only be made after biopsy reveals neutrophilic microabscesses in the dermal papillae. An increased number of mast cells in the absence of other inflammatory cells (except eosinophils) around blood vessels should prompt investigation for mastocytosis.[4] Fiberglass fragments may be found in normal-looking itchy skin in affected individuals.[5] Edema in the dermis with a few or rare eosinophils suggests urticaria.

**Table 5-1 Histologic diagnoses
for clinically normal itchy skin**

Drug hypersensitivity
Urticaria
Papular urticaria
Infestation (e.g., scabies incognito)
Pemphigoid
Dermatitis herpetiformis
Linear IgA dermatosis
Mastocytosis
Fiberglass dermatitis

HISTOPATHOLOGY OF ITCHY SKIN

The histopathologic findings in secondary lesions associated with itching are
shown in Table 5-2. Some further points of emphasis are as follows. Eosinophils in the dermis of an ulcer, chronic dermatitis, or prurigo should alert
the clinician to a possible allergic cause such as a drug eruption, arthropod
reaction, or infestation. Changes of lichen simplex chronicus may be su-
perimposed on atopic dermatitis or an allergic hypersensitivity reaction. Del-
icate superficial dermal fibrosis with loss of the rete ridges and separation
of the epidermis from the dermis suggests a healing excoriation that may
overlie a pathologic process in the dermis (e.g., drug hypersensitivity, papular
urticaria, pemphigoid).

In itchy skin that appears clinically normal, biopsy may reveal characteristic findings (Table 5-3).[6-11] In some cases, confirmatory perilesional immunofluorescence biopsy may be needed (dermatitis herpetiformis, linear
IgA dermatosis, pemphigoid). In other instances, special stains (i.e., napthol
chloroacetate (NCA), toluidine blue, or giemsa for mast cells) may be indicated.

In yet other instances, biopsy of clinically normal itchy skin may produce
normal findings. This information might be helpful to the clinician to eliminate
the possibility of other diseases, drug hypersensitivity or other allergic cause,
and to reassure the patient.

IMMUNOFLUORESCENCE AND ITCHY SKIN

Perilesional skin biopsy adjacent to an excoriation or other nonspecific
lesion for direct immunofluorescence may yield better results in some

Table 5-2 Histopathology of secondary lesions in itchy patients

	Erosion	Ulcer	Prurigo nodularis	Lichen simplex chronicus	Post-inflammatory pigmentary alteration	Scar
Epidermis	Superficial necrosis Scale-crust ± bacteria	Absent Inflammatory crust ± bacteria	Irregular hyperplasia Hyperkeratosis Focal scale-crust	Regular hyperplasia Marked hyperkeratosis ± spongiosis	Variable increased melanin in basal layer	Loss of rete ridges
Dermal–epidermal junction	Fibrin	N.A.	Normal	Normal	Normal	Defective—Epidermis may detach
Dermis	Neutrophils within and around blood vessels	Neutrophils within and around blood vessels	Perivascular lymphoid infiltrate Superficial fibrosis	Vertically oriented capillaries Papillary dermal fibrosis Perivascular lymphoid infiltrate	Melanophages around blood vessels and in superficial dermis Perivascular lymphoid infiltrate	Increased number of parallel arranged fibroblasts Vertically oriented capillaries Perivascular mixed infiltrate

Table 5-3 Histopathologic features of selected causes of itchy skin

	Drug hypersensitivity	Urticaria	Papular urticaria	Infestation	Pemphigoid	Dermatitis herpetiformis	Masto-cytosis	Fiberglass dermatitis
Epidermis								
spongiosis	+	–	+	+	+	–	–	±
exocytosis	++ (L,E)	–	–	+ (L,E)	+ (L,E)	–	–	–
other				Mites or products		acantholytic cells		fiberglass fragments
Dermal–epidermal junction								
vacuolar alteration	±	–	–	–	++	+	–	–
inflammatory cells	+ (L,E)	– (L,E,N)	–	± (L,E)	++ (L,E)	+ (N)	–	–
Dermis								
Papillary								
edema	+	+	++	+	+	+++	–	+
infiltrate	++ (L,E)	+ (L,E,N)	++ (L,E)	++ (L,E)	+++ (L,E,N)	+++ (N)	+ (M, ±E)	+ (L)
Reticular								
edema	+	+	++	+	+	+	+	±
infiltrate	+ (L,E)	± (L,E,N)	++ (L,E)	++ (L,E)	++ (L,E,N)	+ (L,E,N)	+ (M, ±E)	± (L)

L = lymphocytes, E = eosinophils, N = neutrophils, M = mast cells clinical instances than routine histology. This is primarily pertinent in the vesiculobullous diseases which, on occasion, can present only with generalized itch and excoriations. When the age of the patient or the history put dermatitis herpetiformis or pemphigoid at the head of the list of differential diagnoses, immunofluorescence testing will be helpful and is the diagnostic gold standard. The specimen can be obtained on the same visit as that for routine histology and temporarily stored pending results of histopathology. Immunofluorescence may also yield positive results in drug eruptions in which there are immune deposits (i.e., hypersensitivity vasculitis).

CONCLUSION

A skin biopsy is often extremely helpful in the evaluation of the patient with generalized pruritus and no discernible rash or a nonspecific one. However, the information obtained from a biopsy is dependent on the selection of an appropriate lesion for biopsy. Results from a skin biopsy will help the clinician to eliminate some possibilities, to streamline a differential diagnosis, and to direct further evaluation and treatment of the patient, as discussed throughout this book and particularly in Chap. 24. On occasion, histologic examination of what was thought to be a nonspecific or secondary lesion may point to a specific diagnosis such as psoriasis or cutaneous T-cell lymphoma.

REFERENCES

1. Bernhard JD: Invisible dermatoses versus nonrashes. *J Am Acad Dermatol* 9:599, 1983.
2. Brownstein MH: Invisible dermatoses versus nonrashes. *J Am Acad Dermatol* 9:599–600, 1983.
3. Bernhard JD, Haynes H: Nonrashes. 1. The Koebner non-reaction. *Cutis* 29:158–164, 1982.
4. Lever WF, Schaumberg-Lever G: *Histopathology of the Skin,* 7th ed. Philadelphia, Lippincott. 1990, pp 90–93.
5. Cuypers JMC, Hoedemaker J, Nater JP, et al: The histopathology of fiber-glass dermatitis in relation to von Hebra's concept of eczema. *Cont Derm* 1:88–95, 1975.
6. Kligman AM: The invisible dermatoses. Arch Dermatol 127:1375–1382, 1991.
7. Lever WF, Schaumberg-Lever G: *Histopathology of the Skin,* 7th ed. Philadelphia, Lippincott. 1990, p 242.
8. Ackerman AB, Jacobson M, Vitale P: *Clues to the Diagnosis in Dermatopathology.* Chicago, ASCP Press, 1991, pp 373–375.

9. Ackerman AB, Niven J, Grant-Kels JM: *Differential Diagnosis in Dermatopathology.* Philadelphia, Lea and Febiger, 1982, pp 42–43.
10. Ackerman AB, Troy JL, Rosen LB, et al: *Differential Diagnosis in Dermatopathology II.* Philadelphia, Lea and Febiger, 1988, pp 38–39.
11. Ackerman AB: *Histologic Diagnosis of Inflammatory Skin Diseases.* Philadelphia, Lea and Febiger, 1978, pp 295–303.

TABOO TO BOOT

One bliss for which
There is no match
Is when you itch
To up and scratch.

Yet doctors and dowagers deprecate scratching,
Society ranks it with spitting and snatching,
And medical circles consistently hold
That scratching's as wicked as feeding a cold.
Hell's flame burns unquenched 'neath how many a
    stocking
On account of to scratch in public is shocking!

'Neath tile or thatch
That man is rich
Who has a scratch
For every itch.

Ho, squirmers and writhers, how long will ye suffer
The medical tyrant, the social rebuffer!
On the edge of the door let our shoulder blades rub,
Let the drawing room now be as free as the tub!
Avid ankles appeased by the fingernail's kiss
Will revel in ultimate intimate bliss.

I'm greatly attached
To Barbara Fritchie.
I bet she scratched
When she was itchy.

by Ogden Nash

From *Verses From 1929 On* by Ogden Nash. Copyright 1933, 1938 by Ogden Nash. By permission of Little Brown and Company and Curtis Brown, Ltd.

SCRATCHING

Jeffrey D. Bernhard

... At 1:32, she turned her head to the right. At 1:33 she turned it to the left. The crowd roared. "She moved!" At 1:35, heavy action. Yong Yong rolled over on her back and extended a left leg into the air. At 1:35 she scratched it with a right paw. At 1:37 she scratched her bottom with a left paw. From 1:38 to 1:42 she scratched everything she could get her paws on. At 1:43 she presented her left profile to the crowd. Another roar.

from "The Laziest Gal in Town,"
The New York Times, May 3, 1987

Scratching in public is not usually met with so much attention or enthusiasm; in fact, it can get you thrown in jail.[1] But Yong Yong was a panda from Beijing on loan to the Bronx Zoo, and scratching was one of the few things she did at all. Despite the notion that there are no established, specific models for itching, there can be no argument that scratching occurs in the majority of mammalian species. This should come as no surprise; scratching must serve an extremely basic and essential function of integumental protection in the removal of undesired materials, parasites, and undesired visitors from the environment. It is entirely reasonable to suspect that the sensation that triggers scratching in man—itch—is the same sensation that triggers scratching in other animals, but that is an unprovable assumption. The nearly total absence of preclinical research in itching is at least partly the consequence of the intellectual trap inherent in the failure to accept that assumption. Woodward and colleagues have reviewed the various animal models in which scratching can be provoked by chemical or electrical stimulation, as well as their limitations.[2]

The other major intellectual impediment to progress in itch research has been the long-prevalent notion that itching is merely a variety of pain.[3] The evidence that itching is a distinct sensory modality, and not a variety of pain, is reviewed in Chap. 1. Certain similarities and relationships between pain and itching cannot be ignored, but even if itch were a form of pain, the assumption of an identity relationship has not had a productive effect on itch research, and could be jettisoned merely on the hope that the "separate primary sensory modality" position would be more fruitful.

Scratching is the final event in a series of neuronally mediated events: (1) stimulation of cutaneous itch receptors, (2) signal conduction from the receptor by afferent peripheral nerve fibers, (3) central processing in the spinal cord and brain, and (4) the motor scratch response. What is known about the neuroanatomy and neurophysiology of this sequence is dealt with in Chap. 1. The extent to which scratching may occur as a spinal reflex,[4] as opposed to being a purposeful reaction to the perception of itching in the brain, may vary depending on the species and on other circumstances, such as attention and sleep versus wakefulness. Sinclair stated that scratching in man may be "a reaction rather than a reflex, demanding the integrity of at least some part of the brain for its performance."[5] This seems a rather tentative proposition for something that seems to be confirmed by daily experience.

HOW DOES SCRATCHING RELIEVE ITCHING?

> . . . scratching is one of the sweetest gratifications of nature, and as ready at hand as any.
>
> Montaigne[6]

Exactly how scratching relieves itching is not known.[7] One possibility is that scratching provides a neural stimulus that breaks up reverberating circuits in the segment of the spinal cord into which impulses from an itchy site pass.[8] Scratching may work by sensory counterstimulation or may substitute other sensations (e.g., pain) for itching. Indeed, pain is more tolerable than itching in some cases. Pin-pricks, pinching electrical stimulation, and noxious levels of radiant heat may act in similar ways.[9–11] Other physical stimuli, including vibration,[12] transcutaneous nerve stimulation,[13] pressure, heat, cold,[14] and ultraviolet radiation can also inhibit or diminish itching.[15] The "gate theory" provides one attractive explanation for how scratching and other stimuli may relieve itching.[16,17] According to this theory, scratching would stimulate afferent neurons which would inhibit neurons carrying the itch signal, or which would "close" neural "gates" through which itch signals must pass. Additional levels of complexity can be imagined. For example, itch could occur when certain neural centers are released from tonic inhibition; scratching could then work by reestablishing the inhibitory state.

In the 1950s Cornbleet studied scratching and found that the length of scratch strokes roughly coincided with the minimal distance between two simultaneous stimuli that can be distinguished separately, and that this distance varies from one part of the body to another.[18] He also found that the length of scratch strokes increased on the extremities centripetally, and that scratch strokes were shorter across a limb than along the line of its long axis. In areas where the minimal or "liminal" distance for two-point distinction is smallest, such as the fingertip, the length of scratch strokes was shortest as well. In areas such as the middle of the back, where the liminal distance for two-point discrimination is long, scratch strokes are longer. He concluded

> that to extinguish an itch at any site, an important factor must be the scraping, rubbing or pressing of a somewhat similar number of tactile end organs. Where they are sparse, a larger area must be encompassed, while in regions of heavy tactile organ concentration, corresponding smaller areas need be stimulated to gain satisfaction and relief from itching.[18]

One of his most fascinating observations was that

> When the skin is scratched or stroked in a line parallel to the free edges of the nails, scratch strokes are much longer than when the nail scrapes the skin in the usual manner.[18]

This observation is consistent with his proposition that a certain number of "tactile end organs" must be stimulated to extinguish itching at a given site by scratching.

WHY DOES SCRATCHING BEGET MORE ITCHING AND SCRATCHING?

> One scratch is too many, a thousand are not enough.

How scratching leads to more itching is not entirely known, but several different mechanisms may contribute to the so-called "itch–scratch cycle." It is highly likely that scratching the skin causes injury and direct release of inflammatory mediators that enhance or cause itching themselves.[19,20] Neurogenic inflammation probably contributes as well.[20a] Neural proliferation may occur as a consequence of chronic trauma from scratching, as is seen in the lesions of prurigo nodularis.[21,22] Neural hyperplasia is sometimes, but not necessarily seen in prurigo nodularis as well.[23] (See also Chap. 7.) Proliferation and hyperplasia of nerves may lead to lower itch thresholds.

Another mechanism that may contribute to the itch–scratch cycle is the paradoxical increase in liminal distances for tactile discrimination induced by scratching. Cornbleet noted that "rubbing and scratching the skin may raise the liminal stimulus for a given site of the skin as much as three times," and that "this accounts for the relief of itching by these measures."[18] I would suggest that the downside of this is the prediction that succeeding scratch strokes would tend to lengthen if one scratch does not extinguish the itch: This prediction holds for my own experience with mosquito bites. It also provides some basis for the observation that itchy foci often tend to enlarge. In this respect, itch may be analogous to pain, in which an area of secondary hyperalgesia occurs outside the area of injury, evidently as a consequence of reversible changes in central processing of signals from mechanoreceptive fibers which normally evoke nonpainful tactile sensations.[24] Nonneural mechanisms contribute to the expansion of itch foci as well because scratching and the local damage it causes must increase "the quantities of chemical irritants liberated in the skin."[25] Finally, scratching and rubbing can lead to dermographism, which, when it is "symptomatic," itches as well.[26] For any one or more of a number of reasons, then, the natural tendency of an itchy spot is to enlarge, especially if it is scratched. In clinical practice I have never encountered the complaint that an itchy spot started out big and got smaller.

Itchy skin as first described by Bickford in 1938,[27] or alloknesis, as it has been called by Simone and LaMotte and colleagues,[28] is a phenomenon wherein mild mechanical stimulation of an area surrounding an experimental itch stimulus also produces itching. This effect is analogous to secondary hyperalgesia in pain. As mentioned, local effects as well as alterations in central processing may be involved. Interference with the phenomenon of alloknesis (itchy skin) in the area surrounding an itch stimulus must be at play in the observation that stroking, rubbing, or otherwise stimulating the area around an itchy spot like a mosquito bite often provides relief.[8] Similarly, Graham, Goodell, and Wolff found that the application of pinpricks in the area of a histamine-induced flare, or even in the same dermatome, could abolish experimentally induced itching.[29] This might explain the effect of acupuncture and transcutaneous electrical nerve stimulation in itching.[30,31,32]

THE MEASUREMENT OF SCRATCHING AND SOME OF ITS LESSONS

Itching itself is difficult to measure and in the last analysis depends on the subjective response and report of the subject. Wahlgren has reviewed this subject in detail.[33] The visual analogue scale, which requires that the subject estimate the degree of itching by placing a mark somewhere along a 100mm line with "no itch" at one end and terrible itch at the other, is currently a popular tool but still depends on subjective interpretations and responses. Based on the proposition that the measurement of scratching should be a reasonable quantitative reflection of the amount of itching, a number of techniques for measuring scratch have been developed. Savin and colleagues pioneered in this field with the measurement of electroencephalograms, electro-oculograms, submental electromyograms, and muscle potentials from both forearms combined with all-night closed-circuit television observation of all movements, including scratching.[34,35] Taking another tack, Felix and Shuster pioneered the use of motion sensitive limb meters by modifying self-winding wrist watches.[36] Summerfield and Welch then developed a sensitive electromagnetic movement detector to measure nocturnal scratching motions.[37] Another group has gone even further by developing a radar method for measuring scratching activities.[38] Bergasa and colleagues have used a vibration (scratch) transducer taped to the middle fingernail of the dominant hand to record scratching activity in their studies of naloxone infusion for the treatment of chronic cholestatic pruritus.[39]

For some reason most investigators have concentrated on itching and scratching during sleep, which is undoubtedly important and bothersome to patients, but not necessarily more troubling than itching while awake. A final concern is that the measurement of scratch to assess itch may be a bit like measuring pain by recording how loudly or often one says "ouch." Itch and pain can both be suffered in silent immobility.

In any event, the study of nocturnal scratching has led to several important observations. First, Savin and colleagues demonstrated that scratching occurs during all stages of sleep but is more frequent during stages 1 and 2 than it is in stages 3 and 4.[35] Scratching also occurs during paradoxical (REM; rapid eye movement) sleep. The pattern of scratching seems to be more closely related to sleep stage than it does to particular skin diseases, and the duration of scratching bouts is not related to the sleep stage in which they start. Scratch bout duration is longer when patients are awake; from these observations investigators have concluded that scratching is probably a reflex action during sleep but that additional conscious, "deliberate," or cognitive aspects come into play during wakeful itching and scratching.

Aoki and colleagues joined Savin in further studies of nocturnal scratching in which hand movement was monitored by using paper strain gauges attached to the backs of the hands.[40] They confirmed that scratching episodes occurred during all stages of sleep but were most numerous in stage 1. They also found that although their subjects tended to remain in a single sleep stage for the 40 seconds immediately preceding a bout of scratching, they often moved to a more superficial sleep stage by the time the bout had ceased. The observation that sleep tends to lighten after scratching bouts, but remains stable just before they begin, suggests that "scratching itself can lead to lightening of sleep," and helps to account for why "the sleep of itchy patients tends to be superficial and broken." As discussed in Chap. 3, however, psychologic factors may also impact nocturnal wakening in pruritic skin diseases such as psoriasis.[41,42] Furthermore, scratching in chronic itchy skin diseases can take on conditioned aspects.[43]

Studies in children with atopic dermatitis and their parents indicate that behavioral factors can be very important determinants of scratching activity.[44] Gil and colleagues found that verbal or physical actions by parents designed to interfere with scratching seemed to backfire, and they concluded that "attention supplied when the child is not scratching, but engaged in some other behavior, may serve to reduce the overall level of child scratching through differential reinforcement of other behavior."[44] Scratching in children with atopic dermatitis can be reduced when parents ignore it and when they deliver token reinforcement for scratch-free periods.[45] Distraction and structured activities also seem to diminish scratching. How much distraction operates at the behavioral level of scratching as opposed to how much it actually alters the perception of itch is not known; Edwards and colleagues clearly demonstrated that psychological factors such as stress can influence the itch sensation.[46] Behavioral therapy has also been effective in the treatment of adults with so-called "neurotic" or stress-related excoriation.[47]

DELETERIOUS EFFECTS OF SCRATCHING

There was a young belle of old Natchez
Whose garments were always in patchez.
When comment arose
On the state of her clothes
She drawled, When ah itchez, ah scratchez.

("Requiem," Ogden Nash)

From *Versus From 1929 On* by Ogden Nash. Copyright 1933, 1938 by Ogden Nash. By permission of Little Brown and Company and Curtis Brown, Ltd.

It is obvious that scratching can injure the skin. In psoriasis, such injury can lead to the extension of existing lesions and the provocation of new ones. This is known as the Koebner reaction or isomorphic response. In atopic dermatitis, scratching is the agent that converts what might otherwise be itching alone to a rash that itches. Even in nonatopics, scratching can lead to secondary eczematization, secondary infection, lichenification, lichen simplex chronicus, and prurigo nodules. In the 1950s Goldblum and Piper built a scratching machine, and used it to demonstrate that lichenification (thickening of the skin with accentuation of skin markings) could be induced experimentally.[48]

Perhaps the most deleterious effect of scratching is that scratching often begets more itching and scratching: the so-called itch–scratch cycle, which was discussed earlier.

DIAGNOSTIC UTILITY OF SCRATCH MARKS (EXCORIATIONS)

The location, length, nature, and even absence of scratch marks can be helpful in diagnosis. Professor Haxthausen pointed out that scratch marks in pediculosis corporis are often several centimeters long, while those in scabies are usually quite short.[49] Deep, gouged-out excoriations may be present in neurotic excoriation and in delusional parasitosis.[50,51,52] Gouged out excoriations of the face may be a clue to psychosis, although facial excoriations are also seen in acne excorieé (supposedly "*des jeunes filles*" but also seen in *les jeunes hommes*), in which even minimal acne lesions cause so much distress that patients press, squeeze, and excoriate them with fingernails or other sharp implements. Neurotic or obsessional features may be present, and we have seen at least one patient with acne excoriee cured by the use of newer antiobsessive–compulsive psychotropic medication.

In a general way, scratch marks testify to the discomfort of the patient, and their severity and extent provide some measure of the degree of itching present. Their localization (distribution) may also provide a clue to the role of external factors such as fiberglass exposure; to certain diseases such as atopic dermatitis, contact dermatitis, and dermatitis herpetiformis; to infestations; and to arthropod assault. One sign of rubbing instead of scratching is the burnished fingernail.[53] The degree to which evidence of rubbing and scratching correlate with the patient's complaint should also be considered; dramatic divergence may point toward a psychogenic etiology.[53]

DOES SCRATCHING HAVE A "MEANING?"

> If your right elbow itches it is a sign of good luck, if the left one itches it is bad luck—to prevent it knock the right one against something.[54]

In his classic book, *Touching: The Human Significance of the Skin,* Ashley Montagu touched on the folklore, functional, developmental, and psychosomatic aspects of itching and scratching. Montagu argues that "an 'itch' in the mind, as it were, will often express itself as an itch in the skin."[55] Noting that Thomas Carlyle had remarked that "The height of human happiness is to scratch the part that itches," he goes on to state that "the erotic quality of much scratching is fairly obvious." Anyone who has ever scratched a mosquito bite will have observed, along with Montagu, that "scratching may be simultaneously a source of pleasure and of displeasure ..." How often "guilt and a tendency toward self-punishment," or "disturbances in sexuality and hostility" are present in patients with certain chronic itches is widely variable and may be a matter of some debate, which is also addressed in Chap. 25. In discussing psychosomatic pruritus, Montagu states that "angry emotions may be converted infra-symbolically into itching and scratching," that psychosomatic itching may "represent the unconscious striving to obtain the attention that was denied in early life," and that "unexpressed feelings of frustration, rage, and guilt, as well as the strong repressed need for love may find symptomatic expression in the form of *scratching even in the absence of itching,*" (italics added).[55] Erotic and psychologic aspects of itching and scratching are also addressed in Chaps. 11 and 25.

In a 1964 treatise entitled *Itching and Scratching, Psychodynamics*

in Dermatology, Musaph examined itching and scratching as "derived activities."[56] In a wide-ranging review, he discusses cases in which itching results from "the thwarting of an emotion," in which scratching occurs without itching as a compulsion or as an expression of "certain autoerotic,
aggressive and sexual impulses," or as an expression of "feelings of em-
barassment, anger, resentment, joy, tense expectation, sexual excitement,
anxiety and fear." He also examines cases of atopic dermatitis, chronic urticaria, and psychogenic pruritus from a psychodynamic perspective. The
mind and emotions may presumably lead to itching, or may lead to scratching
with or without an itch. Arnold has examined "paroxysmal pruritus," which
may lead to scratching to the point of ulceration and pain, as a reaction to
stressful emotions and situations.[57] It is estimated that about 10 percent of
patients with neurotic excoriation have never experienced a primary itch.[58]

To take fancy and analogy to the extreme, one might argue that a
psychological obsession is like a mental itch, or an idea that itches, and the
compulsions that may stem from such an obsession are analogous to scratching
it. To such mental itches mankind may owe the general theory of relativity,
The Brothers Karamazov, Beethoven's ninth symphony, and the Mona Lisa.
Based on the observation that people often scratch their heads when thinking
or perplexed, the fanciful notion that "thinking itches" has been put forward
as well, and Descartes's maxim has been revised to "I think, therefore I
scratch. I scratch, therefore I am."[59] (*"Je pense, donc je me gratte. Je me
gratte, donc je suis."*)

Napoleon's famous pose is said to have been a clandestine scratch.
Many have argued that Napoleon had an epic case of scabies, others that it
was merely a pompous mannerism. Friedman has elaborated a theory that
he had dermatitis herpetiformis.[60] Murphy has studied the impact of Jean-
Paul Marat's itching, which was probably related to eczema, on the course
of the French revolution.[61] The impact of individual itches, such as Napoleon's and Marat's, or of massive ones, such as pediculosis and scabies in
armies, on the course of history is regrettably beyond the scope of this edition
of this book.

Superstitions, folklore, and sayings about itching and scratching reveal
that our psyche has taken their symbolic significance seriously for ages.
Some poetic license is required here, in that "itching" and "scratching" are
sometimes used interchangeably in common speech, or because a superstition about itching may not be verbalized until someone is seen scratching.
An itchy foot signifies that a journey will be taken, or "the itch to go." An
itchy nose signifies a curious variety of things: "If your nose itched it was a
sign that you would be kissed, cursed, or vexed, run against a gatepost, or
shake hands with a fool."[54] It might also mean a surprise, or impending
anger. Almost any part that itches has been given meaning; an itching ear,
to hear something new. Even parts that itch rarely, if ever, lend themselves
to metaphorical figures of speech; the tongue itches to repeat gossip.[62]

In *Julius Caesar,* (Act IV, scene 3), an itchy palm signifies greed, when Brutus tells Cassius: "Let me tell you Cassius, you your selfe Are much condemn'd to have an itching Palme, To sell, and Mart your Offices for Gold to Undeservers." The itchy palm also intersects with the superstition of touching wood; "When the palm of your hand itches, rub it against oak, as it is a sign of money coming," or, "Scratch on wood, Sure to come good. Scratch on arse, Sure to come farst."[54] Or take the eyes, "If your right eye itches, you will cry; if your left you will laugh; but left or right is good at night."[54]

In times passed scratching or stroking the skin had fatal consequences when it led to urticarial dermographism (skin writing). In the Middle Ages dermographism was considered a sign of the devil, and people afflicted with the disposition to it were burned alive.[63] "Old Scratch" is an alias for the devil.

Henry David Thoreau referred to the "seven-years's itch" but did not explain what it was. The 1952 Broadway play by George Axelrod, entitled "The Seven Year Itch," and later made into a movie starring Marilyn Monroe, is the source of its present significance, "the desire of a married person to stray from his or her spouse after seven years of marriage."[64]

"To start from scratch" has nothing to do with itching, (although some rashes seem to start from scratching!). The expression comes from the sporting world,

> from a race in which *scratch* designates the line or mark that is to be the starting point. Hence, he who starts from scratch starts from nothing; he has no preliminary impetus beyond his own ability, genius, or determination to carry him through the race.[62]

"To come up to scratch" comes from the same source in footracing, and signifies conformance to the rules or to standards of discipline. In racing it has been replaced by "Take your marks."

In medical folklore, the complaint of "itchy teeth" is indicative of a positive review of systems (as the teeth do not itch), and Austen has formulated the following maxim: "If a *positive systems review* includes itching of the teeth, the sedimentation rate will probably be within the normal range."[65] The linguistic "itch to" do this, that, or the other thing is encountered daily in English and in other languages as well. In French, *cela me demange de . . .* conveys an even more intense, irresistible itch to do something than it does in English. The itch to play on words has even been given a name, "paronomastic pruritus," as has the itch to name things, "logodaedalian pruritus."

Montagu's observations on back scratching bring some of these threads together. Noting that the old saying, "'You scratch my back, and I'll scratch yours,' conveys something more than a metaphor," he goes on to say:

> The pleasures of back scratching are phylogenetically very old; even invertebrates are soothed by gentle back rubbing, and it is well known that all mammals enjoy it. Also, like man, other mammals enjoy back scratching in the absence of itching even more than

they do in its presence. The instrument known as a back scratcher or scratch-back is a very ancient device.... Thus, the sheer pleasure-giving qualities of the appropriately stimulated skin testify to its need for pleasurable stimulation....

As the old proverb goes, "Tis better than riches to scratch where it itches."

"God bless the Duke of Argyll."

REFERENCES

1. Weinstein BW, Bernhard JD: Incarceration for excoriation. *Cutis* 45:240, 1990.
2. Woodward DF, Conway JL, Wheeler LA: Cutaneous itching models, Maibach H, Lowe N (eds) *Models in Dermatology,* Basel, Karger. 1985, vol 1, pp 187–195.
3. Bernhard JD: Itching in the nineties. *J Am Acad Dermatol* 24:309–310, 1991.
4. Sherrington CS: Observations on the scratch-reflex in the spinal dog. *J Physiol (Lond)* 34:1–50, 1906.
5. Sinclair DC: In Jarrett A (ed) *The Physiology and Pathology of the Skin,* London, Academic Press. 1973, vol 2, p 495.
6. Montaigne: Of Experience. In: *The Complete Essays of Montaigne,* translated by Donald M. Frame. Stanford, Stanford University Press. 1958, p 841.
7. Wall PD: Why does scratching relieve itching? (abstract) *Skin Pharmacol* 2:219, 1989.
8. Ayres S: The fine art of scratching. *JAMA* 189:1003–1007, 1964.
9. Bickford RG: Experiments relating to the itch sensation, its peripheral mechanism and central pathways. *Clin Sci* 3:377–386, 1937–1938.
10. Graham DT, Goodell H, Wolff HG: Neural mechanisms involved in itch, "itchy skin" and tickle sensations. *J Clin Invest* 30:37–48, 1951.
11. Wright E, McMahon S: The inhibition of itch by noxious, but not innocuous, sensory counterstimulation. *J Physiol* 446:480P, 1992.
12. Melzack R, Schecter B: Itch and vibration. *Science* 147:1047–1048, 1965.
13. Fjellner B, Hägermark Ö: Transcutaneous nerve stimulation and itching. *Acta Derm Venereol* (Stockh) 58:131–134, 1978.
14. Fruhstorfer H, Hermanns M, Latzke L: The effects of thermal stimulation on clinical and experimental itch. *Pain* 24:259–269, 1986.
15. Winkelmann RK: Pharmacologic control of pruritus. *Med Clin North Am* 66:1119, 1982.
16. Melzack R, Wall P: Pain mechanisms: A new theory. *Science* 150:971–979, 1965.
17. Herndon JH Jr: Itching: The pathophysiology of pruritus. *Int J Dermatol* 14:465–484, 1975.
18. Cornbleet T: Scratching patterns. 1. Influence of site. *J Invest Dermatol* 20:105–110, 1953.
19. Greaves MW, McDonald-Gibson W: Itch: Role of prostaglandins. *Br Med J* 3:608–609, 1973.
20. Hägermark Ö, Strandberg K, Hamberg M: Potentiation of itch and flare responses by prostaglandins E2 and H2 and a prostaglandin endoperoxide analog. *J Invest Dermatol* 69:527–530, 1977.
20a. Ratzlaff RE, Cavanaugh VJ, Miller GW, et al: Evidence of a neurogenic component during IgE-medicated inflammation in mouse skin. *J. Neuroimmunol* 41:89–96, 1992.
21. Runne U, Orfanos CE: Cutaneous neural proliferation in highly pruritic lesions of chronic prurigo. *Arch Dermatol* 113:787–791, 1977.
22. Doyle JA, Connolly SM, Hunziker N, et al: Prurigo nodularis: A reappraisal of the clinical and histologic features. *J Cutan Pathol* 6:392–403, 1979.
23. Lindley RP, Rowland Payne CME: Neural hyperplasia is not a diagnostic prerequisite in nodular prurigo. A controlled morphometric study of 26 biopsy specimens. *J Cutan Pathol* 16:14–18, 1989.

24. Torebjörk HE, Lundberg LER, LaMotte RH: Central changes in processing of mechano-receptive input in capsaicin-induced secondary hyperalgesia in humans. *J Physiol* 448:765–780, 1992.
25. Sinclair D: *Mechanisms Of Cutaneous Sensation.* Oxford. Oxford University Press, 1981, p 257.
26. Wong RC, Fairley JA, Ellis CN: Dermographism: A review. *J Am Acad Dermatol* 11:643–652, 1984.
27. Bickford RG: Experiments relating to the itch sensation, its peripheral mechanism, and central pathways. *Clin Sci* 3:377–386, 1937–1938.
28. Simone DA, Alreja M, LaMotte RH: Psychophysical studies of the itch sensation and itchy skin ("alloknesis") produced by intracutaneous injection of histamine. *Somatosens Mot Res* 8:271–279, 1991.
29. Graham DT, Goodell H, Wolff HB: Neural mechanisms involved in itch, "itchy skin," and tickle sensations. *J Clin Invest* 30:37–49, 1951.
30. Monk BE: Transcutaneous nerve stimulation in the treatment of generalized pruritus. *Clin Exp Dermatol* 18:67–68, 1993.
31. Ekblom A, Hansson P, Fjellner B: The influence of extrasegmental mechanical vibratry stimulation and transcutaneous electrical nerve stimulation on histamine-induced itch. *Acta Physiol Scand* 125:541–545, 1985.
32. Lundeberg T, Bondesson L, Thomas M: Effect of acupuncture on experimentally induced itch. *Br J Dermatol* 117:771–777, 1987.
33. Wahlgren CF: Itch and atopic dermatitis: Clinical and experimental studies. *Acta Derm Venereol Suppl* 165:1–53, 1991.
34. Savin JA, Paterson WD, Oswald I: Scratching during sleep. *Lancet* ii:296–297, 1973.
35. Savin JA, Paterson WD, Oswald I, et al: Further studies of scratching during sleep. *Br J Dermatol* 93:297–302, 1975.
36. Felix R, Shuster S: A new method for the measurement of itch and the response to treatment. *Br J Dermatol* 93:303–312, 1975.
37. Summerfield JA, Welch ME: The measurement of itch with sensitive limb movement meters. *Br J Dermatol* 102:275–281, 1980.
38. Mustakallio KK: Scratch radar for the measurement of pruritus. *Acta Derm Venereol Suppl (Stockh)* 156:44, 1991.
39. Bergasa NV, Talbot TL, Alling DW, et al: A controlled trial of naloxone infusions for the pruritus of chronic cholestasis. *Gastroenterology* 102:544–549, 1992.
40. Aoki T, Kushimoto H, Hishikawa Y, et al: Nocturnal scratching and its relationship to the disturbed sleep of itchy subjects. *Clin Exp Dermatol* 16:268–272, 1991.
41. Gupta MA, Gupta AK, Kirkby S, et al: Pruritus associated with nocturnal wakenings: Organic or Psychogenic? *J Am Acad Dermatol* 21:479–484, 1989.
42. Bernhard JD: Nocturnal wakening caused by pruritus: Organic or psychogenic? *J Am Acad Dermatol* 23:767, 1990.
43. Jordan JM, Whitlock FA: Emotions and the skin: The conditioning of scratch responses in cases of atopic dermatitis. *Br J Dermatol* 86:574–585, 1972.
44. Gil KM, Keefe FJ, Sampson HA, et al: Direct observation of scratching behavior in children with atopic dermatitis. *Behav Res Ther* 19:213–227, 1988.
45. Allen K, Harris H: Elimination of a child's excessive scratching by training the mother in reinforcement procedures. *Behav Res Ther* 4:79–84, 1966.
46. Edwards AE, Shellow WVR, Wright ET, et al: Pruritic skin disease, psychological stress, and the itch sensation. *Arch Dermatol* 112:339–343, 1976.
47. Welkowitz LA, Held JL, Held Al: Management of neurotic scratching with behavioral therapy. *J Am Acad Dermatol* 21:802–803, 1989.
48. Goldblum RW, Piper WN: Artificial lichenification produced by a scratching machine. *J Invest Dermatol* 22:405–415, 1954.

49. Haxthausen H: How are dermatological diagnoses made? *Trans St Johns Hosp Dermatol Soc* 30:3–13, 1951. [This journal is now known as *Clin Exp Dermatol*]
50. Fruensgaard K, Hjortshoj A: Diagnosis of neurotic excoriation. *Int J Dermatol* 21:148, 1982.
51. Lyell A: Delusions of parasitosis. *J Am Acad Dermatol* 8:895–897, 1983.
52. Lyell A: Delusions of parasitosis. *Br J Dermatol* 108:485, 1983.
53. Bernhard JD: Clinical aspects of pruritus, in Fitzpatrick TB et al (eds): *Dermatology in General Medicine*, 3d ed New York, McGraw-Hill. 1987, pp 78–90.
54. Opie I, Tatem M: *A Dictionary of Superstitions*. Oxford, Oxford University Press; 1989.
55. Montagu A: *Touching: The Human Significance of the Skin*, 3d ed New York, Harper & Row. 1986, pp 190–193.
56. Musaph H: *Itching and Scratching. Psychodynamics in Dermatology*. Philadelphia, FA Davis, 1964.
57. Arnold HL: Paroxysmal pruritus. Its clinical characterization and a hypothesis of its pathogenesis. *J Am Acad Dermatol* 11:322–326, 1984.
58. Fruensgaard K: Psychotherapeutic strategy and neurotic excoriations. *Int J Dermatol* 30:198–203, 1991.
59. Bernhard JD: Does thinking itch? *Lancet* 1:589, 1985.
60. Friedman R: Emperor's itch: Legend concerning Napoleon's affliction with scabies. *Bull Hist Med* 8:949–955, 1940.
61. Murphy LC: The itches of Jean-Paul Marat. *J Am Acad Dermatol* 21:565–567, 1989.
62. Funk CE: *Heavens to Betsy and Other Curious Sayings*. New York, Harper & Row, 1955.
63. Siemens HW: *General Diagnosis and Therapy of Skin Diseases*. Translated from German by K. Wiener. Chicago, University of Chicago Press. 1958, p 43.
64. Safire, W: On language. The seven-year itch. The New York Times Magazine, March 29, 1992. pp 16–18.
65. Austen KF: Quoted in Macklis RM, Mendelsohn ME, Mudge GH. *Manual of Introductory Clinical Medicine. A Student-to-Student Guide*. Boston, Little, Brown. 1984, p 20.

SEVEN

PRURIGO NODULARIS

CME Rowland Payne

DEFINITION

Nodular prurigo (NP) is an excoriated eruption characterized by lichenified nodules. It is best regarded as a form of chronic eczema. The use of the term *prurigo* in conditions other than the distinctive entity of NP is discussed in Chap. 4.

INTRODUCTION

In 1909, J. Nevins Hyde (Fig. 7-1) described prurigo nodularis.[1] He wrote "the eruptive symptoms were firm pea to finger nail sized nodules occurring . . . chiefly over the extremities. . . . As they grew older they became rough, acquired a horny consistency, and often developed, at the summit, a suggestion of a verrucoid process. After scratching, which was practiced in all cases, the surface of the nodules became furrowed, fissured and, at times, haemorrhagic. In some instances the nodules became fused in a plaque of infiltration; in others they were isolated throughout. . . . The pruritus was sometimes of the severest degree. . . . The disease is of exceedingly slow career lasting from 15 to 20 or more years. . . ." and "the prognosis is in a high degree unfavourable, as regards the comfort of the patients."

Since Hyde, NP has been studied by many authors and five substantial investigations deserve special attention.

Using Masson's stain Pautrier[2] described "l'hyperplasie colossale du tissu nerveux" which later came to be known as the "Pautrier neuroma." Pautrier demonstrated similarities between lichenification and NP.

Iijima[3] studied 33 Oriental patients with NP, in 12 of whom the eruption followed insect bites. Miyauchi and Uehara[4] studied 17 NP patients without a history of insect bites; two thirds of biopsies revealed a hair follicle at the center of the nodule.

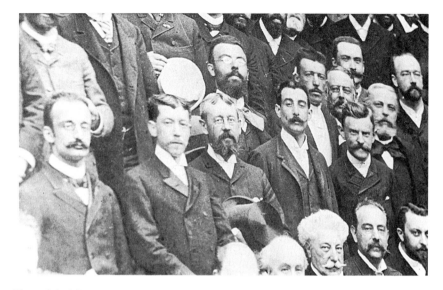

Figure 7-1 J Nevins Hyde, seen here holding a black silk top hat.

Doyle et al.[5] studied 14 patients and Vaalasti et al.[6] studied 8 patients. Both groups noted some degree of neural as well as epidermal and vascular hyperplasia but they, like Iijima and many other workers, were unable to find evidence of frank neuroma formation. They also remarked on increased eosinophil and mastocyte numbers in the dermis and, at the ultrastructural level, degenerative changes in the dermal nerves. Increased levels of sensory neuropeptides in nodular prurigo lesions have been detected by quantitative immunohistochemical analysis.[6a]

In a series of 46 patients 77% were atopic.[7] Potential metabolic causes of pruritus were found in half of patients and focal causes in one third. In one third of patients, psychosocial disorders were considered relevant. This study led to a more detailed investigation of 67 cases of NP (including some of the original 46 patients).[7] The findings are here published for the first time.

EPIDEMIOLOGY

NP affects all ages and the sex ratio is equal. Of 67 patients, 30 were female and 37 male. Age at onset varied from 1 to 82 years, with a mean of 39 years and a median of 39 years (Fig. 7-2). Mean disease duration was 10 years. Disease duration was less than 5 years in one third and exceeded 10 years in 40%. All social classes were affected, with a preponderance among those of a higher socioeconomic status. In Britain, all racial groups are

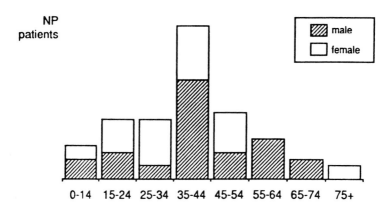

Figure 7-2 Nodular prurigo. Age at onset and sex of 67 patients.

affected, with more Asian, black and Oriental patients than might be expected. Pigmented skins seem to lichenify more readily than Caucasian skin.

ETIOLOGY

NP is always characterized by chronic and severe scratching. This scratching is usually (but not always) a consequence of itching. In most cases the cause of the prurigo is identifiable. In half of patients it is due to a cutaneous disorder (usually atopic dermatitis), in one third the cause is metabolic and in the remainder psychological (usually depression), (Table 7-1).

Table 7-1 Causes of nodular prurigo

Cutaneous
    Atopic dermatitis
    Other eczemas (e.g., contact dermatitis)
    Pemphigoid
    Insect bites
    Onchocerciasis

Metabolic
    Nutritional (including malabsorptions and dietary deficiency)
    Hepatic dysfunction
    Uremia
    Hyercalcemia
    Cerebrovascular disease
Other systemic disease (e.g., Hodgkin's disease[7a])

Psychological
    Depression
    Anxiety

Cutaneous Causes

Of 67 NP patients, cutaneous causes were responsible for prurigo in 35 patients: 20 with atopic dermatitis, 4 with stasis eczema, 3 lichen simplex, 1 nummular eczema, and 2 with other forms of constitutional eczema as well as 2 with insect bites, 1 with lupus erythematosus–lichen planus overlap syndrome, 1 boat builder in whom itching was due to fiberglass and 1 patient with psoriasis who had induced prurigo nodule formation by using a loofah to try to rub away his psoriasis.

NP has also been associated with the sowdah form of onchocerciasis, with leech bites,[8] bullous pemphigoid,[9–12] reactive perforating collagenosis,[13] and multiple cutaneous granular cell tumor of Abrikossoff.[14] Allergic contact dermatitis may contribute to some cases of prurigo nodularis.

NP of cutaneous cause needs to be distinguished from NP that is simply precipitated or localized by an external factor. Cutaneous disorders, such as urticaria, insect bites, venous stasis, actinic keratoses or an episode of infestation may sometimes precipitate or localize NP of metabolic or psychological cause.

Metabolic Causes

Of 67 NP cases, a metabolic cause was found in 20. Eight were classed as nutritional deficiency: four with malabsorption (two following extensive surgery for Crohn's disease, one coeliac disease and one CRST syndrome), two with profound dietary deficiency (including one vegan with coexisting osteomalacia), one with iron deficiency anemia of women, and one with peptic ulceration. Hepatic dysfunction caused seven: two with alcoholic hepatitis and one each with infectious mononucleosis, sarcoidosis, tuberculosis, chronic active hepatitis, and congestive cardiac failure. Chronic renal failure caused two, hypercalcemia due to sarcoidosis one, an adverse drug reaction to antituberculous therapy one, and in one patient (Fig. 7-3) unilateral NP developed during the resolving phase of a cerebrovascular accident (transient unilateral itching provoked unilateral scratching which resulted in unilateral NP. Further resolution of the stroke was accompanied by loss of itching, cessation of scratching and resolution of the prurigo.) Disease duration was shorter in the 20 metabolic cases of NP then in the other 47 cases (p = 0.041). Of the 67 NP cases, three had malignant disease: one with carcinoma of the esophagus, one carcinoma of uterus, and one patient had a history of cured melanoma and cured cutaneous squamous cell carcinoma. Each of these malignancies was considered incidental to the prurigo.

The many diverse metabolic disorders that caused prurigo probably induced itching by a small number of shared mechanisms most important of which seemed to be nutritional deficiency, hepatic derangement, renal failure, neurological damage, and hypercalcemia.

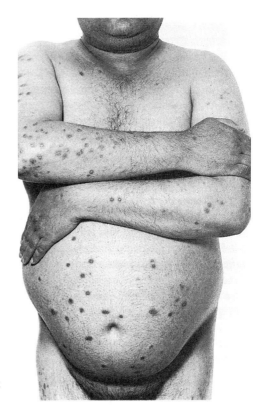

Figure 7-3 Unilateral NP in a patient with a resolving left hemiplegia.

Nutritional deficiency is a clinical finding common to almost half of patients with NP due to metabolic disturbances. Nutritional deficiency occcurs in patients with malabsorption states, gastrointestinal bleeding, peptic ulceration (who suffer from chronic bleeding and a diet determined by indigestion), iron deficiency anemia of women (in which an otherwise possibly adequate diet does not keep pace with recurrent blood loss) and dietary deficiency of various causes whether cultural (vegan) or psychological (the anorectic diet of the depressive, the unvaried diet of the isolated, the unbalanced diet of the alcoholic).

The association between NP and malabsorption is well established. Six cases of NP with gluten enteropathy have been reported;[15–19] although none had dermatitis herpetiformis, all improved with gluten-free diet. The association of NP with malabsorption is not restricted to gluten-sensitive malabsorption. Postgastrectomy malabsorption has occurred with NP.[20] The patient studied, who was never treated by gluten-free diet, responded to treatment of the malabsorption and the NP cleared. NP has also occurred with hookworm infestation[21] and, in the current series, with CRST syndrome and following extensive surgery for Crohn's disease. In so far as development of NP is concerned, the diverse causes of malabsorption seem less important than their common effects. The principal effects of malabsorption are nutritional deficiency and it seems most probable that nutritional deficiency is the shared mechanism by which these various disorders lead to itching. In all cases of nutritional deficiency, there is an imbalance between needs and intake. The most frequently observed net result is sideropenia with or without anemia. Presumably, deficiencies also develop in other trace metals or nutritionally important elements that are not so easily measurable.

Hepatic dysfunction is the next most frequent metabolic cause of NP. Its hallmark is derangement of liver function with elevation of transaminases, gamma-glutamyl transpeptidase or alkaline phosphatase but seldom bilirubin. Alcohol abuse, congestive cardiac failure, viral or bacterial hepatitis, chronic active hepatitis, sarcoidosis, adverse drug reactions, and hepatic metastases are potential hepatic causes. Hepatic prurigo has a good prognosis. In this series, transient hepatitis was associated with transient prurigo in alcoholism, congestive cardiac failure, adverse drug reaction, tuberculosis, and infectious mononucleosis.

Chronic renal failure sufficient to cause severe pruritus is rare in Britain because relatively few patients are dialyzed. In this series both such patients were seen in Oklahoma City, in the United States (by kind permission of Professor Mark Allen Everett). The pathogenesis of the pruritus of renal failure is still controversial.[22] Parathyroidectomy did not stop itching in one case in this series. Uremic anemia of 7–10 g/dl occurred in both. Hypercalcemia and derangement of many other elements also accompanies renal failure. (Also see Chap. 15.)

Other metabolic causes include sarcoidosis by the mechanisms of either hepatic dysfunction or hypercalcemia. Itching may be attributable to Alzheimer's disease and also cerebrovascular accidents. Hypothyroidism probably also causes NP. Diabetes mellitus type II does not.

Psychological Causes

The cause of prurigo was deemed psychological in 11 of 67 patients. Four had depression, five anxiety–depression, and two anxiety states. In five others, psychological disturbances appeared to precipitate NP. Patients with prurigo of psychological origin usually have a background of profound domestic disturbance. They may be polysymptomatic or describe bizarre symptoms. Their excoriations may be of biopsic severity. Sometimes they have an incongruous affect, "la grande satisfaction." Nevertheless metabolic causes always need exclusion.

Atopy

Atopy is common in NP. Of 67 NP patients, 76% were atopic. Numbers of prurigo nodules were related to atopy. The more atopic individuals having more prurigo nodules. However, as one quarter of NP patients are not atopic prurigo nodules are not simply an atopic reaction pattern. Furthermore as atopy, unlike prurigo, is inherited and lifelong, a diagnosis of atopy is not enough to explain a case of prurigo. Atopy facilitates the development of NP but it is not its cause.

HLA and Nodular Prurigo

HLA typing was performed in 23 Caucasian NP patients. When divided into atopics (65%) and nonatopics (35%), HLA A2 phenotype was expressed by 10 of 15 atopics and 0 of 8 nonatopics ($p > 0.01$ Fisher's 2-tail test). Similarly, HLA A19 or its close cross-reactive antigenic group (A29, 30, 31 & 32) was expressed by 1 of 15 atopics and 6 of 8 nonatopics ($p > 0.01$ Fisher's 2-tail test).

These HLA studies are in keeping with the concept that susceptibility to prurigo nodule formation may be genetically determined. HLA A2 phenotype may distinguish the subset of atopics susceptible to NP and A19 may mark the intriguing subset of NP patients who are not atopic.

CLINICAL FINDINGS

Typically, the eruption begins on the distal part of a limb (Fig. 7-4). The initial lesion may follow an insect bite, folliculitis or eczema of various types, usually atopic dermatitis but sometimes nummular eczema. Pruritus is episodic, often provoked by heat and sometimes by anxiety. Itching is usually very severe and in half of cases it is exclusively localized to lesions. Excoriations take the form of scratching rather than picking or rubbing in the majority of patients.

Characteristically, the eruption is symmetrical and grouped, and favors the extensor surfaces and distal parts of the limbs (Figs. 7-5 and 7-6). The limbs are affected in all cases, with lesions being most numerous on periarticular skin (Fig. 7-7). The face and scalp are usually spared. The sacrum, abdomen, and posterior cape area are involved in half of patients. Palms are seldom affected but no part of the body is exempt: in one case nodules were limited to palms, soles, and vulva (Figs. 7-8 and 7-9).

Nodules are usually numerous. However, some patients may have as few as one or two nodules while others exhibit more than 100. Papules are a constant finding. Nodules and papules are characteristically firm and

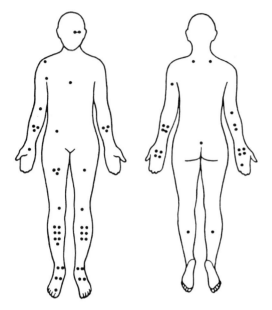

Figure 7-4 Nodular prurigo. Site of initial lesion.

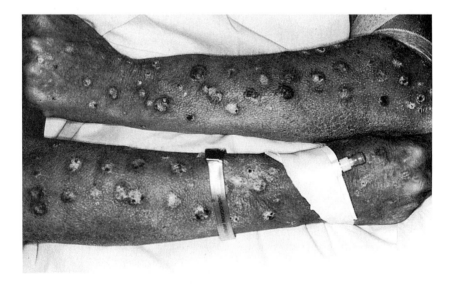

Figure 7-5 NP is symmetrical and favors the distal parts of the limbs.

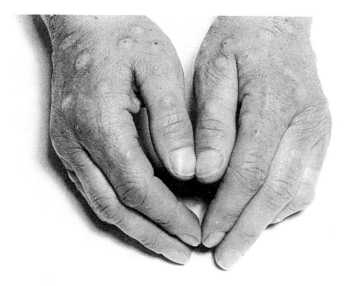

Figure 7-6 NP is symmetrical and favors the extensor surfaces.

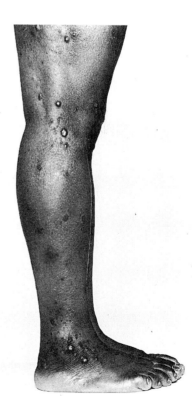

Figure 7-7 In NP, lesions sometimes favor periarticular skin.

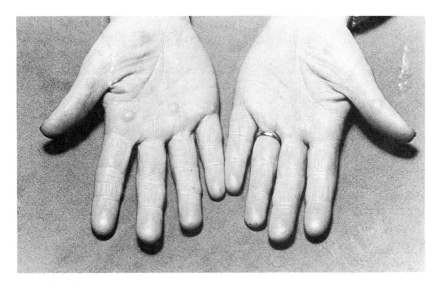

Figure 7-8 NP spares no part of the body. In one patient, prurigo nodules were limited to palms, soles . . .

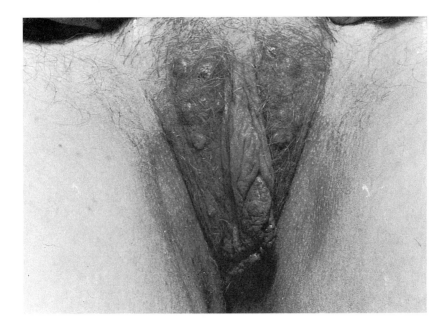

Figure 7-9 . . . and vulva.

lichenified, pink and dome-shaped usually with an excoriated summit and often surrounded by a halo of postinflammatory pigmentation (Fig. 7-10). Where lesions resolve, hypopigmented macules are seen, sometimes with scarring. Intervening skin is commonly xerodermic and sometimes slightly lichenified, feeling thickened and leathery to the touch. Morphology varies with time but topography is fixed (Fig. 7-11a and b). Three-quarters of NP patients exhibit signs of eczema, most commonly lichenified plaques or other elements of atopic dermatitis.

It is hazardous to draw etiologic conclusions from the physical signs of the eruption. Prurigo of metabolic or psychological origin may present in similar ways, the physical signs being more a reflection of the atopic or eczematous nature of the patient's skin than a reflection of the cause of the pruritus.

MICROSCOPIC FEATURES

Hyperkeratosis and large acanthosis are the microscopic hallmarks of NP. Some specimens show claw-like pseudoepitheliomatous hyperplasia. Appearances overlap with chronic eczema (lichen simplex chronicus). Other findings include epidermal eosinophilia even within a few cells of the basal layer (evidence of early keratinization) and dermal fibrosis with vertical collagen banding in the papillary dermis. Less constant findings include

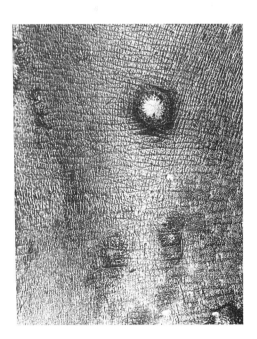

Figure 7-10 Prurigo nodules are lichenified. Perilesional pigmentation and intervening lichenification are common.

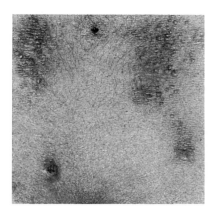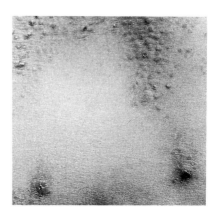

Figure 7-11a and b In nodular prurigo, topography of lesions is constant (a, April 1983 and b, August 1985) and in even the most classical cases of NP the eruption is polymorphic.

hyperplasia of dermal and vascular tissue, an upper dermal infiltrate, and subepidermal fibrin or amyloid deposition.

Neural hyperplasia is variable. Numbers of nerves, notably in the reticular dermis, are statistically increased in NP but obvious neural hyperplasia is neither common nor a diagnostic prerequisite.[23] When it occurs, it does not warrant the term neuroma. In a morphometric study, in which both positive and negative controls were employed, neural hyperplasia was only present in 5 of 26 NP specimens.[23] In the same study it was shown that eosinophil numbers are increased in NP when compared with normal skin, but not when compared with positive controls. Mast cells may be normal in number and electron microscopic morphology. Perez and colleagues recently found an increase in mast cell numbers and evidence of eosinophil degranulation in a study of eight skin biopsy specimens from patients with NP.[23a]

Immunofluorescence is unhelpful in NP except to exclude underlying dermatitis herpetiformis or prepemphigoid.

LABORATORY INVESTIGATIONS

The diagnosis of NP is straightforward but the explanation of its etiology requires a full history, a physical examination, and a number of special investigations (Table 7-2).

In NP, the possibility of malabsorption needs to be considered, especially if there is wasting, anemia, or sideropenia.

Patch testing for allergic contact dermatitis may be helpful in selected cases.[23b]

Table 7-2 Investigation in nodular prurigo*

CBC = complete blood count
ESR = erythrocyte sedimentation rate
Fe/TIBC = iron/total iron binding capacity
Immunoglobulin electrophoresis
BUN = blood urea nitrogen
LFT = liver function tests
Calcium/albumin
TSH = thyroid stimulating hormone
BMZ = basement membrane zone and other autoantibodies
CXR = chest x-ray

*see also Chap. 24.

DIFFERENTIAL DIAGNOSIS

NP is a clinical diagnosis. Its excoriated lichenified nodules should be differentiated from other excoriated nodular eruptions that are not lichenified (Table 7-3).

MANAGEMENT

Symptomatic therapy is essential and very effective but cure only follows treatment of the underlying cause. Duration of NP is no guide to subsequent response to treatment.

Symptomatic Therapy

"For this mater ordeyne a good payre of nayles and rent the skyn and teare the fleshe and let out water and bloude" wrote Borde in 1542,[25] and 450 years later scratching is still the simplest response to itching. Nevertheless, the damage it brings about is usually undesirable. Patients may be helped

Table 7-3 Differential diagnosis of nodular prurigo

Hypertrophic lichen planus
Scabetic nodules
Generalized eruptive histiocytomas[24]
Actinic prurigo
Hyperkeratotic squamous cell carcinoma
Keratoacanthomas of Ferguson-Smith
Cutaneous metastases

to restrain themselves by cutting their nails to the quick, by wearing mittens, and by occlusive bandaging or even plaster of Paris casts.

Emollients can be added to bath water and applied to the skin after bathing. Oral sedative H_1 antihistamines, such as promethazine or trimeprazine are essential. Local photochemotherapy (trioxsalen bath and UVA) was successful in 13 of 15 NP patients.[26] Anecdotal successes have been achieved with PUVA and UVB,[27] etretinate,[28,29] corticosteroids, ACTH,[30] benoxaprofen,[31] erythromycin,[32] cryotherapy,[33] topical capsaicin cream,[33a] and intralesional triamcinolone, with or without lignocaine.[34] Clofazimine is ineffective and probably dangerous.[35]

Thalidomide has been used with success in NP.[36] In our experience, 6 of 10 NP patients improved but none cleared completely. Adverse effects occurred in all 10 and led to discontinuation of treatment in 5. Adverse effects are common, serious, and unpredictable and thalidomide cannot therefore be recommended as a safe treatment for NP in anything but exceptional circumstances.

Etiologic Therapy

Each specific etiology requires its own specific treatment. There is no panacea.

When atopic dermatitis is the cause of NP, treatments aimed at atopic dermatitis are likely to be the most successful. These would include sedative antihistamines and potent or very potent topical corticosteroids, sometimes under occlusion with steroid impregnated adhesive tape or tar bandages. This regimen is most effective when administered on an in-patient basis.

In NP of metabolic origin, hepatic cases carry the best prognosis: when liver function tests return to normal, a successful outcome can be expected. Nutritional deficiency is common and usually secondary to post-surgical malabsorption, dietary insufficiency, or peptic ulceration. Although this is often associated with iron deficiency anemia, iron supplements alone are not always helpful. If those deficient of iron are also deficient of other blood-borne nutrients, it may be more logical to advise eating 200 gms of animal liver each week.

In patients who scratch for psychological reasons, treatment depends on the underlying disturbance. The most frequent is depression and this often responds to tricyclic antidepressants such as dothiepin. (Also see Chap. 25.)

To consider NP as an idiopathic distinct entity is unhelpful. It encourages the hope that some empirical therapeutic agent might be successful in all cases. This approach can be hazardous if serious and correctable underlying pathology is overlooked or if potentially toxic treatments, such as thalidomide, are attempted unselectively.

In NP, remission can be expected when there is good patient compliance with symptomatic measures. However, cure is dependent on resolution of the underlying disorder. Follow-up is needed, not only to monitor therapy, but also, in therapy-resistant cases, to review the underlying diagnosis.

SUMMARY

Nodular prurigo (NP) is defined as an excoriated eruption characterized by lichenified nodules. Experience in 67 patients is reported.

NP affects all ages and the sex ratio is equal. Pruritus is episodic and severe. The eruption is polymorphic and favors the periphery. Topography is constant but morphology varies with time. NP has many clinical and histological similarities with eczema. Neural hyperplasia is minimal or absent.

NP usually has an identifiable cause. In half of patients it is due to a cutaneous disorder (usually atopic dermatitis), in one third the cause is metabolic, and in the remainder the cause is psychological (usually depression). The diverse metabolic disorders that cause NP induce itching by a small number of shared mechanisms, most commonly nutritional deficiency, hepatic dysfunction, and uremia. Nutritional deficiency sometimes results from malabsorption (more often post-surgical than gluten-sensitive).

NP is best regarded as a form of chronic eczema rather than a disease sui generis. Most often affected are atopics of HLA phenotype A2, also susceptible are nonatopics of phenotype A19 (or its close cross-reactive group). Numbers of nodules are related to severity of atopy. Whatever the underlying cause, NP is always characterized by chronic and severe scratching (Fig. 7-12).

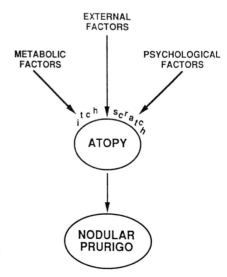

Figure 7-12 Schematic representation of the pathogenesis of nodular prurigo.

Treating the prurigo or the nodules symptomatically is of temporary benefit. Lasting improvement follows resolution of the cause.

REFERENCES

1. Hyde JN: Prurigo nodularis, in Hyde JN, Montgomery FH (eds): *A Practical Treatise on Diseases of the Skin for the Use of Students and Practitioners*, 8th ed. Philadelphia, Lea & Febiger. pp 174–175, 1909.
2. Pautrier L-M: Le névrome de la lichenification circonscrite nodulaire chronique (lichen ruber obtusus corné, prurigo nodularis). *Ann Dermatol Syphil* (Paris) VII:897, 1934.
3. Iijima S: Prurigo nodularis. *Tohoka J Exp Med* 54:73, 1951.
4. Miyauchi H, Uehera M: Follicular occurrence of prurigo nodularis. *J Cutan Pathol* 15:208, 1988.
5. Doyle JA, Connolly SM, Hunziker N, et al: Prurigo nodularis: A reappraisal of the clinical and histological features. *J Cutan Pathol* 6:392, 1979.
6. Vaalasti A, Soumalainen H, Rechardt L: Calcitonin gene-related peptide immunoreactivity in prurigo nodularis: A comparative study with neurodermatitis circumscripta. *Br J Dermatol* 120:619, 1989.
6a. Adabia Molina F, Burrows NP, Russell Jones R, et al: Increased sensory neuropeptides in nodular prurigo: A quantitative immunohistochemical analysis. *Br J Dermatol* 127:344–351, 1992.
7. Rowland Payne CME, Wilkinson JD, McKee PH, et al: Nodular prurigo—A clinicopathological study of 46 patients. *Br J Dermatol* 113:431, 1985.
7a. Shelnitz LS, Paller AS: Hodgkin's disease manifesting as prurigo nodularis. *Pediat Dermatol* 7:136–139, 1990.
8. Braun-Falco D, Marghescu S: Prurigo nodularis Hyde-artige Reaktion durch Blutegelbiss. *Hautarzt* 18:112, 1967.
9. Provost TT, Maise JC, Ahmed AR: Unusual subepidermal bullous diseases with immunologic features of bullous pemphigoid. *Arch Dermatol* 115:156, 1979.
10. Zone JJ, Provost TT: Bullous diseases, in Moschella SL (ed): *Dermatology Update*. New York, Elsevier. 1979, pp 361–389.
11. Massa MC, Connolly SM: Bullous pemphigoid with features of prurigo nodularis. *Arch Dermatol* 118:937, 1982.
12. Roenigk RK, Dahl MV: Bullous pemphigoid and prurigo nodularis. *J Am Acad Dermatol* 14:944, 1986.
13. Henry JC, Jorizzo JL, Apisarnthanarax P: Reactive perforating collagenosis in the setting of prurigo nodularis. *Int J Dermatol* 2:386, 1983.
14. Noppakun N, Apisarnthanarax P: Multiple cutaneous granular cell tumours simulating prurigo nodularis. *Int J Dermatol* 20:126, 1981.
15. Wells GC: Skin disorders in relation to malabsorption. *BMJ* iv:937, 1962.
16. MacKie RM: Intestinal permeability and atopic disease. *Lancet* 2:155, 1981.
17. Howell R: Exudative nummular prurigo with idiopathic malabsorption syndrome. *Br J Dermatol* 79:357, 1967.
18. Goodwin PG, Levene GM: Nodular prurigo associated with gluten enteropathy. *Proc Roy Soc Med* 70:140, 1977.
19. Suarez C, Pereda JM, Monero LM, et al: Prurigo nodularis associated with malabsorption. *Dermatologica* 169:211, 1984.
20. Howell R: Nodular prurigo with post-gastrectomy malabsorption syndrome. *Br J Dermatol* 79:357, 1967.
21. Kolyadenko VG, Svirid AA, Shupenko NM: Prurigo nodularis Hyde. *Vestnik Dermatologii Venereologii* 1:44, 1980.

22. Greer KE: Prurigo nodularis and uremia. *South Med J* 68:138, 1975.

23. Lindley RP, Rowland Payne CME: Neural hyperplasia is not a diagnostic prerequisite in nodular prurigo. A controlled morphometric microscopic study of 26 biopsy specimens. *J Cutan Pathol* 16:14, 1989.

23a. Perez GL, Peters MS, Reda AM, et al: Mast cells, neutrophils, and eosinophils in prurigo nodularis. *Arch Dermatol* 129:861–865, 1993.

23b. Zelickson BD, McEvoy MT, Fransway AF: Patch testing in prurigo nodularis. *Contact Dermatitis* 20:321–325, 1989.

24. Ashworth J, Cream JJ: Generalized eruptive histiocytomas in an atopic: Presentation to the Derm Sec, Roy Soc Med, 21 May 1987.

25. Borde A: Introduction and dyetary, 1542 in Furnivall (ed): Early English Text Society, London, 1870.

26. Vaatainen N, Hannuksela M, Karvonen J: Local photochemotherapy in nodular prurigo. *Acta Derm Ven* 59:544, 1979.

27. Anderson TF, Waldinger TP, Vorhees JJ: UVB phototherapy: An overview. *Arch Dermatol* 120:1502, 1984.

28. Gip L: Prurigo nodularis (Hyde) treated with Tigason. *Dermatologica* 169:260, 1984.

29. Rowland Payne CME: Etretinate and nodular prurigo. *Br J Dermatol* 118:136, 1988.

30. Crosnier-Servaye A, Couteaux-Dumont C, Lapière CM: Evolution favourable de deux "prurigo nodulaire" sous traitement par ACTH synthétique et corticostéroïdes. *Arch Belges Dermatol Syphil* 4:413, 1971.

31. Hindson TC: Treatment of nodular prurigo with benoxaprofen. *Br J Dermatol* 107:369, 1982.

32. Shelley WB: *Consultations in Dermatology II.* Philadelphia, Saunders, 1974, p 47.

33. Stoll DM: Treatment of prurigo nodularis: Use of cryosurgery and intralesional steroids plus lidocaine. *J Dermatol Surg Oncol* 9:922, 1983.

33a. Tupker RA, Coenraads PJ, van der Meer JB: Treatment of prurigo nodularis, chronic prurigo and neurodermatitis circumscripta with topical capsaicin. *Acta Derm Venereol* (Stockh) 72:463–465, 1992.

34. Waldinger TP, Wong RD, Taylor WR, et al: Cryotherapy improves prurigo nodularis. *Arch Dermatol:* 1598, 1984.

35. Belaube P, Devaux J, Pizzi M, et al: Small bowel deposition of crystals associated with the use of clofazimine (Lamprene) in the treatment of prurigo nodularis. *Int J Leprosy* 51:328, 1983.

36. Winkelmann RK, Connolly SM, Doyle JA, et al: Thalidomide treatment of prurigo nodularis. *Acta Derm Ven* 64:412, 1984.

EIGHT

PRURITUS IN CHILDREN

Karen F. Rothman

INTRODUCTION

Although itching is a common malady in children, a literature search from 1965 to the present revealed no articles specifically dealing with this topic. In this chapter, I focus on the causes, physical manifestations, and treatment of itching in children.

There are no pruritic skin disorders that are unique to children. However, the frequency of certain diseases is different in patients of various ages, and the clinical appearance of some disorders may have special characteristics in children. For example, in scabies in children bullous lesions, involvement above the neck, and burrows on the feet seem to be more common than in adults.

It is useful to approach the differential diagnosis of the itchy child based on the morphology of the lesions (see Tables 8-1—8-4). Skin disorders may cause lesions of more than one morphology and thus may be listed in more than one table. Although there are characteristic locations for most rashes, it is important to keep in mind that, just as in adults, the morphology of the lesion is more likely to lead to the correct diagnosis than its location. Most of the diagnoses in Tables 8-1 to 8-3 can be made clinically; specialized tests may be unnecessary for the experienced physician.

Certain diseases deserve special mention, either because itching is a major component of the child's distress or because the diseases are rarely seen outside of the pediatric population.

Table 8-1 Pruritic scaly eruptions in children

Disease	Skin manifestations	Usual locations	Diagnosis	Associated findings
Atopic dermatitis	Ill-defined, red, scaly plaques	Depends on age of child	Clinical	Allergies, asthma, family Hx
Icthyosis	Polygonal scales	Extremities → trunk	Clinical	Family Hx
Lichen Planus	Planar, polygonal, purple, papules	Wrists, ankles, trunk	Clinical; Biopsy	—
Psoriasis	Well-defined, red scaly plaques	Elbows, knees, scalp	Clinical	Family Hx, arthritis
Pityriasis rosea	Oval scaling plaques	Trunk	Clinical	—
Pityriasis lichenoides et varioliformis acuta	Small scaly plaques heal with pigment changes	Trunk → extremities	Clinical; Biopsy	—
Tinea	Rings or serpiginous scaly plaques	Anywhere contacted	Potassium hydroxide prep	Hair loss if on scalp
Xerosis	Scale without erythema	Extremities, trunk	Clinical	—
Lichen simplex	Lichenified scaling plaques	Groin, lower legs	Clinical	—
Prurigo nodularis	Scaly nodule, often has hemorrhagic crust	Anywhere	Clinical; Biopsy	—
Contact dermatitis	Geometric oozing scaly plaques	Anywhere contacted	Clinical	—
Scabies	Excoriations, vesicles	Web spaces, intertriginous areas; scalp in infants	Scabies prep	Contacts itchy
Nonbullous impetigo	Honey-colored scale/crust	Face, extremities	Clinical; Bacterial cx	Crowded living conditions

Note: Hx = history, cx = culture

Table 8-2 Vesicular & pustular pruritic eruptions in children

Disease	Skin manifestations	Usual location	Diagnosis	Associated Findings
Varicella	"dew drop on a rose petal"	Generalized	Tzank, culture	Hx of exposure; pneumonia
Herpes simplex	Grouped vesicles on erythematous base	Anywhere contacted	Tzank, culture	—
Zoster	Groups of vesicles in a dermatome	Dermatomal	Tzank, culture	Hx of chicken pox
Coxsackie A	Papules and vesicles	Palms, soles, palate	Clinical	Fever, diarrhea
Bullous impetigo	Bullae, usually without surrounding erythema	Extremities	Culture, gram stain	Fever, malaise
Folliculitis	Perifollicular pustules	Extremities	Clinical; culture, gram stain	—
Candidiasis	red macules, peripheral vesicles, & pustules	Groin	Clinical, KOH	Oral thrush: Rare, mucocutaneous candidiasis
Scabies	Vesicles, pustules, excoriations	Web spaces, intertriginous areas, scalp in infants	Scabies prep	Family members itchy
Dermatitis Herpetiformis	Hemorrhagic crusts & erosions	Elbows, knees, buttocks	Biopsy-immunofluorescence	Diarrhea-celiac sprue
Bullous disease of childhood	groups of annular erosions	Thighs, trunk	Biopsy-immunofluorescence	—
Insect Bites	Occurs only with certain insects in certain children	Extremities	Clinical	—
Mastocytosis	Red-brown macules—may blister after trauma	Anywhere	Darier's sign; biopsy	Occasional: generalized urticaria
Erythropoietic Protoporphyria	Erythema, edema, or symptoms alone	Dorsum of hands, face	Blood, urine, stool porphyrins	Family Hx

Note: Hx = history

Table 8-3 Erythematous nonscaling pruritic eruptions in children

Disease	Skin manifestations	Location	Diagnosis	Associated findings
Perianal/perivaginal strep	Tender, intense erythema	Genital region	Culture	—
Candida	Red macules, peripheral pustules, & vesicles	Groin	Clinical; KOH	Oral thrush rare: mucocutaneous candidiasis; may scale
Urticaria	Smooth red papules and plaques	Anywhere	Clinical	Occasional anaphylaxis
Mastocytosis	Brown, red macules which urticate after stroking	Anywhere	Darrier's sign; biopsy	Occasional anaphylaxis
Insect bites	Red papules, often grouped	Extremities → trunk	Clinical	—
Papular Urticaria	Crops of red papules w/hemorrhagic crusts	Nonclothed areas	Clinical	Exposure to Pets and/or insects
Viral Exanthem	morbilliform	depends on virus	Clinical	Fever, cough, myalgias, diarrhea
Drug eruptions	moribilliform	Trunk → Extremities	Clinical	Occasional multisystem involvement
Polymorphous light eruption	Red macules, papules	sun exposed areas, especially arms	Clinical, biopsy	—

Table 8-4 Pruritus without rash in children: differential diagnosis

Hepatic failure
Renal failure
Underlying malignancy
Diabetes
Hyperparathyroidism
Pseudohyperparathyroidism
Erythropoietic protoporphyria
Iron deficiency anemia
Hyperthyroidism
Aquagenic pruritus
"Subclinical" variants of scabies

ATOPIC DERMATITIS

Atopic dermatitis is seen in approximately 12 percent of children. Although Dennie–Morgan pleats near the eyes and hyperlinear palms may be present in newborn infants with an atopic diathesis, symptoms rarely begin before 6 weeks of age. In infants, ill-defined erythematous plaques are most commonly seen on the cheeks and trunk as well as the extensor surfaces of the extremities. As the child grows older, atopic dermatitis usually begins to involve the flexural areas as is characteristically seen in adults with this disease. The incessant quality of the pruritus seen in this disorder is not unique to atopic dermatitis, but is quite characteristic. Children scratch or rub their plaques constantly. Many parents report that this behavior is so frequent they feel that it has become a habit, even after the plaque has apparently improved. The atopic's skin may be unusually sensitive to certain types of fabrics, especially wool. Removal of clothing may cause frenzied attacks of itching, which may, or may appear to be due to exposure to the air.[1]

SCABIES

Scabies in infants may appear identical to the disease in adults. However, urticarial and bullous lesions, lesions in the scalp and on the face, and/or large eczematous plaques may occur. The diagnosis should be suspected in infants and children who have a rash involving the intertriginous areas and web spaces of the fingers and toes, as is seen in adults. Itching is usually most pronounced in the areas where most lesions are, and is characteristically most intense at night.

URTICARIA (hives)

This is a problem commonly encountered by pediatricians and dermatologists. The clinical manifestations as well as common underlying causes vary with the age of the patient. In children less then 24 months of age, angioedema, and hemorrhagic lesions resembling erythema multiforme are common.[2] In approximately two thirds of patients less than 24 months of age, an identifying cause can be found. For infants less than 6 months old, cows milk allergy is the most common cause of hives. Drug ingestion and viral infections make up the majority of known causes of urticaria in children 6 to 24 months of age. Other studies have looked at urticaria in children up to age 12 or 16 years.[3–5] For older children, the underlying cause can be determined in 15 to 87 percent of patients.[4] Physical urticaria, particularly from the cold, food allergies and additives, and viral and streptococcal infections, are common etiologic factors. Children with chronic urticaria have a better overall prognosis than adults with chronic urticaria: Approximately 55 percent are symptom free within a year.[3,4] Although children old enough to express their feelings will usually say they are itchy when they have hives, most children I have seen with hives do not seem to be as itchy as adults with this disorder. Young children with hives may appear uncomfortable, finding it difficult to sit still, but most seem relatively symptom free.

INSECT BITES AND STINGS

Insect bites and stings may cause pruritic papules, urticarial wheals, or blisters, depending on the specific insect and the host response. *Papular urticaria* (also known as strophulus, prurigo simplex acuta, and lichen urticatus) is a cutaneous reaction to bites and stings that is most commonly seen in children. (See Chaps. 4 and 9.) Five to ten millimeter erythematous papules occur in crops. Central puncta may be present in occasional lesions, but hemorrhagic crusts secondary to excoriations are more common. Lesions usually occur in crops and are generally most prevalent on the unclothed areas of skin. Some or most of the lesions may be due to actual bites, but others may be due to an autosensitization phenomena.[6,7] Bedbugs, fleas, certain mites, mosquitoes, and other insects may be responsible.

ERYTHROPOIETIC PROTOPORPHYRIA

Children with erythropoietic protoporphyria (EPP) may be irritable when placed in the sun as infants. As they grow older and are able to verbalize their symptoms, children with this disease characteristically complain of a burning or itching sensation when exposed to the sun. Acute changes include erythema and edema; shallow, waxy scars occur later. Blisters and erosions, although sometimes present on the dorsum of the hands and face, may be absent. However, the unusual (if not somewhat bizarre) nature of the symptoms, combined with a positive family history in some cases (as the disease is autosomal dominant), may help the clinician to suspect the correct diagnosis.

PERIANAL OR VAGINAL STREPTOCOCCAL INFECTION

This is a recently recognized cause of pruritus and pain in children.[8,9] It is commonly recurrent. A culture swab of the area will grow group A beta-hemolytic strep, but the lab must be told to culture the specimen in an appropriate culture medium so that it does not become overrun with coliforms.

MASTOCYTOSIS

Mastocytosis refers to a group of disorders in which affected tissues are infiltrated by large numbers of mast cells. Two thirds of affected patients are children[10] but the disease may begin at any age. Virtually any organ can be affected, but symptomatic and clinically relevant organ involvement is rare in children, particularly in those who manifest the disease prior to age 2 years.[10,11] Nearly all patients with mastocytosis have cutaneous lesions. Dermatographism is also usually present. Tan macules that urticate after stroking the skin (Darier's sign) are characteristically seen. When the mast cell infiltrates are degranulated by chemical or physical stimuli, widespread flushing of the skin may occur. Vesicles and bullae over the lesions may appear after rubbing the skin, particularly in young children with mastocytosis. Occasional patients may anaphylax from the sudden massive release of histamine that occurs when the mast cells degranulate.

Several different clinical patterns may be seen in children with mastocytosis. In urticaria pigmentosa, which is the most commonly seen variant, children have multiple tan macules ranging in size from a few millimeters to one to two centimeters. Children with urticaria pigmentosa usually develop the disease prior to age 2 years. Ten to fifteen percent of patients with mast cell disease have solitary mastocytomas. These children have one or a few tan macules, which may be up to several centimeters in size. They may be present at birth and virtually always appear within the first 6 months of life. Diffuse cutaneous mast cell infiltration is the least common variant of this disorder. In patients with this disorder, the integument may appear normal in color or slightly red, light brown, or yellow. A thickening of the skin with an increase of normal skin markings is common. Vesicles and bullae commonly appear after mild skin rubbing. Massive release of histamine with resultant shock can occur on a recurrent basis.[11] Although lesions of mastocytosis are comprised of histamine-containing mast cells, in my own experience it is rare for children with urticaria pigmentosa or solitary mastocytomas to complain of significant pruritus and excoriations are rarely present. Patients with diffuse cutaneous mastocytosis may be extremely pruritic; their frequent rubbing and scratching of the lesions may make the symptoms even more pronounced.

BLISTERING AND PUSTULAR PRURITIC LESIONS

These are commonly seen in the pediatric population. The differential diagnosis of these lesions is listed in Table 8-2. Although the experienced clinician can usually distinguish these entities based on the clinical presentation, a few bedside diagnostic techniques that are easy to perform are necessary in some cases. The Tzank smear is useful for confirming the diagnosis of a herpes infection. It is performed by scraping the base of a blister onto a slide, staining the slide with Geimsa or Wright's stain, and looking for virus-infected multinucleated giant cells. The Tzank preparation cannot distinguish between the varicella-zoster virus and herpes simplex virus. If this distinction cannot be made on clinical grounds, culture or immunofluorescence testing can be performed. Gram stain is useful for patients with bullous impetigo or folliculitis. Culture may be useful in occasional patients to determine the most appropriate antibiotic therapy. A mineral oil preparation is useful in diagnosing scabies; a lesion is scraped off the skin and its contents placed on a slide. A drop of mineral oil is added and a cover slip is placed over the preparation. Scabies mites, feces, and/or eggs may be seen. Potassium hydroxide preparation is useful for patients with possible fungal infection. Scale and/or fluid is placed on a slide. One to two drops of 10 to 20 percent potassium hydroxide is added and a cover slip is placed. The material is heated for 5 to 10 seconds. Hyphae and/or spores may then be visualized. Although all of the above preparations are useful in proving a diagnosis if they are positive, a negative preparation does not rule out the possibility of any of the listed infections or infestations.

METABOLIC CAUSES OF PRURITUS

Children with liver, renal, or endocrine dysfunction or failure may develop pruritus just as their adult counterparts do. In nearly every case symptoms of organ failure precede pruritus, so the cause of pruritus is not difficult to determine. Metabolic aspects of itching are discussed in Chap. 18.

MALIGNANCY

Like adults, children occasionally present with pruritus with or without a rash as the first symptom of an underlying malignancy.[12,13] The association of generalized pruritus with occult malignancy is covered in detail in Chap. 21.

MANAGEMENT

The management of pruritus in children depends on the underlying disease. Space does not permit a detailed description of the management of each disease, but some general points and a discussion of the management of some of the uncommon causes of childhood itching are presented.

Infants and young children do not possess the vocabulary to tell us they are itchy. Although infants can certainly accidentally scratch themselves, purposeful scratching does not occur in the first few weeks of life. Therefore, we must learn and develop skills for assessing the subtle signs and symptoms that young children with itching have. Itchy infants may have difficulty falling asleep and may waken more frequently at night. I have seen infants as young as 4 to 6 weeks of age with scabies or atopic dermatitis who move constantly when laid down, rubbing against the sheets, apparently uncomfortable in any position. Itchy infants may be extremely fussy and difficult to satisfy. One $2\frac{1}{2}$ year old child that I cared for with severe atopic dermatitis had speech delay for no apparent reason. Two weeks later, when the itching was well controlled, she began speaking in full sentences and interacting more with others! While this is an extreme example, young children with pruritus may interact much better with others once their itching is well controlled.

ANTIHISTAMINES

Antihistamines are of major importance in the treatment of pruritic children. Diphenhydramine, hydroxyzine, and clemastine fumarate are available in liquid form; chlorpheniramine is available in chewable tablets. Dosages required in children are based on weight, but therapeutic dosages vary widely.[7] Guidelines for proper use of antihistamines in children can be found in the Harriet Lane handbook.[14] As with adults, large doses of antihistamines may be required to control itching. This may result in profound sedation, making it difficult for the child to carry out his or her normal daily activities. I generally advise parents to give low enough doses of antihistamines during the day on a regular 4- to 6-hour schedule (except for clemastine fumarate, which is administered twice daily) so that the child can function normally and yet is not uncomfortable with itching. At night, I recommend giving 2 to 3 times the daytime dose, which, it is hoped, will enable the child and his family to sleep through the night. Hyperactivity occurs in 10 to 15 percent of children given any specific antihistamine; if this occurs, the parents should be advised to stop its use and an antihistamine of a different class should be used. Nonsedating antihistamines may be very useful in children with histamine-mediated disorders who are old enough to swallow pills, but as of this writing, are not available in liquid form. Antihistamines are discussed in detail in Chap. 29. In nonhistamine mediated disorders, their major mode of action is probably related to sedation or their soporific effect.

TOPICAL AGENTS

Baking soda, colloidal oatmeal, and tar-containing preparations may be useful additives to the bath for children with pruritus. Although bath oils may be safely applied to the child following a bath, I vigorously discourage adding oil to the tub. The oil makes the tub slick, which may result in slipping accidents. Cleaning of the tub after oil is added increases parental work. Thirdly, oil is insoluble and is inadvisable for patients whose homes have septic tanks.

Emollients

They may be useful for any condition in which the skin is dry. For infants, I most frequently recommend Vaseline® petroleum jelly. It is easy to find, spreads easily, is inexpensive, and contains no alcohol or preservatives. Older children and adults may object to the greasy feel of petrolatum so more expensive, cosmetically elegant preparations may be required. Examples include: Moisturel®, Lubriderm®, Theraplex®, and DML®. Creams should be used in preference to lotions because they are better at increasing and maintaining skin hydration. Parents should be cautioned that for some pruritic children, particularly those with atopic dermatitis, any lotion or cream may sting on application. For these children, petrolatum is the best moisturizer. For some children and parents, the application of any topical preparation turns into a battle, even if it doesn't hurt. Allowing the child to apply the moisturizer may decrease the number of fights in some households, although parents must be prepared for a potential mess! Several moisturizers are available in pumps, spray foams, and mousses, all of which may make application more fun for the child. Examples include Lubriderm® cream (in a pump), Johnson's baby oil body moisturizing mousse®, and Sarna® foam.

Topical steroids

These are very important in the treatment of pruritus in children when a steroid-responsive dermatosis is present. Because of concern about adrenal suppression[15-17] from absorption of topical steroids and localized skin atrophy, the weakest preparation that will get the job done is the most appropriate steroid to use. The use of ultra-potent steroids should be avoided in children. Potent topical steroids, such as hacinonide and fluocinonide, should be avoided in most infants. These potent topical steroids may be necessary for short courses (i.e., less than 2 weeks) for children over 6 months of age, but less potent medications should generally be tried first. Potent topical steroids should be avoided on the face and in skin folds, particularly under the diaper, as steroid atrophy and adrenal suppression may occur under these circumstances.[15-17] Children who require long term administration of potent topical steroids should have their growth parameters monitored regularly and should also have tests of adrenal cortical function performed periodically. Children with atopic dermatitis are often of shorter stature than nonatopic individuals, and chronic topical steroids probably have some role in this.[18]

Miscellaneous

Topical nonsteroidal agents, such as Sarna® and Prax®, may also be useful in the control of itching in children. These are discussed in Chaps. 26 and 27. Frequent clipping of finger nails and wearing mittens to bed at night may decrease the damage that the pruritic child can do to his or her skin. Behavioral modification techniques[19] as well as transcutaneous electrical nerve stimulation [20] may be useful in older children with chronic pruritus. Ultraviolet phototherapy and photochemotherapy (PUVA) for atopic dermatitis is addressed in Chap. 28. The decision to utilize a treatment such as PUVA in children must be weighed against the known risks. Atherton and colleagues reported that growth rates in atopic dermatitis patients returned to normal after successful PUVA treatment.[21]

Children with chronic renal failure suffering from intractable pruritus may be treated with ultraviolet therapy if they are able to safely stand alone in the phototherapy box.[22] Children with cholestatic liver disease may also suffer from intractable, disabling pruritus.[23,24] Phenobarbital is helpful in some patients. Cholestyramine resin is distasteful, so it is difficult for children to take. Furthermore, cholestyramine may cause constipation, acidosis, and hypernatremia.[23] In these children, surgical bile diversion[23] and/or oral rifampin may provide relief.[24] Pruritus associated with renal and hepatic disease is discussed in greater detail in Chaps. 15 and 16.

Children with cutaneous mastocytosis may be asymptomatic and not require therapy. For those with itching, topical steroid preparations may decrease the episodic urtication of the lesions and/or may help the lesions resolve more quickly.[25] For infants and children with severe systemic symptoms, ketotifen may be useful, [26] although it is not currently available in the United States. Oral disodium cromoglycate[27] or photochemotherapy[28] may be useful in some cases.

The parents of the chronically pruritic child may feel overwhelmed, exasperated, exhausted and helpless. Unaffected siblings may feel ignored and unloved. As physicians caring for an itchy child, we must realize the stresses placed on other family members. We should acknowledge the difficulties faced by the family and help to educate and emotionally support them as we try to make the child more comfortable.

REFERENCES

1. Bernhard JD: Nonrashes 5. Atmoknesis: pruritus provoked by contact with air. *Cutis* 44: 143–144, 1989.
2. Legrain V, Taieb A, Sage T, et al: Urticaria in infants: A study of forty patients. *Pediatr Dermatol* 7:101–107, 1990.
3. Harris A, Twarog FJ, Geha RS: Chronic urticaria in childhood: Natural course and etiology. *Ann Allergy* 51:161–165, 1983.
4. Kauppinen K, Juntunen K, Lanki H: Urticaria in children. *Allergy* 39:469–472, 1984.
5. Bonifazi E, Meneghini CL, Ceci A: Pathogenetic factors in urticaria in children. *Dermatologica* 154:65–72, 1977.
6. Mroczkowski TF, Milikan LE: Pruritus and prurigo, in Ruiz-Maldonado R, Parish LC, Beare JM (eds): *Textbook of Pediatric Dermatology*. Philadelphia, Grune and Stratton. 1989, pp 611–615.
7. Lynch PJ: Vascular reactions, in Schachner LA, Hansen RC, (eds) *Pediatric Dermatology*, vol 2. New York, Churchill Livingstone. 1988, pp 959–1014.
8. Krol AL: Perianal streptococcal dermatitis. *Pediatr Dermatol* 7:97–100, 1990.
9. Kokx NP, Comstock JA, Facklam RR: Streptococcal perianal disease in children. *Pediatr* 80:659–663, 1987.
10. Kettelhut BV, Metcalfe DD: Pediatric mastocytosis. *J Invest Dermatol* 96:15S–18S, 1991.
11. Stein DH: Mastocytosis: A review. *Pediatr Dermatol* 3:365–375, 1986.
12. Summers CG, MacDonald JT: Paroxysmal facial itch: A presenting sign of childhood brainstem glioma. *J Child Neurol* 3:189–192, 1988.
13. Shelnitz LS, Paller A: Hodgkin's disease manifesting as prurigo nodularis. *Pediatr Dermatol* 7:136–139, 1990.
14. Greene MG: The Harriet Lane Handbook, 12 Ed. St. Louis, Mosby Year Book, 1990.
15. Munro DD: Topical corticosteroid therapy and its effect on the hypothalamic-pituitary-adrenal axis. *Dermatologica* 152:173–180, 1976.
16. Munro DD: The effect of percutaneously absorbed steroids on hypothalamic-pituitary-adrenal function after intensive use in in-patients. *Br J Dermatol* 94:67–76, 1976.
17. Feiwel M, James VHT, Barnett ES: Effect of potent topical steroids on plasma-cortisol levels of infants and children with eczema. *Lancet* I:485–487, 1969.
18. Kristmundsdottir F, David TJ: Growth impairment in children with atopic eczema. *J Royal Soc Med* 80:9–12, 1987.
19. Melin L, Frederiksen T, Noren P, et al: Behavioral treatment of scratching in patients with atopic dermatitis. *Br J Dermatol* 115:467–474, 1986.
20. Bjorna H, Kaada B: Successful treatment of itching and atopic eczema by transcutaneous nerve stimulation. *Acupunt Electrother Res, Internat* J 12:101–112, 1987.
21. Atherton DJ, Carabott F, Glover MT, et al: The role of psoralen photochemotherapy (PUVA) in the treatment of severe atopic eczema in adolescents. *Br J Dermatol* 118:791–795, 1988.
22. Gilchrest B, Rowe JW, Brown RS, et al: Relief of uremic pruritus with ultraviolet phototherapy. *N Engl J Med* 297:136–138, 1977.

23. Whitington PF, Whitington GL: Partial external diversion of bile for the treatment of intractable pruritus associated with intrahepatic cholestasis. *Gastroenterology* 95:130–136, 1988.

24. Cynamon HA, Andres JM, Iafrate RP: Rifampin relieves pruritus in children with cholestatic liver disease. *Gastroenterology* 98:1013–1016, 1990.

25. Barton J, Lavker RM, Schechter NM, et al: Treatment of urticaria pigmentosa with corticosteroids. *Arch Dermatol* 121:1516–1523, 1985.

26. Czarnetzki BM: A double-blind cross-over study of the effect of ketotifen in urticaria pigmentosa. *Dermatologica* 166:44–47, 1983.

27. Soter NA, Austen F, Wasserman SI: Oral disodium cromoglycolate in the treatment of systemic mastocytosis. *N Engl J Med* 301:465–469, 1979.

28. Smith ML, Orton PW, Chu H, et al: Photochemotherapy of dominant, diffuse, cutaneous mastocytosis. *Pediatr Dermatol* 7:251–255, 1990.

ITCHING DUE TO BITES, STINGS, AND INFESTATIONS

Mark J. Scharf

Whether on land or sea, we share our world with a host of arthropods and other invertebrate species whose bites, stings, and infestations may result in injury or disease. This chapter will focus on the diagnosis, treatment, and prevention of encounters with those organisms which typically produce itching when they contact human skin. Readers who are interested in pursuing these topics in great detail are referred to monographic sources listed in references.[1–6] The concept of *papular urticaria* from arthropod assaults is also discussed in Chap. 4.

ARTHROPODS

Scabies, Lice, And Other Mites

Scabies

> "It's impossible to have scabies and not scratch."[7]
> P. Levi

Etiology. Scabies in humans is due to an infestation by the itch mite, *Sarcoptes scabiei,* var *hominis.* The adult female mite, measuring only 40 μm (1/16 in.) and barely visible to the unaided eye, initiates the infestation when she finds a suitable site on the skin of her human host and begins digging a burrow between the layers of the stratum corneum and the stratum granulosum.[3p9,8,10] Along the length of the burrow, which she enlarges at a rate of 0.5 to 5.0 mm per day, she lays 2 to 3 oval-shaped eggs daily as she feeds on nutrients oozing from the cells on which she has chewed.[3p10] In addition to laying eggs, the burrowing mite also passes behind her the waste products of digestion, which appear as little brownish pellets known as scybala. Less than 10% of the eggs gives rise to adult mites, which must go through a larval stage and one or two nymph stages before reaching maturity in 10 to 14 days.[3pp13–14] The average number of adult mites that could be found in patients with scabies was observed to be 11.3 in a study involving 886 cases.[4p12] This number may vary widely depending on the bathing habits and immune status of the patient and whether topical or systemic steroids have been employed prior to adequate scabecidal treatment.

Epidemiology. In this century there have been three recorded upsurges in the incidence of scabies. The first two coincided with the first and second world wars, and the third began in the 1970s. Whether these increases were due to factors relating to war, changes in social or sexual habits, a reduction in immunity in the host populations, or changes in the infectivity of the mite are not known.[3pp105–107] In general, spread of the mite requires close personal contact with an infested individual; however, in cases of crusted or Norwegian scabies more casual contact or fomites may be sufficient to transmit the mite. The scabies mite is very sensitive to extremes of temperature and humidity. From several studies it appears that the adult mite can survive at room temperatures of 21 to 25°C with 60% to 90% humidity for up to 3 days.[3p17.9] Although fomites are not usually considered a major factor in the spread of scabies, I have diagnosed several cases in which the disease was transmitted when college roomates shared a sweatshirt, or when a patient slept over in the bed of (but was not and had not been intimate with) a person who was later diagnosed with scabies. In addition to articles of clothing and bedding, scabies mites have been recovered from the dust found on bedroom and bathroom floors and upholstered furniture from the houses of patients diagnosed with scabies.[10] Dust samples from 44% of infested patients' homes contained scabies mites, and in 64% of those cases in which mites were recovered, they were alive at the time they were analyzed.[10] It is therefore possible that infested fomites may be more significant in the spread of scabies or in treatment failures than was previously believed.[10]

HIV infection may also affect the epidemiology and clinical manifestations of scabies.[10a] (See also Chap. 20.)

Clinical manifestations. There are two distinct types of itching seen in scabies, localized and generalized.[2p229] Generalized pruritus may range from mild to severe and is observed 4 to 6 weeks after mite infestation has begun.[5p72] Generalized itch is attributed to the development of allergic sensitization against components of the mites, eggs, or scybala.[3p36,5p72] Localized itching in scabies has been described as having a burning character and is caused by a local reaction to the presence or activity of the mite.[2p229]

Physical examination. The primary lesion in scabies is the burrow, which is found primarily on the sides or webspaces of the fingers, wrists, elbows, penis, and scrotum. Burrows may also be found on the buttocks, breasts, and anterior axillary folds.[3p23] In infants the face, neck, and soles may be involved. Burrows appear as short S-shaped or straight greyish lines with a small vesicles at the distal end overlying the site of the female mite.[11]

With experience, sharp-eyed observers may be able to spot the mite, which appears as a small greyish speck, and remove it by scraping with a blade and placing it on a microscope slide. A hand lens may be helpful for spotting small intact burrows that are likely to yield positive scrapings.[12] Covering the burrow prior to scraping with a drop of mineral oil (which can also be placed on the slide) helps to immobilize the mite and will not dissolve the scybala.[9] The burrow then can either be scraped vigorously six to seven times until the entire top of the papule has been removed, or the blade can be used to perform a superficial epidermal shave biopsy.[6,9] The scraping can then be covered with a coverslip and viewed at low power. The presence of adult or immature mites, eggs, or scybala is diagnostic for scabies.

Another technique for visualizing the burrows is to apply a water washable ink or topical tetracycline to the suspected area, wash off the excess, and then look for retained ink (which stains the burrows) or tetracycline, which also concentrates in the burrows and fluoresces under Wood's lamp exam.[8]

In addition to the burrow, which may be very difficult to identify in many cases, scabetic patients exhibit a variety of skin changes including inflammatory and "noninflammatory vesicles, erythematous urticarial papules, excoriations, and eczematous patches."[5p71] Several cases of scabies with pemphigoid-like bullae have also been reported.[13]

Many cases of scabies are complicated by secondary infections due to scratching that may result in the formation of pustules and bullae (especially in children), as well as furuncles, abscesses, and cellulitis.[3pp23,36] Ordinary urticaria is occasionally seen as a consequence of an allergic hypersensitivity reaction to scabies infestation.[14]

Norwegian or crusted scabies is a rare variant of the disease most commonly seen in the immunocompromised, severely debilitated or mentally retarded host. Norwegian scabies is clinically manifested by a crusted psoriasiform dermatosis of the hands and feet with dystrophic nails and varying degrees of an erythematous scaling eruption that may be generalized.[3p28,4p27] In crusted scabies the affected areas are literally teeming with mites, which makes these cases highly communicable. Most of the patients who are at risk for crusted scabies are either hospitalized or institutionalized, and there have been a number of case reports of nosocomial outbreaks of scabies that were traced back to these unfortunate patients. There have been several cases of Norwegian scabies occurring in patients with AIDS, which resulted in outbreaks of scabies in hospitals.[15,16]

There are a number of well described clinical variants of scabies in addition to Norwegian scabies that are also worth noting. They are summarized in Table 9-1.

Differential diagnosis. Scabies has been described as a great imitator of other pruritic dermatologic diseases and its differential diagnosis can be extremely broad (see Table 9-2). It is, therefore, not uncommon for patients with scabies to be diagnosed and treated for one form or another of eczematous dermatitis without ever being questioned or examined for scabies. In order to make the diagnosis of scabies the practicing physician must first consider the diagnosis, and then continue to maintain a high degree of suspicion for the disease.

Table 9-1 Clinical variants of scabies[2,3]

Type	Predisposing factors	Clinical findings
Scabies Incognito	Prior use of topical or systemic steroids, immunosuppressed patients	Increased number and extent of burrows, less itching than expected
Scabies in the clean patient	Frequent bathers	Itching with very few papules or burrows
Nodular scabies	Previous exposure to scabies may result in localized delayed type hypersensitivity reaction, more common in children	Firm reddish brown intensely pruritic dermal nodules of the penis, scrotum, axilla
Urticarial scabies	Immediate type hypersensitivity response to antigenic components of scabies mite	Urticarial wheals and papules may obscure burrows and other diagnostic features of scabies
Vasculitic scabies	Arthus-like reaction develops in sensitized individuals(?)	Palpable purpura of the lower extremities, occasionally generalized
Scabies in infants	Recent adoptions from foreign countries with high incidence of scabies	Atypical distribution involving head, neck, palms, and soles
Scabies in the aged patient	Elderly patients, often hospitalized or institutionalized, often bedridden	Severe itch with minimal inflammatory response, may involve back
Scabid[17]	Id reaction to scabies	Widespread papulovesicles of the trunk, arms, legs, and face
Bullous scabies	High level of sensitization to scabies antigens, increased skin fragility in youth or old age(?)	Pemphoid-like blisters (vesicles and bullae)
Norwegian scabies	Immunocompromised, severely debilitated, or mentally retarded patients	Hyperkeratotic, crusted psoriasiform dermatitis of the palms and soles, may be generalized; nail dystrophy

Table 9-2 Differential diagnosis of scabies[2-5]

Atopic dermatitis
Allergic and irritant contact dermatitis
Seborrheic dermatitis
Neurodermatitis
Dyshidrotic eczema (pompholyx)
Prurigo (See Chaps. 4 and 7.)
Papular urticaria (See Chap. 4.)
Pyodermas (impetigo, furunculosis)
Pityriasis rosea
Pruritic dermatoses of pregnancy (See Chap. 19.)
Infectious eczematoid dermatitis
Insect bites
Other mites (Cheyletiella, Canine scabies, etc.)
Lichen planus
Psoriasiform dermatoses of the palms and soles
Dermatitis herpetiformis
Mastocytosis
Histiocytosis X
Lymphoma
Urticaria
Vasculitis
Pediculosis pubis and corporis
Delusions of parasitosis (See Chap. 25.)
Sabra dermatitis (prickly pear dermatitis)[2]
Syphilis
Keratosis follicularis (Darier–White disease)
Pemphigoid[13]
Pruritus related to underlying systemic disease

In addition to a complete examination of the skin and a careful search for burrows, the patient should be questioned with regard to itching at night especially on retiring; itching of the hands, breasts, or genital areas; a history of friends or family members who are itchy; or a history of exposure to scabies in the home or workplace. When any of these are answered in the affirmative, they may help to prompt the correct diagnosis. Scabies should also be considered (along with pediculosis pubis and other venereal diseases) in the pruritic patient with a history of sexual promiscuity.

Management. Making the diagnosis of scabies can be a very satisfying experience for the clinician. It can also be one of the most distressing diagnoses a patient can hear. After weeks or months of torment from itching, secondary infections, and sleepless nights, patients can hardly be blamed if they appear less than grateful when given this diagnosis. They may be anxious or embarrassed about the social stigma surrounding scabies, and they may be frustrated and angered by prior consultations from physicians whose explanations and prescriptions didn't alleviate their suffering. Obviously, understanding and reassurance on the part of the physician are invaluable in the approach to these patients.

Once the diagnosis of scabies has been firmly established (preferably by positive scraping, but also when there is a history of close exposure to a known scabetic patient, or when the physical examination and history of itching are highly suggestive of scabies) the patient and his or her close contacts must be treated. While it may not be possible or practical to achieve positive scrapings in every case, I always strive to confirm the diagnosis through a microscope before treating with scabecidal medications, for if the treatment fails to relieve the patient's itch within the expected time frame (2–4 weeks on average), I know that if the diagnosis was accurately established I am either dealing with a prolonged hypersensitivity reaction against residual elements of the dead mites, or with a partially treated or reinfested patient. If the diagnosis was not established definitively before treatment for scabies was begun, and the patient continues to have itching, the clinical situation becomes more difficult. The diagnostic possibilities must then include not only treatment failure, reinfestation, and postscabietic pruritus, but also the entire differential diagnosis of pruritus.

Drug therapy. For many years the treatment of choice for scabies was 1.0% gamma-benzene hexachloride lotion (lindane) applied for 8 to 12 hours at night. While still a highly effective scabecidal agent, concerns have been raised about its potential for acute central nervous system (CNS) toxicity. When applied in large amounts to the skin of young children, or when overused or overapplied to inflamed or damaged skin, lindane has caused seizures and deaths.[18] In most cases one application of lindane (if applied correctly) is sufficient, however a second application may be prescribed as a precaution in case of inadequate use.[2p268]

Permethrin 5% cream (Elimite) has been shown in several studies to have a higher cure rate and lower toxicity than lindane, and has also proved to be more effective than 10% crotamiton cream (Eurax) in the treatment of children.[19–21] Based on these studies, the Medical Letter now considers Permethrin 5% cream the drug of choice for the treatment of scabies.[18] Side effects with permethrin 5% cream are limited to itching erythema and edema.[18] No systemic reactions have been reported with permethrin 5% cream and it has not been shown to have teratogenic effects in animals.[18] For all these reasons permethrin 5% cream can be recommended for the treatment of premature infants and small children, patients with seizures and neurological complications, in pregnant woman and nursing mothers, in cases of treatment failures with lindane, and in crusted scabies.[20]

In addition to lindane and permethrin, other scabecidal agents available in the United States at the present time include 10% crotamiton cream and 5% or 10% precipitated sulfur in petrolatum or a water-washable base.[8] Eurax may have some antipruritic properties, but it is generally considered less effective than lindane and must be applied twice and left on the skin for a 48-hour period.[8,18] Precipitated sulfur is an effective treatment for scabies, but it requires multiple nightly applications, has a disagreeable odor, stains clothing, and has produced serious complications and death in infants.[5p77,8]

When treating scabies, it is extremely helpful for patient compliance to send the patient home with written instructions for how to apply the medication, who to treat, and what to do with clothing and linens. These guidelines are summarized in Table 9-3.

Most scabietic patients will require some treatment for symptomatic relief of itching. Antihistamines, colloidal baths, topical antipruritic creams or lotions, and topical steroids may all be beneficial. Some general measures for symptomatic relief of itching in this setting (and for other bites and infestations as well) are listed in Table 9-4.

Itching may also result from secondary infections, which should be treated with the appropriate antibiotics. Patients with itching that persists beyond several weeks after treatment should be reexamined for the possibility of treatment failure or for reinfestation that could have occurred if a previously unidentified scabietic contact went untreated.

Treatment of Norwegian scabies is more difficult than standard cases of the disease because the dystrophic nails and thick hyperkeratotic crusts may shield some of the mites from the scabicidal medication. Patients with crusted scabies are highly infectious and treatment failure in these cases is likely to have serious consequences for other patients and staff who may become infested from these patients. There have been many suggestions

Table 9-3 Instructions for patients with scabies

1. Apply the medication (lindane lotion or permethrin cream) from the neck down to the toes. Do not miss any areas. Be sure to treat under the arms, breasts, and genital area; between the buttocks; and in any skin folds. Trim and clean the nails and apply the medication under the nails. In infants, also apply to the head and face.
2. Apply the medication at night to dry skin and leave it on for 8 to 12 hours, then wash off. If instructed by your physician, you may reapply the medication in 1 week. Do not apply the medication more frequently than instructed because this can cause further skin irritation.
3. Itching may continue for several days to several weeks after treatment has been completed. This does not mean that the treatment was unsuccessful. Most patients have some degree of itching for a period of time after treatment because of a continued allergic reaction to the mites that have been destroyed by the treatment. Follow the instructions given by your physician for relieving the itch. If the itching persists beyond 3 or 4 weeks after treatment you must return for a follow-up visit.
4. All family members, anyone living in the house, any close personal contacts, and frequent visitors such as relatives or babysitters should be treated.[2]
5. Clothing, linens, bedcovers, and towels should be washed in hot water or dry cleaned. Clean or vacuum the floors in the bathrooms and bedrooms as well as any upholstered chairs or couches.[10]

Table 9-4 General measures for the symptomatic treatment of itching due to bites and infestations

1. Cooling colloidal baths in tepid water (e.g., colloidal oatmeal, baking soda)
2. Cooling lotions (such as Sarna[R])
3. Topical anesthetic gels creams, lotions, or sprays containing pramoxine (Prax[R], PrameGel[R])
4. Combination agents such as 1% hydrocortisone plus pramoxine (Pramosone[R] 1% cream or lotion)
5. Cool compresses
6. Calamine lotion
7. Topical corticosteroids
8. Oral antihistamines

See also Chap. 26 and 27

for the treatment of Norwegian scabies over the years. Recently O'Donnell, O'Loughlin, and Powell suggested a regimen that is both reasonable and effective and that is summarized in Table 9-5.[22]

The diagnosis and management of scabies in patients with HIV disease can present special challenges.[10a] (See also Chap. 20.)

The question of scabies mites resistant to various scabecidal drugs, including lindane, has been raised repeatedly over the years and has yet to be answered conclusively.[23-25] In the majority of cases, "when infestation persists, only inadequate treatment or reinfestation can be blamed."[5p78]

Mites from pets and domesticated animals

Animal scabies. Canine scabies and scabies infestations from other pets are not uncommon and should be investigated when scabies is suspected but scrapings from the patient are negative. Symptoms of canine scabies tend to be more localized than for human scabies, with multiple pruritic papules (which may have a punctum) appearing in areas of skin that are in contract with the animal harboring the mites, typically the forearms, lower chest, abdomen, and anterior thighs.[5p76,26] The papules may enlarge and develop excoriations with pustules and crusts.[26] A history that reflects improvement of the condition in the pet owner or family member when away

Table 9-5 Management of crusted scabies[22]

1. Isolate the index case.
2. Apply lindane lotion to unbathed skin from the neck down and wash off after 8 hours.
3. Treat the face and scalp if there is proof or high likelihood of scabies above the neck.
4. Trim the nails daily and scrub subungual areas daily with lindane.
5. Apply lindane daily to the hyperkeratotic crusts.
6. Reassess the patient weekly for the presence of mites on both the skin and nails.
7. Examine and treat both direct and indirect patient contacts.

Adapted from O'Donnell, O'Loughlin & Powell[22]

from the animal for several weeks, and return of symptoms on re-exposure to the animal is highly suggestive of animal scabies and other pet-born mite infestations.

In addition to canine scabies, there are a number of other types of scabies mites that may infest livestock and domesticated animals and attack unwary human hosts. They include equine, camel, goat, sheep, pig, cattle, and monkey scabies.[2pp283–285] With the exception of monkey scabies, which is indistinguishable clinically from human scabies, almost all of these mites are of the "bite and run"[27] variety, which means that they do not burrow or live for any appreciable time on the human host.[2p285] This makes identifying the cause of the bites much more challenging, because by the time the rash is symptomatic, the mite has left the skin (except in the cases of monkey scabies as noted above and in camel scabies where the mite may remain hiding within the hair follicle of an inflamed follicular papule).[2p285] Patients must be questioned closely regarding contact with pets or other animals, whether in the home or in their travels.

In order to arrive at a diagnosis, the suspected pet must become the patient. With the help of a knowledgeable veterinarian the afflicted animal (often an undernourished puppy) should be inspected for signs of sarcoptic mange, which presents with scaling and denuded areas on the face, ears, elbows, and intertriginous folds.[5p76,28] The affected areas on the· dog begin as pale reddish papules that progress to excoriated, lichenified, crusted areas with matted hair.[2p282] These areas should be scraped and the scales or crust examined for mites, which appear very similar to human scabies.

Once diagnosed, the animal should be treated under veterinary supervision by steps to remove the crusts and by the application of lindane lotion or sulfur ointment.[2p282] Animal scabies tends to be a self-limited disease in humans in most cases. In some patients, symptoms may improve more quickly when they are treated with scabecidal regimens; however, it is not clear if this is due to a prophylactic action of the drug (which may make the human host less inviting to further attack), or to a direct effect on mites that may still be wandering around on the patients skin or clothing. A placebo effect must also be considered, as many patients will find it difficult to believe that the mites are not somehow still on their skin. Treatment of itch is symptomatic once the affected animal has been treated or avoided.

Chyletiella. Chyletiella dermatosis, also known as "walking dandruff," is another mite infestation associated with cats, dogs, and rabbits that can affect humans. It may offer an even greater diagnostic challenge than animal scabies.[26–30] Often there is very little sign of skin disease in the affected pet, but the patient may be afflicted with an intensely pruritic, macular, papulo-vesicular, and eventually pustular and crusted eruption on the flexor surfaces of the arms, chest, abdomen, and thighs, which correspond to areas of contact with the pet.[26,29] The diagnosis is made by placing the suspected animal on a large piece of black paper and then combing the center of the back vigorously for "walking scales," which must be collected and examined in order to identify the mite.[28p331]

The affected animal should be treated with insecticidal shampoos, sprays, or powders two to three times at weekly intervals and the animal's environment should be cleaned as well to prevent reinfestation.[29–33] As in animal scabies, the disease in humans is self limited, requiring only symptomatic treatment once the infested animal is either avoided or treated.

Other mites in the environment. In addition to animal scabies and cheyletiella, there are a number of other mites in the environment the bites of which may produce clinically significant pruritic syndromes in humans. A partial listing of these mites includes: harvest mites, fowl or avian mites, murine mites, food mites, and grain mites. In general they produce clinical symptoms and findings similar to those due to harvest mites, which will be discussed in the following section.

Harvest mites. Harvest mites are among the best known cause of mite bites.[11] They are found throughout the world in a variety of habitats.[26,34] In the United States they are commonly referred to as chiggers, red bugs, or mower mites.[11,26] The six-legged larval form of the harvest mite (which is responsible for the majority of bites) attaches itself to its host while the victim is traveling through open fields or is in contact with vegetation infested with the mites.[26] The bites occur predominantly in constrictive areas of clothing, such as the elastic bands of socks or undergarments.[26] Initial exposure to these mites may result in minimal or no symptoms, but with re-exposure, sensitization results and patients present with small, intensely pruritic papules at the bite sites, which may be accompanied by urticarial wheals.[11,26] Secondary excoriations lead to a progression of pustules and crusting. In extremely sensitized individuals vessicles, bullae, fever, granulomatous reactions, and lymphadenopathy may result.[11,26]

Diagnosis is made by history of exposure, history of the rash, and clinical exam. Occasionally a tiny bright red mite that has not yet left or been scratched away can be identified in fresh bites.[11] Treatment is symptomatic. Prevention can best be achieved by applying DEET (Diethyl toluamide) to all areas of potential skin and clothing exposure.[26,35] Pyrethrin, which is available as a clothing spray and is marketed in the United States as a Permanone Tick Repellant® may also be useful for application to clothes before venturing into harvest-mite-infested areas.[36] Although it has only been tested against mosquitoes and tick bites, studies have shown that the repellant effects of clothing treated with pyrethrins may be additive to those of DEET.[37]

Pediculosis (Lice). In addition to scabies, there are only a few other dermatologic diseases the mere mention of which can make the skin of even the most experienced clinicians crawl and itch. If it is impossible to have scabies without scratching, it is nearly impossible to make the diagnosis of pediculosis without feeling itchy. To make matters worse, the body louse is the vector for typhus, trench fever, and relapsing fever.

Etiology. *Pediculosis humanus* and *Pthirus pubis* are the two species of lice that are obligate human parasites. There are two forms of *P. humanus, P. humanus corporis,* the body louse, which lives in the seams of clothing and fomites, and *P. humanus capitis,* which infests the human scalp. *Pthirus pubis,* also known as the crab louse or pubic louse, lives on the short thick hairs of the pubic region, chest, abdomen, and legs, and occasionally on the beard area, eyelashes, and eyebrows.

Epidemiology. The incidence of *P. corporis* infestations increases with wars and other calamities that cause overcrowding and poor hygiene and sanitation. Homeless people who may not have the opportunity to change or wash their clothing are susceptible. Spread of the lice occurs primarily through contact with infested clothing or bedding.

Head lice infestations are common in school children, more often in girls than boys.[5p128] In adults the condition is also more common in women, and any age group may be affected.[38] Head lice may be transmitted by close personal contact or by the sharing of hats, combs, or brushes used by an infested individual.

The incidence of pubic lice is increased with sexual promiscuity, and the majority of infestations are spread by intimate physical contact. Outbreaks of pubic lice can occur in families, especially when there is bed sharing between parents and children or among siblings.[2p52]

Diagnosis. While the diagnosis of pediculosis is generally not as difficult to make as it is in scabies, the infestation will remain undiscovered and untreated if lice are not considered among the causes of chronic pruritus. Pruritus of any hairy area should suggest the diagnosis of pediculosis.[5p134]

In *P. corporis* it is rare to find lice or nits on the body; they must be searched for in the seams of clothing. In *P. capitis* infestations, nits are relatively easy to find if you look for them especially above the ears and in the suboccipital areas of the scalp. They appear as "small, oval whitish, semitranslucent nodules" which are firmly cemented to the scalp hairs.[5p128] Nits found on hairs within one quarter of an inch from the scalp indicate ongoing infestation and are probably viable.[5p130,39] Adult lice or immature nymphs are only rarely found in head lice infestations. Infestations with pubic lice, *P. pubis,* are diagnosed by finding the adult louse or nits attached to short thick body hairs. They appear as "small 1 to 2 mm brownish grey specks" that when viewed with a hand lens can be seen to be grasping a hair on either side with their claws.[2p51]

Clinical manifestations. The universal symptom of pediculosis is itching. In the initial stages of all of these infestations the pruritus may be mild, but as sensitization develops, the pruritus increases. Itching is more generalized in body louse infestations. It is localized to the head and neck with head lice. With pubic lice the pruritus is limited to the infested areas of the body, those containing thick, short hairs.

In *P. corporis,* bite areas initially appear as evanescent tiny 3 to 4 mm papules with a central red punctum.[2p35,40,41] After a week or more of infestation the bite sites may develop urticarial wheals or more pruritic, persistent papules.[42] Secondary infections due to scratching then complete the picture. In patients with longstanding infestations with body lice, scattered pigmentation of the lower trunk in areas of frequent bites is characteristic.[2p36] In patients with heavy infestations, a brownish-bronze diffuse pigmentation may develop over the genitalia, groin area, upper inner thighs, and axillae.[2p36]

The bite sites from head lice are not readily apparent in most cases. Itching of the head and neck accompanied by recurrent pyodermas and cervical or occipital adenopathy is characteristic of head lice infestations.[5p130]

The bite sites of the pubic louse are innocuous in most cases; however, nonblanching slate-grey or bluish grey macules known as maculae caeruleae, which are unique to *P. pubis,* can occasionally be seen in fair-skinned individuals in bite sites where the louse has been feeding in one place for a long time.[2p52,5p133,43] Pruritus, excoriations, and occasionally lymphadenopathy in the pubic area, or other hair-bearing areas of the trunk and thighs should prompt a search for pubic lice. In preadolescent children whose parents or siblings are infested, the eyelashes and eyebrows are commonly involved.[5p134]

Treatment. In cases of body lice the patient's clothing (not the patient) must be treated.[44] Clothing and linens must be washed and dried with the washer and dryer adjusted to the hottest settings.[44] Alternatively clothes may be dry cleaned, treated with insecticidal sprays, or placed in sealed plastic bags for 2 weeks (as the lice or hatching nymphs cannot survive this long off the host without a blood meal).[5p135,44p250]

For head lice and pubic lice any number of preparations are effective if used properly; however gels or liquids containing pyrethrins plus piperonyl butoxide (e.g., RID[R], A-200 Pyrinate[R] or permethrin 1% cream rinse (Nix Creme Rinse[R]) are superior to lindane shampoo in their ability to kill lice and have similar ovicidal capacity.[8p96,45,46] After shampooing and drying the hair with a towel, Permethrin 1% creme rinse is applied and left on for 10 minutes, then rinsed out with water. A single treatment is sufficient.[44p250] Pyrethrins plus piperonyl butoxide are rubbed into the hair and scalp or pubic area and left on for 10 minutes, then rinsed out with water, and the treatment is repeated in 7 to 10 days.[8p96] Lindane 1% shampoo should be massaged into the hair and scalp or pubic area and left on for 4 to 5 minutes and then rinsed out with a repeat treatment in 7 to 10 days.[5p135] For pubic lice lindane cream or lotion can be applied to the affected hairy areas and left on for 8 to 12 hours, and then repeat treatment in 1 to 7 days.[5p136] Removal of nits (which is probably optional once the above medications have been used correctly) can be facilitated by soaking the hair in 3% to 5% acetic acid solution for 15 minutes, and then combing out the nits with a fine toothed comb.[44p250]

Family members and sexual contacts should also be treated. Treat secondary infections with antibiotics and follow the guidelines in Tables 9-5 for relieving pruritus. Combs and brushes can be soaked in 2% Lysol or a pediculocidal shampoo for an hour, or in hot water (149°F) for 5 to 10 minutes.[8p97]

Eyelash infestations with *P. pubis* can be treated with the twice daily application of petrolatum for 8 days with mechanical removal of the nits, or with 0.025% Physostigmine opthalmic ointment applied with a cotton-tipped swab.[8p97]

Bedbugs. There are two types of bedbugs that primarily parasitize man, *Cimex lectularius* (the common bedbug) and *C. tropica* (the tropical bedbug).[47] Bedbugs generally feed at night or an hour before dawn. When not feeding they hide themselves in the bed and other furniture, in the walls of old houses, under loose wallpaper and in any other darkened crevice they can find.[28p332,47] The bite of the bedbug is generally painless and is likely to appear in groups of oval wheals with central puncta. They often occur in groups of three or so, "breakfast, lunch, and dinner."[47p413] As sensitization develops, the reaction to the bites becomes more pronounced, and can occasionally be bullous.[47p413] Secondarily infected and excoriated eczematous eruptions occur frequently in children.[47p413] Treatment is similar to other bite reactions previously described. Professional exterminators are required in order to eradicate these unwelcome pests.

Fleas. Fleas are a common cause of insect bites, especially in households with pets. The most common species that infests not only cats and dogs but also humans is the cat flea, *Ctenocephalides felis*.[48] *Ctenocephalides canis* (the dog flea) is also quite common and is also not particular about which host (dog, cat, or human) it feeds on.[48] Patients suspected of having flea bites who do not have pets should be questioned as to whether they visit the homes of friends who keep pets, or whether they have recently moved into a house in which pets were previously kept. (See also Chap. 4.)

Depending on the individual, flea bites may range from asymptomatic to intensely pruritic papules, which in the most sensitized patients may appear vasculitic. It is therefore not unusual for only one member of a family to complain of bites. Flea bites are often found on the lower extremities in groups of urticarial papules, often in groups of three.[48p243] They also may be seen along the belt line or waist line of undergarments. Fleas are probably responsible for some cases of so-called "itchy red bump disease," which is discussed in Chap. 4.

The suspected dog or cat must be examined for fleas, eggs, and concretions of flea feces adhering to their fur.[28p331] In addition to the pet, fleas must be eradicated from the pet's bedding by washing and drying with high heat, and from the rest of the house by vacuuming carpets and furniture before and after spraying with flea sprays and foggers.[48p242] Physicians should not hesitate to recommend that patients employ a professional exterminator for this task.

Flea bites in the hypersensitive individual may require topical steroids and antihistamines, as well as the other measures outlined in Table 9-4.

BITES AND STINGS OF OTHER INSECTS AND ARACHNIDS

There are a seemingly endless variety of mosquitoes, flies, ants, wasps, hornets, bees, ticks, and spiders, the bites and stings of which may cause itching. In general however these bites and stings do not present the clinician with the same degree of difficulty in diagnosis as those discussed in the preceding sections. Some of these bites are more painful than itchy (i.e., wasp or bee stings), while others may cause a great deal of necrosis (i.e., Brown recluse spider bites).[48a] Hypersensitivity to hymenoptera stings can result in anaphylaxis and death, and patients who are known to be highly allergic may need to undergo desensitization treatments by an allergist or immunologist.

Most pruritic insect bite reactions can be treated in the manner described in Table 9-4. For those patients who develop persistent bite reactions intralesional steroid injections may be needed.

PRURITIC MARINE DERMATOSES

When humans venture from the land into the lakes and seas they enter a new world filled with incredible life forms, some of which may cause itching. While most patients will have some recollection of being stung by a jellyfish or handling a firesponge, they will have no recollection of silent encounters with several organisms that are capable of causing pruritic papular eruptions long after they have left the water.

The diagnosis of cercarial dermatitis must be considered in the patient presenting with itchy papules predominantly on exposed areas of skin who went swimming in a lake, pond, or coastal water several days beforehand. More commonly known as "swimmers' itch" or "clam diggers' itch," this condition is due to the penetration of the skin by the cercarial forms of nonhuman schistosomes. These organisms require small warm-blooded mammals or birds to complete their life cycles and are unable to cause human schistosomiasis. Initial exposures to cercarial dermatitis may cause mild to moderate itching. With increasing exposure the reaction is increasingly pruritic and may be complicated by secondary infection, fever, and malaise. Human forms of schistosomiasis may also result in a similar eruption in areas of the world where the disease is endemic.[49] Treatment of cercarial dermatitis is symptomatic (see Table 9-4), and prevention consists of avoiding infested waters or by wearing protective clothing.[50]

"Sea bather's eruption" is another marine dermatosis that is often confused with cercarial dermatitis. It differs from swimmers' itch in that the areas involved are predominantly areas covered by the bathing suit worn at the time of exposure. The two conditions also differ in that sea bathers' eruption only occurs in salt water, whereas swimmers' itch has been reported in both fresh and salt water. The lesions begin as erythematous macules within 24 hours of exposure to seawater and progress to wheals and papules that itch and burn. Until recently the cause of seabather's eruption was unknown, but new research implicates the larval forms of a Thimble jellyfish, *Linuche ungiculata,* as one etiologic agent.[51] The tiny larvae become trapped under swimming garments and their stings result in a papular dermatitis. As in swimmers' itch, sensitization increases with continued exposure in some patients. Seabather's eruption may also be caused by the planula larvae of the sea anemone, *Edwardsiella lineata.*[52] Outbreaks caused by this organism have occurred as far north as Long Island, NY. Treatment of the itch from sea bathers' eruption is again symptomatic. Physicians and pharmacists in the Caribbean who are not familiar with this condition have on occasion mistakenly prescribed lindane for it because it is often referred to as "sea lice." Prevention involves wearing of wet suits or lycra body suits that seal tightly at the cuffs, although lesions may occur at the cuff edges.[51]

Pseudomonas folliculitis or "hot tub folliculitis" is the final condition to be considered here in patients with itchy papules arising from an aquatic environment. Macules, papules, and pustules develop on the trunks of patients who have bathed in contaminated hot tubs. The condition is caused by a superficial infection of the skin by species of Pseudomonas bacteria that multiply in hot tubs that are not kept at consistently high temperatures, or in which the levels of chlorine or other antibacterial agents have not been properly maintained. In most cases the disease is self limited, and all that is required in healthy individuals is the application of antipruritic lotions and the avoidance of further exposure to or repair of the hot tub in question.

REFERENCES

1. Goddard J: *Physician's Guide to Arthropods of Medical Importance.* Boca Raton, CRC Press, 1993.
2. Alexander JO: *Arthropods and Human Skin.* New York, Springer-Verlag Berlin Heidelberg, 1984.
3. Orkin O, Maibach HI: *Cutaneous Infestations and Insect Bites.* New York, Marcel Dekker, 1985.

4. Orkin M, Maibach HI, Parish LC, et al: *Scabies and Pediculosis*. Philadelphia, Lippincott, 1977.

5. Parish LC, Nutting WB, Schwartzman RM: *Cutaneous Infestations of Man and Animal*. New York, Praeger Publishers, 1983.

6. Peter W: *A Colour Atlas of Arthropods in Clinical Medicine*. London, Wolfe Publishing Ltd, 1992.

7. P. Levi: *Moments of Reprieve*. New York, Penguin, 1987, p 60.

8. Arndt KA: Infestations: Pediculosis, Scabies, and Ticks, in Arndt KA: *Manual of Dermatologic Therapeutics*, 4th ed. Boston, Little, Brown and Company, 1989, pp 94–100.

9. Sokolova TV: Survival of human itch mites of *Sarcoptes Scabiei* de Geer (Acariformes, Sarcoptidae) in the environment. *Vestn Dermatol Vene* 7:21–26, 1992.

10. Arlian LG, Estes SA, Vyszenski-Moher MS: Prevalence of *Sarcoptes scabiei* in the homes, and nursing homes of scabietic patients. *J Am Acad Dermatol* 19:806–811, 1988.

10a. Funkhouser ME, Omohundro C, Ross A, et al: Management of scabies in patients with human immunodeficiency virus disease. *Arch Dermatol* 129:911–913, 1993.

11. Rees RS, King LE: Arthropod bites and stings, in Fitzpatrick TB, Eisen AZ, Wolff K, et al (eds): *Dermatology in General Medicine*, 3d ed. New York, McGraw Hill, 1987, Chap 208, pp 2495–2505.

12. Muller G, Jacobs PH, Moore NE: Scrapings for human scabies, a better method for positive preparations. *Arch Dermatol* 1007:70, 1973.

13. Ostlere LS, Harris D, Rustin MHA: Scabies associated with a bullous pemphigoid-like eruption. *Br J Dermatol* 123:217–219, 1993.

14. Chapel TA, Krugel L, Chapel J, et al: Scabies presenting as urticaria. *JAMA* 1:246:1440–1441, 1981.

15. Rostami G, Sorg TB: Nosocomial outbreak of scabies associated with Norwegian scabies in an AIDS patient. *Int J of STD & AIDS* 1:209–210, 1990.

16. Sorera G, Ruis F, Romeu J, et al: Hospital outbreak of scabies stemming from two AIDS patients with Norwegian scabies. *Lancet* 335:1227, 1990.

17. Wolf R, Landau M: Scabid: An unusual id reaction to scabies. *Internat J Dermatol* 32:128, 1993.

18. The Medical Letter, Permethrin for scabies, 32:21–22, 1990.

19. Schultz MW, Gomez M, Hansen RC: Comparative study of 5% permethrin cream and 1% lindane lotion for the treatment of scabies. *Arch Dermatol* 126:167–170, 1990.

20. Haustein UF, Hlawa B: Treatment of acabies with permethrin versus lindane and benzyl benzoate. *Acta Dermato-Venereologica,* 69:348–351, 1989.

21. Taplin D, Meinking TL, Chen JA, et al: Comparison of crotamiton 10% cream (Eurax) and permethrin 5% cream (Elimite) for the treatment of scabies in children. *Pediatr Dermatol* 7:67–73, 1990.

22. O'Donnell BF, O'Loughlin S, Powell FC: Management of crusted scabies. *Internat J Dermatol* 29:258–266, 1990.

23. Hernandez-Perez E: Resistance to antiscabietic drugs (letter), Taplin D: (Reply). *J Am Acad Dermatol* 8:121–123, 1983.

24. Purvis RS, Tyring SK: An outbreak of lindane-resistant scabies treated successfully with permethrin 5% cream. *J Am Acad Dermatol* 25:1015–1016, 1991.

25. Witkowski JA, Parish LC: Lindane resistant scabies (letter). *J Am Acad Dermatol* 27:648, 1992.

26. Millikan LE: Mite infestations other than scabies. *Semin Dermatol* 12:46–52, 1993.

27. Shelley ED, Shelley WB: The diagnostic challenge of nonburrowing mite bites *Cheyletiella yasguri, JAMA* 251:2690–2691, 1984.

28. Shelley WB, Shelley ED: Bites and stings, in Shelley WB, Shelley ED (eds): *Advanced Dermatologic Diagnosis*. Philadelphia, Saunders, 1992, pp 330–357.
29. van Bronswijk JEMH, de Kreek EJ: *Cheyletiella* (Acari:Cheyletiellidae) of dog, cat and domesticated rabbit: A review. *J Med Entomol* 13:315–327, 1976.
30. Rivers JK, Martin J, Pukay BA: Walking dandruff and Cheyletiella dermatitis. *J Am Acad Dermatol* 15:1130–1133, 1986.
31. Fox JG, Reed C: *Cheyletiella* infestation of cats and their owners. *Arch Dermatol* 116:435–437, 1980.
32. Hewitt M, Turk SM: *Cheyletiella* sp. in the personal environment. *Br J Dermatol* 90:679–683, 1974.
33. Kunkle GA, Miller WH: *Cheyletiella* infestation in humans. *Arch Dermatol* 116:1345, 1980.
34. Yates VM: Harvest mites—A present from the Lake District. *Clin Exp Dermatol* 16:277–278, 1991.
35. Wright RH: Why mosquito repellants repel. *Sci Am* 233:104–111, 1975.
36. The Medical Letter, 31:45–47, 1989.
37. Lillie TH, Schreck CE, Rahe AJ: Effectiveness of personal protection against mosquitoes in Alaska. *J Med Entomol* 25:475–478, 1988.
38. Mellanby K: The incidence of head lice in England. *Med Officer*, 65:39–43, 1941.
39. Juranek OD: The nuisance diseases: Pediculosis and scabies. *USHEW* 4:1, 1976.
40. Duffy DM: Ectoparasitic infestations. *Cutis* 7:161–168, 1971.
41. Lloyd L: *Lice and Their Menace to Man*. London, Henry Frowde, Oxford University Press, 1919.
42. Rook A: Skin diseases caused by arthropods and other venomous or noxious animals, in Rook A, Wilkinson DS, Ebling FJG (eds): *Textbook of Dermatology*, 3d ed. Oxford, Blackwell, 1979.
43. Maunder JW: The appreciation of lice. *Proc R Inst Great Britain* 55:1–31, 1983.
44. Kramer EM, Honig PJ: Severely pruritic lesions, in Bondi, EE, Jegasothy BV, Lazarus GS (eds): *Dermatology Diagnosis and Therapy*, 1st ed. Norwalk, Appleton & Lange, Chap 12, pp 248–250, 1991.
45. The Medical Letter, Permethrin for Head Lice, 28:89–90, 1986.
46. Taplin D, et al: Permethrin 1% creme rinse for the treatment of *Pediculosis humanis* var *capitis, Pediatr Dermatol* 3:344–348, 1986.
47. Crissey JT: Bedbugs: an old problem with a new dimension. *Internat J Dermatol* 20:411–414, 1981.
48. Hutchins ME, Burnett JW: Fleas. *Cutis* 51:241–243, 1993.
48a. Wilson DC, Leyva WH, King LE: Arthropod bites and stings, in Fitzpatrick TB, Eisen AZ, Wolff K, et al (eds): *Dermatology in General Medicine*, 4th ed. New York, McGraw Hill, 1993, pp 2810–2826.
49. Gonzalez E: Schistosomiasis, cercarial dermatitis and marine dermatitis. *Dermatol Clin* 7:291, 1989.
50. Scharf MJ, Baker AS: Bites and stings of terrestrial and aquatic life, in Fitzpatrick TB, Eisen AZ, Wolff K, et al: (eds): *Dermatology in General Medicine*, 4th ed. New York, McGraw Hill, 1993, pp 2789–2810.
51. Tomchik RS, Russell MT, Szmant AM, et al: Clinical perspectives on seabather's eruption, also known as "Sea Lice," *JAMA*, 269:1669–1672, 1993.
52. Freudenthal AR, Joseph PR: Seabather's eruption. *N Engl J Med 329*:542–544, 1993.

ITCHING IN SCARS

Lori E. U. Herman

INTRODUCTION

Most wounds and all surgical incisions heal with scar formation. Patients frequently report itching in and around healing wounds, including maturing burn wounds,[1] yet there is little written on the symptomatology of itching in wounds and even less attention to the pathophysiology of this phenomenon.

NORMAL AND ABNORMAL HEALING

Itching associated with normal healing is common but is usually mild and resolves quickly. Occasionally pruritus and discomfort associated with wound healing may be prolonged. This usually occurs when wounds are subject to factors that delay wound healing or lead to abnormal healing, such as that which occurs in hypertrophic or keloidal scarring.

MEDIATORS OF THE ITCH RESPONSE THAT MAY BE INVOLVED IN SCARS

The sensation of itching can be elicited directly by both physical and chemical stimuli. Physical factors include mechanical and electrical excitation, heat, and negative pressure or suction.[2] Early investigations of chemical stimuli employed naturally occurring plants such as cowhage, the barbed spicules of which form a protective cover for the pods of the legume *mucuna pruriens*. In the mid-1950s Shelly and Arthur characterized the pruritogenic agent in cowhage as an endopetidase.[3] Subsequent experiments with various other endopeptidases such as papain, trypsin, and chymotrypsin demonstrated the effectiveness of these agents in producing pruritus either directly or through enhanced release of histamine.[4] Of the chemical substances known to trigger itching, histamine is by far the most important but various other vasoactive polypeptides such as bradykinin and proteolytic enzymes, including kallikrein, appear to act either independently or as potentiators of the itch response. Several of these pruritogenic substances also actively participate in the early and late phases of wound healing, as discussed later.

Histamine

Histamine is a common mediator of itching in many skin disorders. While experimental injection of histamine into the dermis causes pain, intraepidermal administration causes itching.[5] Histamine appears to be involved in a much broader spectrum of physiological and pathological events within the skin than was once thought, however, including regulation of growth and repair.[6]

The role of histamine in the inflammatory phase of wound healing is well documented. Changes in histamine levels and metabolism are characteristic of healing wounds.[7] Studies performed in rats have demonstrated that histamine plays an important role in the early phases of wound healing. Histamine depletion from the skin retards wound healing. In contrast, administration of histamine intraperitoneally has been shown to advance the rate of healing of wounds incised on the backs of rats.[8]

Additional studies in rats, conducted by Nilsson and co-workers as well as others, similarly showed that histamine is produced at a high rate in cutaneous wounds as a result of increased histidine decarboxylase and that the rate of healing can be augmented or diminished by artificially increasing or decreasing the histamine-forming capacity of these wounds.[7,9] In addition, in vitro studies on strains of normal human fibroblasts and fibroblasts derived from keloids show that histamine stimulates the growth of fibroblasts.[10] Keloids and hypertrophic scars contain increased numbers of histamine-containing mast cells.[11] The increased histamine content in keloids and hypertrophic scars appears to parallel the rate of collagen synthesis.[12] Russell and his fellow investigators found that the growth plateau of a high percentage of fibroblast strains grown in histamine-enriched media was elevated from 50 to 300 percent over control cultures and that strains derived for keloid tissue were more responsive to histamine than strains derived from normal skin.[10]

In addition, Topol et al. demonstrated growth suppression of keloidal cell strains exhibiting augmented growth in the presence of histamine when pharmacologic doses of the class I antihistamine diphenhydramine were added to the medium containing histamine.[13]

In view of evidence that histamine plays an important role in healing, it is easy to postulate that increased levels of histamine in wounds, normal scars, keloids, and hypertrophic scars may also account, at least in part, for the itching reported by patients.

Other Mediators Involved in Both Scar Metabolism and Itching

It has also been demonstrated that other vasoactive peptides including kinins and prostaglandins of the E series (PGE) are involved in the acute inflammatory phases of wound healing. These may contribute to the itching symptomatic of early scars as well. Both bradykinin and prostaglandin E_1 and E_2 promote vasodilation. In addition, PGE helps mediate the effects of histamine via cyclic AMP.[14,15]

Several of the vasoactive compounds produced at sites of tissue injury have the capacity to induce itch. Intracutaneous injection of both kallikrein and bradykinin into human subjects produces itch. The itch induced by bradykinin but not by kallikrein can be inhibited by the antihistamine levomepromazine.[16]

In separate studies, both PGE_1 and PGE_2 have been shown to have an effect on histamine-induced itch. Greaves and McDonald-Gibson studied the effects of topicaly applied prostaglandin E_1 on the itch threshold in 23 subjects and demonstrated increased sensitivity to itching evoked by histamine in 20 of the 23 subjects studied.[17] In a study by Hägermark and Strandberg, intradermal injection of PGE_2 resulted in itching that was alleviated by pretreatment with the antihistamine chlorcyclizine, indicating that at least part of the PGE_2 response may be mediated via histamine release. However, when PGE_2 was given together with histamine, the itch and flare response produced by the mixture was potentiated more than could be accounted for by simple additive histamine effects.[18]

Thus it appears that a variety of molecules active during wound healing also have the capacity to initiate or potentiate itching.

NERVE REGENERATION AND ITCHING

Although we have an ample understanding of the structure of peripheral nerves, the task of classifying the many variants of nerve endings and assigning them to specific modalities has not been fully worked out. This is especially true for the several types of receptors innervated by thinly myelinated and unmyelinated C fibers in the skin. These fibers transmit sensations of pain, cold, warmth, itch, and tickle. The receptor structures associated with each of these modalities have only been partially identified.[19]

Evidence indicates that the sensation of itching is a primary sensory modality separate from pain and not, as was once thought, a subthreshold variety of pain.[2,20] A specific subset of C fibers exists that appears to encode the itch sensation separately from other sensory modalities.[21] Although itch can frequently coexist with pain in the same area, it is associated with a scratching reflex as opposed to a withdrawal response.[22]

Nerve regeneration occurs in all healing wounds and the specificity of these regenerating nerves appears to be preserved.[23] Recent work by LaMotte et al. suggests the existence of chemonociceptive afferent fibers that respond to intradermal injection of histamine and capsaicin but not to thermal or mechanical noxious stimuli.[24] Growing evidence suggests that histamine acts directly on these nerve endings independent from its wheal and flare effect on the integument.[25–27] Further studies in brain tissue suggest that biogenic amines, including histamine, may potentiate the response of neurons to depolarizing agents, and that this augmentation may operate by elevating intraneuronal levels of the ubiquitous second messenger, cyclic AMP.[27]

Increased levels of chemical mediators such as histamine, bradykinin, and prostaglandins, present in early wounds and abnormal scars, may account for a "chemogenic itch" that is separate from the itching elicited from mechanical stimulation. The observation that itching associated with wound healing gradually subsides in parallel with scar maturation and normalization of these chemical mediators supports this postulate.

In addition to chemical stimulation, the manner in which nerves regenerate may contribute to abnormal itching. Myelinated nerve fibers regenerate along myelin tubes but peripheral nerves are demyelinated and have no structure to guide the direction of their regenerative growth. Sensation is restored by a combination of forward extension into the denervated area and collateral sprouting of neighboring undamaged nerve endings. Regenerating nerves do not respect previously adhered to boundaries and readily pass into domains once innervated by unrelated peripheral nerves. Competition can occur between nerves, and this can determine the eventual pattern of nerve regeneration that is established.[28]

A disproportionate number of thinly myelinated and unmyelinated C fibers present in immature or abnormal scars could contribute to the increased perception of itching experienced by many patients.

Lastly, production of itch from mechanical stimulation has been well documented. Scar remodeling lasts from 6 months to up to 2 years and involves changes in the arrangement of collagen, in the content of vessels, and in the overlying epidermis. Diamond has demonstrated that nerve regeneration has no spatial or time constraints.[28] It is likely that direct mechanical stimulation of nerve endings during scar remodeling accounts at least in part for the sensation of itch experienced by patients with immature, abnormal, or elevated scars.

THERAPY

The pruritus generated by healing wounds and scar formation appears to respond similarly to treatment of itching from other causes. Antihistamines, emollients, topical antipruritics, and anti-inflammatory agents such as topical and intralesional corticosteroids have all been proved to be beneficial in relieving the discomfort caused by itching in some patients.

Antihistamines ameliorate the burning and itching associated with keloids and hypertrophic scars. As discussed previously, these abnormal scars contain significantly more histamine than normal skin.[12]

Topical application of aloe vera, a tropical cactus plant, has a wide following as a folk remedy especially in the treatment of burn patients. Aloe vera concentrated extract inhibits thromboxane A2, an essential component of the prostaglandin cascade.[29] In addition, a protease inhibitor that interferes with the actions of bradykinin has been found in various Aloe species.[30,31] The combined anti-inflammatory effects of these substances may indeed be beneficial in the treatment of itching in scars.

Topically applied retinoic acid has also been used to treat keloids and hypertrophic scars. It was first suggested as a possible treatment because of its ability to decrease DNA synthesis of fibroblasts in tissue culture.[32] In a clinical trial of 28 patients with keloids or hypertrophic scars De Limpens reported a favorable response in 77 percent of the abnormal scars in which a 0.05 percent solution of retinoic acid was applied.[33] Although additional studies have not yet been done, this treatment modality offers a safe approach in single or combination therapy.

Topical vitamin E has been prescribed for the treatment of wounds on the basis that it may, like corticosteroids, impede scar formation. Like cortisone, it functions as a membrane stabilizer and helps to preserve the integrity of lysosomes.[34] When given to rats, vitamin E results in wounds with decreased tensile strength compared to controls.[35] There is no evidence, however, that this is of therapeutic benefit in the treatment of raised or pruritic scars and application of topical vitamin E may, in fact, be at times detrimental as patients may become allergic to any number of components used in these preparations.

The effects of topical vitamin E on early postoperative surgical scars was reported by Jenkins and colleagues in 1986 in a prospective, randomized study of 159 operative procedures. They found no beneficial effect with respect to scar thickness, range of motion, change in graft size, or final cosmetic appearance. In addition, 19.9 percent of the patients studied developed adverse reactions in the form of rash or pruritus necessitating discontinuation of therapy.[36] In general, topical therapy with vitamin E of early wounds or abnormal scars is not beneficial and should be avoided.

Since Conway and Stark, in 1951, first reported that ACTH relieved the pain and itching associated with keloids, physicians have been experimenting with various ways to use steroids in the treatment of abnormal scars.[37] Corticosteroids are known to decrease the rate of protein synthesis and thereby inhibit collagen synthesis. They also diminish the inflammatory reaction that may be abnormal and prolonged in hypertrophic and keloidal scarring. In addition, scars pretreated with steroids postoperatively show an inhibition of fibroblast migration to the pretreated site. Cohen[38] and Ceilly[39] and their coworkers have proposed that corticosteroids specifically act by inhibiting alpha-globulin collagenase inhibitor, which is elevated in keloidal scars.

Regardless of the mechanism, injection of intralesional steroids appears to be superior to other modalities employed in the treatment of abnormal scars. I recommend this as a first line of therapy and also suggest daily massage of the scar to my patients as a supplement to intralesional corticosteroid injections. I find that this helps to soften the scar and enhances the response to steroids. Although this approach usually leads to clinical improvement in appearance and symptoms, total resolution is rare. Fortunately, much of the residual discomfort resolves with time.

SUMMARY

Whether as part of normal or abnormal healing, mediators such as histamine, kallikrein, bradykinin, and prostaglandins may contribute to the abnormal sensation of itching in scars. A disproportionate number of regenerating nerves may be programmed to detect itching and may be more sensitive to the chemical and mechanical stimuli inherent in healing wounds and immature or abnormal scars. Although several therapeutic modalities may provide some symptomatic relief, further studies are needed before we can hope to comprehend the complexities of this common and annoying complaint.

REFERENCES

1. Warden GD: Outpatient care of thermal injuries, in Boswick JA Jr. (ed) *Surg Clin N Amer* Philadelphia, Saunders. 67(1):147–157, 1987.
2. Herndon JH: Itching: The pathophysiology of pruritus. *Int J Dermatol* 14:465–484, 1975.
3. Shelley WB. Arthur RP: Studies on cowhage (mucuna pruriens) and its pruritogenic proteinase, mucunain. *Arch Dermatol* 72:399–406, 1955.
4. Hägermark O. Rajka G. Bergqvist U: Experimental itch in human skin elicited by rat mast cell chymase. *Acta Dermatovener* 52:125–128, 1972.

5. Keele CA, Armstrong D: *Substances Producing Pain and Itch.* London, Edward Arnold, Ltd. 1964 p 125.
6. Davies MG, Greaves MW: Sensory responses of human skin to synthetic histamine analoques and hisamine. *Br J Clin Pharm* 9:461–465, 1980.
7. Kahlson G, Rosengren E: Histamine formation as related to growth and protein, in Blum JJ (ed): *Biogenic Amines as Physiologic Regulators.* Englewood Cliffs, NJ, Prentice Hall. 1970, p. 223–238.
8. Boyd JF, Smith AN: The effect of histamine and a histamine-releasing agent (compound 48/80) on wound healing. *J Path Bact* 78:379–388, 1959.
9. Nilsson K, Rosengren E, Zederfeldt B: Wound healing as dependent of rate of histamine formation. *Lancet* 2:230–234, 1960.
10. Russell JD, Russell SB, Trupin KM: The effect of histamine on the growth of cultured fibroblasts isolated from normal and keloidal tissue. *J Cell Physiol* 93:389–394, 1977.
11. Hakanson R, Owman C, Sjoberg NO, et al: Direct histochemical demonstration of histamine in cutaneous mast cells. *Experientia* 25:854–855, 1969.
12. Cohen IK, Beaven MA, Horakova Z, et al: Histamine and collagen synthesis in keloid and hypertrophic scar. *Surg Forum* 23:509–510, 1972.
13. Topol BM, Lewis VL, Benveniste K: The use of antihistamine to retard the growth of fibroblasts derived from human skin, scar and keloid. *Plast Reconstr Surg* 68(2):227–230, 1981.
14. Bennett RG: Fundamentals of cutaneous surgery. St. Louis, MO. CV Mosby Co. 1988, p 35.
15. Knighton DR, Fiegel VD, Doucette MM, et al: The use of topically applied growth factors in chronic nonhealing wounds: A review. *Wounds* 1:71–78, 1989.
16. Hägermark Ö: Studies on experimental itch induced by kallikrein and bradykinin. *Acta Dermatovener* 54:397–400, 1974.
17. Greaves MW, McDonald-Gibson W: Itch: Role of prostaglandins. *Br Med J* 3:608–609, 1973.
18. Hägermark Ö, Strandberg K: Pruritogenic activity of prostaglandin E2. *Acta Dermatovener* 57:37–43, 1977.
19. Kruger L: Cutaneous sense organs and the role of thin fibers in sensation, with particular reference to reinnervation, in Gorio A, Millesi H, Mingrino S (eds): *Posttraumatic Peripheral Nerve Regeneration: Experimental Basis and Clinical Implications.* New York, Raven Press. 1981, pp 549–561.
20. Tuckett RP, Wei JY: Response to an itch-producing substance in cat. I. Cutaneous receptor populations with myelinated axons. *Brain Res* 413:87–94, 1987.
21. Torbejörk HE, Ochoa JL: Specific sensations evoked by activity in single identified sensory units in man. *Acta Physiol Scand* 110:445–457, 1980.
22. Fjellner B: Experimental and clinical pruritus. *Acta Dermato Venereol Suppl* 97:2–34, 1981.
23. Dykes RW, Terzis JK: Reinnervation of glabrous skin in baboons: Properties of cutaneous mechanoreceptors subsequent to nerve crush. *J Neurophysiol* 42:1461–1478, 1979.
24. LaMotte RH, Simone DA, Baumann TK, et al: Hypothesis for novel classes of chemoreceptors mediating chemogenic pain and itch, in Dubner R, Gebhart GF, Bond MR (eds): Proceedings of the Vth World Congress on Pain. Amsterdam, Elsevier, 1988, pp 529–535.
25. Kiernan JA: The involvement of mast cells in vasodilation due to axon reflexes in injured skin. *J Exper Physiol* 57:311–317, 1972.
26. Scuka M: Analysis of the effects of histamine on the endplate potential. *Neuropharmacology* 12:441–450, 1973.
27. Shimizu H, Creveling CR, Daly JW: Effect of membrane depolarization and biogenic amines on the formation of cyclic AMP in incubated brain slices, in Greengard P, Costa E, (eds): *Advances of Biochemical Psychopharmacology,* vol. 3. New York, Raven Press. 1970, pp 135–154.

28. Diamond, J: The recovery of sensory function in skin after peripheral nerve lesions, in Gorio A, et al (eds): *Posttraumatic Peripheral Nerve Regeneration: Experimental Basis and Clinical Implications.* New York, Raven Press. 1981, pp 533–548.

29. Penneys NS: Inhibition of arachidonic acid oxidation in vitro by vehicle components. *Acta Dermatovener* 62:59–61, 1982.

30. Natow AJ: Aloe vera, fiction or fact. *Cutis* 37:106–108. 1986.

31. Yagi A, Harada N, Yamada H, et al: Antibradykinin active material in *Aloe Saponaria. J Pharmacoceutical Sci* 71:1172–1774, 1982.

32. Christophers E, Lagner A: In vitro effects of vitamin A acid on cultured fibroblasts, lymphocytes, and epidermal cells: A comparative study. *Arch Dermatologische Forschung* 251:147–153, 1974.

33. De Limpens AMPJ: The local treatment of hypertrophic scars and keloids with topical retinoic acid. *Br J Dermatol* 103:319–323, 1980.

34. Bennett RG: Cutaneous structure, function, and repair, in EA Klein (ed): *Fundamentals of Cutaneous Surgery.* St. Louis, CV Mosby. 1988, p 79.

35. Ehrlich HP, Tarver H, Hunt TK: Inhibitory effects of vitamin E on collagen synthesis and wound repair. *Ann Surg* 175(2):235–240, 1972.

36. Jenkins M, Alexander W, MacMillan BG: Failure of topical steroids and vitamin E to reduce postoperative scar formation following reconstructive surgery. *J Burn Care Rehabil* 7:309–312, 1986.

37. Conway H, Stark RD: ACTH in treatment of keloids. *Arch Surg* 64:47–50, 1952.

38. Cohen IK, Beaven MA, Horakola Z, et al: Histamine and collagen synthesis in keloid and hypertrophic scars. *Surg Forum* 23:509–510, 1972.

39. Ceilly RI, Babin RW: The combined use of cryosurgery and intralesional injections of suspensions of fluorinated adrenocorticosteroids for reducing keloids and hypoertrophic scars. *J Dermatol Surg Oncol* 5(1):54–56, 1979.

Acknowledgment: I would like to thank Arnold H. Herman, M.D., FACS, for his insight and patience in the preparation of this chapter.

VULVODYNIA, SCROTODYNIA, AND OTHER CHRONIC DYSESTHESIAS OF THE ANOGENITAL REGION (INCLUDING PRURITUS ANI)

Marilynne McKay

ITCHING VERSUS BURNING

The dermatologist usually has little difficulty distinguishing itchy skin from painful skin: itching is a "hands-on" problem, but burning or pain is a "hands-off" symptom.[1] When patients rub or scratch, they cause visible changes (excoriation, lichenification, even ulceration), and the objective signs of pruritus confirm the diagnosis even if the patient for some reason denies touching the skin. Itchy mucosal surfaces are less likely to show typical changes of lichenification, and rapid cell turnover time makes erosions heal quickly. Nonspecific edema or erythema may be the only evidence of rubbing. Burning, stinging, or rawness is even more difficult to assess, because patients usually avoid contact with the affected skin and mild erythema may be the only visible finding.

Mucous Membrane Symptoms

In general, the description of "burning" seems to be applied more often to mucous membrane symptomatology than that of keratinized epithelium. Because patients often use the term "dryness" as a synonym for irritation, it may confuse the examiner when normal secretions seem to be present in the vaginal, oral, or ocular mucosae. Itching can also occur on mucous membranes, but seems to be much more common on the conjuctiva, nasal mucosa, or genitalia than on oral mucosae. Localized itching on other parts of the body often has a pleasurable component (hence the development of lichenification), but mucosal itching seems to be a more frantic, acute problem. Understanding mucous membrane symptoms is confusing because different medical specialties become involved in the patient's care depending on the location of the discomfort, a situation which makes similarities in epithelial reactions and disorders difficult to assess. Candida, for example, is known to be a factor in oral as well as vaginal burning in the absence of typical white mucosal plaques. It has been proposed that this may represent a localized mucosal hypersensitivity to candida,[2] an association that may have significance to other mucous membrane symptoms as well. Another cause of mucosal burning is endogenous dysesthesia. Specific nerve roots may affect the oral cavity, the entire perineum or localized perineal areas such as the urethra, scrotum, vulva, or anus (or anterior or posterior combinations). Wherever the location, many cutaneous dysesthesias respond well to low-dose tricyclic antidepressants (see following). Oral mucosal burning will be discussed primarily as it relates to other symptom complexes and diagnostic patterns.

Genital disorders induce psychosomatic overlay (and vice versa), but a thorough diagnostic examination by a knowledgeable examiner is essential to accurate diagnosis. This first step is not always simple: there are many diseases that can affect this area, and not every specialist the patient has consulted is guaranteed to be expert in all of them. Dermatology, gynecology, urology, neurology, gastroenterology, colorectal surgery, and psychiatry all have something to contribute to the physician trying to understand the multifactorial nature of chronic anogenital discomfort, but no one specialty seems to have all the answers. It is interesting that women are far more likely to present with perineal symptoms. This undoubtedly relates to pelvic floor structure and the proximity of excretory and reproductive organ systems, as well as other factors, but it is somewhat distressing to note how consistently psychiatric problems have been invoked as "causes" of chronic, poorly understood pain in women.

Acute-onset perineal itching or burning should take the physician through the usual differential diagnosis, including candida infection, irritant and contact dermatitis, urinary tract infection, hemorrhoids, pinworms, and condylomata. It is a different challenge to unravel the complicated skein of chronic cutaneous symptomatology, and that will be the major focus of this chapter (Table 11-1). Because so little is actually understood about the complaint of chronic burning (or non-itch), pain terminology is reviewed and the limitations of evaluating the "chronic pain patient" discussed. A brief overview of the major disorders and their relationships is followed by the diagnostic approach to the patient. A final overview summarizes principles of management.

Endogenous Dysesthesias

There are many different terms that describe a painful sensation. The neurological literature offers neuralgia (a sharp pain in the distribution of a specific nerve), dysesthesia (a disagreeable sensation present with ordinary stimuli), allodynia (sharp pain evoked with light touch), and causalgia (burning pain associated with nerve injury). In my experience, chronic cutaneous symptoms most likely to be evaluated by the dermatologist usually best fit the descriptions for neuralgia or dysesthesia (e.g., postherpetic neuralgia). Terminology can be more specific if an individual nerve is involved, (trigeminal neuralgia, pudendal neuralgia, etc.), but diagnosis can be difficult. Dysesthesia is a useful umbrella term for superficial burning related to nerve distribution; it includes specific neuralgias as well as nonspecific conditions like reflex sympathetic dystrophy, which ongoing investigations may prove to be related.

Perineal innervation is primarily sacral in origin and midline branches may overlap, making symptoms hard to localize. In addition, the close involvement of pelvic organs (urethra, bladder, vagina, cervix, rectum) further confuses the examiner who is unsure of innervation patterns. For example, although patients often complain of "vaginal burning," there are not many nerve endings actually inside the vagina. Discomfort usually originates at the vulvar introitus or vestibule, and stimulation of this area (as in intercourse) can act as a trigger point to spread pain to adjacent areas.[3]

Reflex sympathetic dystrophy. Similar to causalgia, reflex sympathetic dystrophy (RSD) is a term for superficial burning pain thought to be related to sympathetic innervation. It can occur after minor nerve injury, and the resultant hyperesthesia and burning pain of the skin tends to spread beyond its original dermatomal pattern. This might be seen more often than it is diagnosed, especially since its presentation varies among individuals and over time, and its pathophysiology is not completely understood. Experience with RSD effecting the sacral nerves and pelvic floor is very limited. (See also Chap. 12.)

Pudendal neuralgia. The pudendal nerves are the major branches innervating the perineum; this is the nerve that is infiltrated with anesthesia during childbirth. Pudendal neuralgia is typically described as pain radiating from the vulva to the rest of the perineum, groin, or thighs. There may be hyperesthesia in a saddle distribution extending from the mons pubis to the upper inner thighs and posteriorly across the ischial tuberosities.[4] Other symptoms said to be typical of pudendal neuralgia are highly variable, including episodic paroxysmal stabbing discomfort, deep aching, and chronic burning; this variability makes it difficult to recognize a specific syndrome.

Table 11-1 Differential diagnosis of chronic anogenital itching and burning

	Appearance	Pattern	Diagnosis
Itching with objective skin findings			
Pruritus ani Pruritus scrota Pruritus vulvae	Lichenification (leathery thickening of skin from scratching)	Throughout affected area; constant (may be worse at night)	Lichen simplex chronicus (LSC) due to: chronic dermatitis (contact or irritant), tinea, candida, pinworms (p. ani only)
	Atrophy, whitening, loss of skin architecture	Symmetrical periorificial "keyhole"; (penis, not scrotum)	Lichen sclerosus et atrophicus (LS or LSA)
	Flesh-colored or pigmented papules	Grouped or scattered over genital area	Molluscum contagiosum, skin tags, condylomata acuminata (human papilloma virus, HPV), or multifocal intraepithelial neoplasia (carcinoma-in-situ)
	Erythema, erosions, edema, satellite pustules	Intertriginous; from skin folds outward	Candida
	Blisters or eroded papules; location may vary slightly with each episode	Localized; intermittent; ± prodrome	Herpes simplex, recurrent (plus lesions elsewhere, consider dermatitis herpetiformis)
Chronic burning (stinging, irritation, rawness) with minimal skin change			
Rectal burning (pain)	Variable erythema Fissure, papules, or nodules	Usually localized Perianal; worse with bowel movement	Irritant dermatitis, perianal strep cellulitis Perianal strep cellulitis, pilonidal sinus, hemorrhoid, cutaneous Crohn's

Scrotodynia	Erythema common	Usually entire area	History of topical steroid use
Vulvodynia	Intense erythema of vulva; fine papules and sebaceous hyperplasia	Mostly on labia majora, minora may be affected	Rebound dermatitis from withdrawal of potent topical steroids
	Erythema; postcoital irritation, often edema. May have dermatitis with flares	Inner minora, cyclic symptoms, minimal discharge. Flares may involve vulva	Cyclic vulvovaginitis: (+) history candida; Rx long-term anticandidals; associated with antibiotics, estrogens
	Erythema, tenderness at Bartholin's openings (5 and 7 o'clock)	Localized at vestibule, entry dyspareunia	Vulvar vestibulitis: often starts with chronic inflammation, recovery possible in early stages
Urethral burning	Variable erythema	Localized dysuria, increased frequency	Interstitial cystitis (IC): typical urodynamics, objective cystoscopy findings
	Variable erythema	Recurrent, variable; some associated with vulvodynia	Urethral syndrome: urodynamics not typical for IC, cystoscopy normal

Chronic burning or pain without skin change

	No objective skin findings	Constant pain; saddle distribution; most older patients (may have urethral, rectal, or low back pain)	Dysesthesia (pudendal neuralgia, reflex sympathetic dystrophy): responds to tricyclic antidepressants, topical anesthetic (xylocaine 5%)

Further investigation is needed to determine the relationship of sensory input (pudendal neuralgia) to sympathetic nerves (reflex sympathetic dystrophy) or to as yet undetermined factors.

Antidepressants have been shown to be effective in the management of certain types of pain whether or not depression is present, and amitriptyline, a tricyclic, has been used for many years.[5] It is effective in mucous membrane dysesthesias as well as pudendal and postherpetic neuralgias. The recommended dosage for pain management is half or less than needed for treatment of depression, and patients can often discontinue treatment when symptoms are controlled. Although side effects are common (usually dry mouth and an initial "tired" feeling), low dosages of 30 to 50 mg daily are usually well tolerated and effective. In older patients, it is best to begin with only 10 mg at bedtime for the first week or two, and then increase by 10 mg every week to the dosage required for control of symptoms (50 to 75 mg). Alternative medications include desipramine (another tricyclic), trazodone, and clonazepam (a benzodiazepine); unfortunately, fluoxetine, though well tolerated, has not proven useful for neuralgias or dysesthesias. Other neuropharmacologic drugs may also be used; neurologic consultation is recommended.

PSYCHOLOGICAL MANIFESTATIONS

Special care must be taken in interpreting investigations purporting to analyze the personalities of patients with different diseases, because these characteristics can be viewed as either cause or effect in relation to a disease process. In the first case, the patient's psychological traits are seen as the primary influence for a particular disease pattern; in the second, the type of disease influences the patient's attitude and outlook. Discussions of "disease effect" tend to be supportive, and often define coping skills and management strategies for patients. It is much more speculative to characterize "cause," or the type of patient likely to have a certain disease, especially when the etiology of a problem is unknown. If the disorder is clearly psychiatric in nature, then psychological evaluation of patients at risk may be helpful; if the disorder is physical, psychological testing may be less relevant.

Patients with chronic disease of any kind may have psychological difficulties in dealing with certain aspects of their problem; this is especially true with visible dermatologic diseases and with genital disorders leading to impotence or dyspareunia. Patient affect is unquestionably an important factor in the physician's evaluation, but this must be considered in context. It should come as no surprise that in a series of patients with symptomatic vulvovaginitis, the stress levels of those without a diagnosis were found to be much higher than in those patients in whom an etiology had been determined.[6]

Prior to the early 1970s, the medical literature was replete with references to the psychological significance of anal and genital pruritus. Men with pruritus ani were said to have obsessional[7] or depressive[8] personalities, while women with pruritus vulvae were said to suffer primarily from frustration of the sexual drive[8-10] and hysterical personality disorders.[7,11,12] It is interesting that reports of personality-linked pruritus declined markedly after the introduction of topical steroids. These agents have proven to be remarkably effective in treating recalcitrant genital itching, especially when coupled with an empathetic and reassuring approach on the part of the treating physician.[13]

References to the therapeutic management of genital pain and burning prior to 1985 are even more difficult to find and interpret—there was some postwar interest in the sequellae of traumatic injuries to male genitalia, but in general, genital, and especially vulvar, burning was much more likely to be considered to be psychosomatic in nature.[14] Over the past 10 years, descriptions of the physical findings typical of vulvar vestibulitis and other types of vulvodynia (see following) have appeared in various gynecologic and dermatologic publications, and are even finding their way into popular women's magazines. The nonspecialist working with these patients is often unfamiliar with these terms and physical findings, however, and subtle diagnostic criteria may not be appreciated.

The "classic clinical characteristics" of patients with so-called psychosomatic vulvovaginitis (persistent symptoms of longstanding duration, lack of demonstrable pathology, multiple consultations, failure to respond to standard empirical therapies, symptoms out of proportion to objective findings, "allergy" to many common vaginal preparations, reluctance to consider to a psychophysiologic cause, and emotional lability)[6,14,15] are typical of vulvodynia patients, especially those with vulvar vestibulitis, cyclic vulvovaginitis, and dysesthetic vulvodynia or pudendal neuralgia (see following).[16] Interestingly, they are also typical of the description of patients with interstitial cystitis, another poorly understood chronic bladder disorder affecting female patients.

In the past 10 years there has been a renewal of investigative interest in dermatologic, gynecologic, and urologic reasons for genital symptomatology. This new information demands reinterpretation of previous data, especially from the psychiatric and psychological literature. Although remarkable progress has been made, there is much to be learned. There is still a significant lack of understanding of localized hypersensitivity reactions in skin and mucous membranes—not only with regard to nerve endings and pain, but with regard to inflammatory mediators released by organisms such as candida.

ITCHING: PRURITUS ANI, SCROTA, VULVAE

Genital pruritus is an annoying problem for patients, although it is relatively responsive to topical steroids. They often arrive at the office with a long list of medications which have been prescribed by other physicians and the complaint, "Nothing works." When the treatment regimen the physician has recommended has also been pronounced ineffective, the patient's "negative attitude" tends to reinforce the doctor's suspicion that the patient has a psychological problem.

Actually, a major source of dissatisfaction can be the patient's expectations of therapeutic results; these must be discussed early in the physician-patient relationship, or the best possible treatment program will be doomed to failure. Even though a patient may have itched for years, there is always the hope of a "miracle cure." The physician must ask specifically, "Do you mean that the medicine works as long as you use it, or that it doesn't work at all?" Often the patient admits that the medication is effective when applied, but is frustrated that the symptoms return when it is discontinued. Apprising the patient that it will be months before symptoms resolve may come as a surprise, but once the patient accepts the chronicity of the problem and its treatment, therapeutic success is markedly enhanced.

As with evaluating any patient with lichen simplex chronicus (LSC), underlying causes of pruritus must be considered. On the genitalia, maceration and intertriginous rubbing contribute to exacerbation and continuation of symptoms, and infections are particularly likely to initiate itching. Tinea and candida are the most common offenders, and may be primary or secondary to the process. Vigorous scratching can introduce bacterial infection as well, especially if the skin is eczematous. In many cases of LSC, the initiating cause cannot be identified; the patient should be reassured that this is probably of no consequence, because the problem is now only the secondary change that has developed as a result of scratching. If the patient has a history of genital warts (human papillomavirus, HPV) there is a potential risk of carcinoma in situ; multifocal lesions should be biopsied.

In a detailed and well-referenced discussion of pruritus ani, Koblenzer[17] notes that males predominate over females 2 to 4:1 in this disorder. She agrees that it is multifactorial in origin, with seborrhea, maceration, hygienic aspects, dietary indiscretions (causing irritating elements in the feces), and secondary infection with bacteria and yeasts all acting as potential contributors and exacerbators. Another review[18] emphasizes the difference between idiopathic and secondary pruritus ani, stating that an underlying cause can be determined in 60 percent of men and only 30 percent of women with this disorder. Fecal contamination is considered to be the most common problem in pruritus ani,[19] mostly acting as an irritant to perineal skin.

There is real disagreement on the influence of psychogenic factors in the etiology of pruritus ani. Although many authors agree that psychic stresses may be an aggravating or perpetuating factor as they are in other chronic dermatoses, there tends to be less feeling at the present time that anal itching represents a more specific neurosis or psychosis. As mentioned, removal of offending irritants, good perineal hygiene, and topical steroids have provided remarkable relief to a majority of patients.

There is often confusion about the appropriate potency of topical steroids prescribed for genital symptoms. There are no hard-and-fast rules to follow, except to use only the strength necessary to control symptoms and to avoid using fluorinated steroids on erythematous, burning skin. Thickened plaques of LSC may require high-potency steroids, at least initially; betamethasone dipropionate 0.05 percent or clobetasol propionate 0.05 percent may be used on LSC for 6 to 8 weeks without complication. On the other hand, much less potent preparations can set off periorificial dermatitis and rebound burning if used on nonlichenified skin (see Side effects of topical steroids).

In childhood, genital pruritus is often the result of irritant dermatitis. This is especially true for young girls who are more likely to have fecal contamination of the vulva by not wiping front-to-back or who overscrub the genitalia or take irritating bubble baths. Pinworms are more common in childhood and typically involve the anus, but may also be seen at the vaginal opening. The technique of applying cellophane tape to the anus at bedtime and then to a glass slide in the morning may result in collection of ova which can be sent to a laboratory for examination and diagnosis.

Vaginal or rectal discharge in childhood should be evaluated for evidence of possible sexual abuse, and genital lesions should be examined carefully. Lichen sclerosus (see following) can occur in childhood, and friable purpuric lesions may suggest trauma when they are discovered. Labial agglutination occurs relatively frequently in little girls, and does not indicate an erosive dermatosis (such as lichen planus or lichen sclerosus) as it does in the postpubescent female.

BURNING: THE "-ODYNIAS"

When a patient has an unusual complaint and there seem to be few objective physical findings, the physician is challenged to provide an appropriate differential diagnostic workup. Obviously, the examiner's bias can influence findings, especially when there is major psychologic stressor like dyspareunia. The simple process of giving a name to a patient's symptom complex is often a major stress reliever; fear of the unknown can be worse than dealing with a chronic problem. The Greek work "odynia" means pain, and has been used in medicine for many years to indicate localized discomfort (e.g., pleurodynia). Glossodynia, burning tongue, is well known, and because this word also described a localized mucous membrane symptom, "vulvodynia" was coined to describe nonspecific burning of the vulva.[20] (This term replaced "burning vulva syndrome," a less acceptable diagnostic expression for patients).[21] Scrotodynia is a rather specific condition about which little is known, except that overtreatment often plays a major role.

Glossodynia and orodynia. Separation of the symptom of burning tongue from that of burning mouth in general can be helpful in determining the most likely differential diagnosis. The classic patient with glossodynia is re-ported to be female, peri- or postmenopausal, and literature citations prior to the 1970s note the usual "undue emotional disturbance and anxiety"[22,23] found with chronic symptomatology which is difficult to visualize. Recent studies report different incidences of precipitating factors: a British study[24] found denture defects to be the most common cause of glossodynia, but this was not corroborated in a group of American patients. In that series, candida was thought to be the cause of symptoms in 21 percent of patients, geographic tongue in 26 percent, and multiple etiologies were noted in 12 percent. Psychogenic influences were said to be "responsible" in 37 percent and "a factor" in 11 percent (a total of 48 percent, mostly in postmenopausal women). Only 2 percent were considered to be secondary to trauma, and 2 percent to pernicious anemia; none were found to have diabetes mellitus.[25] It is not clear whether habit tic, "busy tongue," or fiddling with dentures were considered to be psychogenic, but this might account for the difference in etiologies reported.

It is important to remember that candida has variable appearances on mucous membranes; organisms can be isolated from areas which clinically appear to be atrophic, as well as from more typical whitish exudative lesions. Candida-related mucosal atrophy has been reported in association with top-ical steroids used in inhalers for asthma[26] as well as from dental appliances.[27] The interested reader is referred to excellent reviews of glossodynia[28] and the multiple manifestations of oral candidiasis[29] (as well as other oral con-ditions) in the "Disorders of Mucous Membranes" issue of Dermatologic Clinics edited by Roy S. Rogers, III, MD in October 1987.

Interstitial cystitis and urethral syndrome. Most physicians think of painful micturition in terms of urinary tract infection, or possibly localized irritant dermatitis. There is a group of patients, whoever, who live with constant pelvic and bladder pain related to urinary frequency and mucosal inflam-mation. Symptoms are often nonspecific and irritable in nature; urine cultures and cytology studies are negative. There is no precise definition for interstitial cystitis (IC), and its etiology and pathogenesis is unknown; it is primarily a diagnosis of exclusion. Inflammation of the bladder wall is often part of the symptom complex, and cystoscopy is performed as part of the workup; if no bladder abnormalities are found, the patient may be given the diagnosis of urethral syndrome.[30] Irritative voiding symptoms are typical of both IC and urethral syndrome, and it has been proposed that the latter may be an early form of IC.[31]

Two-thirds of these patients report dyspareunia, and suicidal ideation has been admitted by 50 percent. It is estimated that there are between 20,000 and 90,000 diagnosed IC patients in the United States,[32] 90 percent of whom are women. Because there are no uniform criteria for diagnosis of the syndrome, it is not unusual for patients to go for years without a diagnosis and to be told that they have a psychological cause for their discomfort. An energetic physician-patient, Dr. Vicki Ratner, has encouraged IC patients to form a large politically active support group, the Interstitial Cystitis Association (ICA) which is currently raising money for its own grants in IC research. Needless to say, the ICA[33] does not consider this a psychiatric disorder and is very interested in psychological coping mechanisms for women with chronic pain. Publicity has encouraged research, and new theories for the etiology of IC and urethral syndrome include neurotransmitters, dysesthesias, a variety of inflammatory mediators, infectious agents, and immunological factors.

Vulvodynia. The International Society for the Study of Vulvar Disease (ISSVD) has defined vulvodynia as "chronic vulvar discomfort, especially that characterized by the patient's complaint of burning, stinging, irritation, or rawness."[21] Patients with the complaint of vulvar burning may describe different patterns of discomfort. These patterns are diagnostic clues to the patient's problem, and when coupled with characteristic physical findings, they enable the physician to choose the therapeutic program that will have the best potential for success.

Cyclic vulvovaginitis. Patients complain of recurrent episodes of vulvar burning, often related to a specific time during each menstrual cycle (during ovulation, for example, or just before menses). Dyspareunia is reported as "irritation after intercourse," and there is often vulvovaginal erythema and the sensation of swelling during cyclic episodes. The introitus may be inflamed and the skin fissures easily. A vaginal discharge is rare, and the patient is symptom-free at other times of the month.[20] This condition is most often seen in women 25 to 45 years of age who produce their own estrogens or are on estrogen replacement therapy after surgery.

Candida has almost always been cultured at some time from the vaginas of these patients, and they will often admit that they improve on anticandidal therapy, although symptoms return rapidly. Whether the problem is some yet undetermined cyclic change in the vaginal ecosystem (lactobacillus has been implicated) or related to candida hypersensitivity, cyclic vulvovaginitis responds best to consistent long-term anticandidal therapy.[34] Either oral ketoconazole (200 mg tablet) or an applicator of imidazole or azole vaginal cream may be used, but treatment must continue for several months. This is usually initiated on a twice daily basis for 2 weeks, then daily for 1 month. After that, half-doses (half a tablet, 100 mg, of ketoconazole; one-half applicator of vaginal cream) are used if possible: daily for 2 months, decreasing to a half-dose Monday-Wednesday-Friday for another 2 months. (If the patient is taking oral ketoconazole, liver function tests should be obtained after the first month and every 2 to 3 months thereafter).

Vulvar vestibulitis. The vestibule is the vulvovaginal mucous membrane; it extends from midway on the inner labia minora to the hymeneal ring and contains the urethra, Skene's and Bartholin's glands, and the minor vestibular glands. Vulvar vestibulitis is a chronic, persistent clinical syndrome characterized by severe pain on vestibular touch or attempted vaginal entry; tenderness to pressure localized within the vulvar vestibule; and physical findings confined to vestibular erythema of various degrees.[35-37] Vulvar vestibulitis is a clinical diagnosis; biopsy is rarely of benefit, since findings are nonspecific.

Pain at or around the vestibular glands is probably the primary cause of entry dyspareunia; the pain is typically chronic and unremitting, often with no other symptom. It is thought to be unlikely that any one infectious agent is the cause (neither candida nor HPV has been consistently identified), but the chronic inflammation often seen on histology probably has a significant role in the local destruction of these glands[38] and damage to nerve endings.

Patients who describe episodic vestibulitis have a better prognosis for recovery; remissions have occurred spontaneously and with conservative therapy. Patients with vestibulitis should avoid local inflammation (by using vaginal anticandidal creams or suppositories when taking antibiotics, avoiding irritating topical medications or potent topical steroids, and maintaining regular use of hydrocortisone cream or ointment). Aggressive destructive therapy for nonspecific findings (e.g., subclinical HPV) is discouraged.

Patients who have had vulvar vestibulitis for more than 1 or 2 years (for whom conservative therapy has failed) are candidates for surgical resection of the affected area. A crescent-shaped portion of the affected vestibule is removed, including the adjacent hymeneal ring; the vaginal mucosa is undermined and advanced to keratinized skin on the perineum where it is closed primarily.

Vulvar vestibulitis is probably the most important element to evaluate in multifactorial vulvodynia, and seems to be the most refractory to treatment.[39] An informal poll of the Committee on Vulvodynia at the 1991 ISSVD Congress confirmed that most experts believe that vulvar vestibulitis is probably preventable, although as yet there is only speculation on etiologic or exacerbating factors. A review[40] of 46 young women with symptoms involving tissues derived from the embryonic urogenital sinus revealed 10 with interstitial cystitis, 25 with focal vulvitis (vulvar vestibulitis), and 11 with both diagnoses, suggesting a possible analogy between certain urethral and vulvovaginal disorders. It is intriguing to speculate that cyclic vulvovaginitis and chronic inflammation may be precursors to vulvar vestibulitis in the same way the urethral syndrome may be related to interstitial cystitis.

Dysesthetic vulvodynia. The patient is typically postmenopausal and often elderly, and she complains of constant unremitting vulvar burning in a diffuse pattern, usually over the entire surface of the inner labia, sometimes extending onto the labia majora.[20,36] There are rarely any cutaneous signs except a variable erythema, often related to the use of topical medications. Dysesthetic vulvodynia was originally proposed as a diagnosis of exclusion ("essential" vulvodynia)[20] to describe a neurological problem which might relate to damaged sensory nerves or an altered perception of sensation. Patients respond to the same low-dose tricyclic antidepressant regimens used to treat postzoster or pudendal neuralgia (see following).[41]

Complaints of urethral or rectal discomfort in addition to vulvar burning are not uncommon. These patients are rarely taking estrogen replacements, and if sexually active, they seldom complain of dyspareunia. Patients describe awareness of a low-grade burning which is "always present;" it is usually not worsened by touch or wiping. Tricyclic antidepressant therapy alone (or in conjunction with topical lidocaine 5% ointment) was rarely helpful in vulvodynia patients under the age of 40 unless they also have symptoms typical of fibromyalgia or urethral syndrome, disorders also reported to respond in some cases to low-dose tricyclic antidepressants.[41]

Scrotodynia. Penile pain may be related to cutaneous disease (lichen sclerosus, lichen planus, candida, phimosis) or to distal urethral inflammation (urethritis, Peyronie's disease, paraurethral abscess), and the urologist is often best equipped to evaluate these problems along with the dermatologist. Lichen simplex chronicus of the scrotum is common and easy to recognize; it is often started by candida infection. The complaint of scrotal burning, however, is usually as nonspecific as burning elsewhere on the perineum. Unfortunately, the patient's ability to examine the affected area may complicate management as he fixates on erythema as the "cause" of his problem. When he applies topical steroids, the erythema improves as a result of the medication's vasoconstrictor effect. However, under the mistaken impression that this is "curing" the problem, the steroids are applied as often as necessary to decrease erythema. In some cases, the patient may wake himself up at night to apply the medication. Genital skin, while susceptible to atrophy, seems to be even more susceptible to rebound dermatitis from overuse of topical steroids. Just as in perioral dermatitis on the face, "periorificial" dermatitis may be seen as the result of chronic topical steroid use on the genitalia.[42] Treatment is with gradual withdrawal of the potent steroid (concomitant oral tetracycline may also help) and counseling to treat symptoms, not erythema. Tricyclic antidepressant therapy may be indicated in dysesthesia doses.

DIFFERENTIAL DIAGNOSIS OF CHRONIC PERINEAL BURNING

A variety of mucous membrane and perineal disorders have been described with general comments on similarities and differences in their presentations.

The remainder of this chapter presents the approach to the patient with perineal symptoms, the elements of differential diagnosis, and principles of management.

Dyspareunia

The complaint of dyspareunia, or painful intercourse, should be explored carefully. Vaginal dyspareunia is a dysfunctional problem with psychological implications similar in some ways to male impotence, but the male physical component (lack of ability to initiate and perform the sexual act) is more easily visible to both partners. While scrotal burning is a recognized clinical complaint, this rarely results in painful intercourse; vulvar burning, on the other hand, may only be apparent when coitus is attempted.

If there have been visible lesions, such as petechiae or tears on the skin or bleeding after intercourse, an erosive dermatosis should be suspected (see following). Patterns of dyspareunia can be helpful in diagnosis. Ask whether there is pain at entry or if the problem is better described as cutaneous irritation after intercourse. Does every coital episode produce discomfort or is it intermittent?[3] Does the patient have symptoms other than with intercourse?

History

The patient should be allowed to describe the sensation of discomfort as accurately as possible, particularly in localizing the area and differentiating the complaint of itch from that of pain. Some find it difficult to explain a dysesthesia: offering a choice of words is sometimes helpful, as is asking how they might recreate the pain for someone else. (Be careful of overinterpretation: the expressions "scalded" or "blistered" are often used by patients to describe a sensation, not a lesion.)

The history of the symptomatic patient should include inquiries about preexisting dermatoses (including oral mucosal lesions), candida, condylomata, methods of cleansing, and the use of topical and systemic medications. Previous treatments should be explored, especially if these were traumatic (CO_2 laser, 5-fluorouracil cream, surgical procedures) or resulted in a clearly allergic response (vesicles or erosions lasting for two weeks) rather than local irritation (stinging and burning on application). The patient should be asked specifically about risk factors: for example, the candida-prone patient may receive frequent rounds of antibiotics for sinusitis, urinary tract infections, or acne; steroids or other immunosuppressants may be prescribed for a variety of disorders. Estrogen deficiency may be important if the patient is perimenopausal.

There is occasionally a clearly recognizable precipitating event for the onset of chronic perineal symptomatology (a fall with injury to the sacrum or coccyx, long-term antibiotic therapy with development of chronic candidiasis), but this is the exception rather than the rule. Chronic problems often begin insidiously, but the patient may not report previous intermittent symptoms on the first visit; it is not unusual, however, for the slow onset of discomfort many months or years before to be recalled on subsequent visits, especially if treatment has been successful.

Often the most important part of history-taking is listening to the patient's theories about what has happened so that these can be addressed directly. It is not unusual for patients to fear an unusual or particularly virulent infection; in this era of AIDS, they have often had themselves tested for HIV. Patients may be overly concerned with *why* they have this problem: this question usually indicates that they believe that it is somehow their fault as a result of something they did or didn't do (sexual activity, cleansing, a certain diet, exercise, or a variety of other factors). The examiner should be patient and reassuring; explaining why a fear is unreasonable is far more helpful than saying that you don't know why the problem began.

Physical Examination

While some patients will describe elements of itching and burning, the two conditions may usually be differentiated on physical examination. Cutaneous changes of lichenification (leathery thickening) or excoriation (scratch marks) are more typical of pruritus, because the patient with burning skin rarely rubs or scratches the affected area. Without evidence of scratching, the patient with cutaneous burning or dysesthesia may appear to have a normal examination.[43]

The physician should become experienced with normal genital anatomy. This is especially important in the evaluation of the vulva, since this is an area not routinely examined by nongynecologists.[42] Although trained vulvologists have little trouble in finding objective signs, patients often comment that their other physicians "never saw anything there," confirming that inexperienced or unprepared clinicians are less likely to discover significant diagnostic clues to treatable causes of vulvar, or indeed any genital discomfort.

The physical examination should be careful and complete. Assessment of painful skin is often best done with a cotton-tipped applicator; dermatomal patterns should be identified and both sides of the body tested for comparison. By using a hand-held mirror, the genital examination can be performed with the patient's assistance; this offers an opportunity for the physician to explain anatomy, answer questions, and reassure the patient about normal findings. Some degree of pinkness or erythema is as normal for the genital and perineal region as it is for the face, and physiologic "blushing" may be a factor in each of these areas. Distinguishing abnormal degrees of erythema is important but may be difficult.

In many cases, the differential diagnosis will include one or more problems. On the genitalia, erythematous papules and pustules develop as a complication of topical steroid use, as well as with cutaneous infections. Bacterial, fungal, and viral infections should all be considered in this area, occurring either as primary or secondary problems.

Diagnostic tests should be directed toward documentation of infection, and the female examination should include a vaginal smear and a culture for candida. Visible changes (plaques, scarring, thickening), should be biopsied, preferably in the thickest portion of a lesion. Acetowhitening (application of vinegar or 3–5% acetic acid for 1–2 minutes) can be used to highlight thickened areas if there is a history of HPV. If HPV infection is found on the vulva, colposcopy of the vagina and cervix is recommended; if on the anus, proctoscopy. Biopsies should be performed on any diagnostically questionable areas, especially if intraepithelial neoplasia is suspected, but biopsies are rarely helpful for nonspecific inflammation or vestibulitis. Findings such as koilocytosis without obvious condylomata should be considered nonspecific; many women with this histology are asymptomatic and others with vulvar burning have no evidence of HPV.

Exogenous (Cutaneous) Etiologies

Dermatoses. Cutaneous disease should be the first diagnostic consideration in evaluating the patient with chronic perineal discomfort. Infectious agents are frequently secondary to a disruption of the skin's normal barrier function.

Inflammatory dermatoses. Papulosquamous or bullous dermatoses can become eroded as the result of maceration in intertriginous areas, or symptoms may be secondary to the patient's scratching or inflammation from infection.[44] Medication intolerance can be primary or secondary; overuse of topicals can cause an irritant dermatitis, or the underlying dermatitis can make the skin sensitive to irritating ingredients in the topical. Young girls are especially likely to be sensitive to bathwater irritants such as detergents, shampoos, or antibacterial soaps; vigorous scrubbing should be avoided.

Erosive vulvovaginitis may represent lichen planus, which is typically chronic. Episodic burning may be due to erosions from herpes simplex, lupus erythematosus, bullous dermatoses, aphthosis, and Behçet's. A biopsy for direct immunofluorescence should be considered in the differential diagnosis of erosive vulvovaginitis.

Lichen sclerosus et atrophicus (LSA). Lichen sclerosus can present with a variety of symptoms, ranging from intense pruritus or burning to the patient's complete unawareness of cutaneous changes. Men are much more likely to notice involvement of the glans penis, especially since phimosis may develop.[45] Erosions are common, especially in uncircumcised males, and candida may be present as well. Atrophic lesions are more likely to be associated with anal fissures or introital tearing during intercourse, whereas hypertrophic LS is more likely to be excoriated.

Therapy with high-potency topical steroids is now considered to be the treatment of choice for lichen sclerosus,[46] especially if lesions are pruritic. Therapy is maintained on a b.i.d. dosage for the first month or so, then decreased to daily until symptoms are controlled. Maintenance with low-dose steroids or testosterone 2 percent ointment is recommended. In prepubertal girls, hydrocortisone cream (1.0% or 2.5%) is usually sufficient for control of symptoms.

Infections. Candida is the most important infectious agent to consider in the evaluation of the patient with perineal burning or itching. Not only is it commonly seen as a primary infection, but secondary invasion of dermatitic skin is very likely.

Fungus: Tinea and candida. Men are more likely to have chronic and recalcitrant tinea infections of the groin (tinea cruris), but this diagnosis should be considered in women with vulvar itching as well. It is not uncommon to find tinea in the hair follicles of the mons pubis in women who have been treated with topical steroids and antibiotics for presumed bacterial folliculitis. Candida infections are more common in uncircumcised males and those with macerated intertrigo; scrotal involvement is a classic (if not very accurate) way to distinguish candida from tinea, which has been said to occur rarely on the scrotum.

Probably as a result of a vaginal reservoir, recurrent candidiasis seems to be more of a problem for women. Predisposing factors for candida include immunosuppression, antibiotic ingestion, and estrogen therapy (oral contraceptives, estrogen replacement). Other infectious causes of vaginitis do not cause chronic burning, although frequent treatment with antibiotics (including metronidazole) may predispose the female patient to unrecognized candida superinfection.

Vaginal candidiasis is a multifactorial problem, and cyclic vulvovaginitis is particularly puzzling. It has been suggested that the host's immune response to the organisms may be critical to disease occurrence, since some women remain symptomatic even when vaginal candida has been eliminated by treatment.[47,48] A localized hypersensitivity has been postulated, with the mucosae exhibiting a persistent allergic reaction which reactivates when only a few candida organisms (or cross-reactive substances) are present.[2,48] Effective treatment for this group of vulvodynia patients is long-term (4–6 months) maintenance therapy with local or systemic anticandidal agents (see previous text). The key to successful management in cyclic vulvovaginitis appears to be consistent low-dose suppression of candida until the inflamed mucosa regains its normal barrier function.

Molluscum contagiòsum. Flesh-colored umbilicated papules often itch on genitalia; patients may excoriate lesions and leave erosions which can confuse the examiner. In most cases these are easily recognized, but tiny lesions may be mistaken for folliculitis and a group may be misdiagnosed as herpes simplex. Local destruction of lesions is generally effective, but repeated visits may be necessary to treat recurrences.

HPV and papillomatosis. Primary or recurrent condylomata acuminata (human papillomavirus infection, HPV) occasionally itch, especially if lesions are extensive around the anus where hygiene may become a problem. A similar problem can occur with secondary candida infection on the scrotum, vulva, or vaginal introitus with multiple lesions, but so-called "subclinical" HPV is often overdiagnosed as a factor in chronic vulvar burning.

In some cases of pruritus vulvae, a thick papillomatous surface of the labia minora is secondary to continuous rubbing and excoriation; these changes gradually resolve with control of the underlying inflammation. Vestibular papillae are normal growths in the vulvar vestibule which may easily be mistaken for condylomata,[35,36,49] and repeated or aggressive therapy should be reserved for cervical or vulvar intraepithelial neoplasia, intractable symptoms, or disease recurrence after successful therapy. Some experts feel that "koilocytosis" is the nonspecific histologic equivalent of "papillomatosis."

Herpes simplex. Episodic burning, localized or with a deep or "aching" sensation, is typical of recurrent herpes simplex virus (HSV) infection. Patients usually describe a prodromal ache or itch, followed by the development of painful grouped papules or vesicles that erode, leaving a tender exposed area which gradually heals over in about 7 to 10 days. Some patients have recurrent lesions within a few-centimeter radius, while others report that lesions skip locations, even crossing the midline (a pattern similar to oral recurrences).

Invisible cervical or vaginal lesions make the diagnosis of herpes more difficult. Symptoms in this case may be typical of that described for pudendal neuralgia (episodic discomfort, dysesthesias of the groin or buttock, or sciatica-like pain extending down the back of a thigh). The pattern of recurrence is a helpful diagnostic clue in nonlesional recurrent HSV; pains which are constant, short-lived, or episodic in cycles less than 2 weeks apart are less likely to be HSV-related. The dosage of acyclovir in a primary HSV infection is 200 mg by mouth every 4 hours, five doses daily for 10 days. Recurrences are treated on the same schedule for only 5 days. Suppression of HSV outbreaks can usually be achieved with 400 mg acyclovir (2 tablets) twice daily; some patients do well on 200 mg three times daily.

Herpes zoster (postherpetic neuralgia). This diagnosis is usually made on the previous history of a unilateral vesicular eruption which often spreads to the thigh or even the leg. This typical pattern may be confounded by extension to adjacent dermatomes (changing unilateral involvement to the entire perineum) or an atypical nonbullous eruption. In some cases, the patient's inability to give an accurate history (senile or AIDS dementia, for example) also makes the diagnosis difficult. Treatment for postzoster neuralgia is the same as that outlined for pudendal neuralgia, beginning with tricyclic antidepressants.

Perianal cellulitis. May present as persistent rectal erythema and irritation, lasting often over a period of weeks or months.[50,51] It is more familiar to pediatricians because it is more likely to occur in childhood. Children or adults may complain of painful defecation, and chronic perianal fissures may be misdiagnosed as candida. Erythromycin is effective, but may require long-term therapy depending on culture results.

Iatrogenic factors

Side effects of topical steroids. "Periorificial dermatitis" is a genital condition that appears to be analogous to perioral dermatitis, a fine papular acneiform facial eruption caused by the use of potent fluorinated steroids. The condition is a rebound inflammatory reaction with erythema and a burning sensation that flares each time the steroid is withdrawn. This begins a cycle of symptomatic vulvar or scrotal dermatitis as the patient treats the burning and erythema with the agent causing the problem. The appearance of tiny pustules may cause rebound dermatitis to be mistaken for acute candidal infection, and vice versa; the history is helpful, but high-potency steroids combined with anticandidals may worsen rather than treat the problem. Potent steroids should be reserved for thick itchy lesions and not used at all on erythematous burning skin.

CO_2 laser. Effectively utilized as a treatment for carcinoma-in-situ (vulvar intraepithelial neoplasia, VIN) and condylomata, CO_2 laser therapy is nonetheless a traumatic procedure. Healing by secondary intention is painful and superficial nerve injuries take time to recover; normally symptoms gradually resolve over several months. In some cases, however, vulvar vestibulitis has apparently been initiated by laser therapy. It is not known how this occurs or how it can be avoided; of course, many cases of vestibulitis occur spontaneously and a few have even been improved with laser therapy, so this does not prove a cause-and-effect relationship. The indications for CO_2 laser are generally serious enough to warrant the limited risk, but this should be considered with caution as a treatment trial for symptomatic burning.

Alcohol injections. Subcutaneous injection of absolute ethyl alcohol has been recommended in gynecologic textbooks as treatment for intractable pruritus vulvae. This was said to be better than vulvectomy or surgical denervation of the vulva (the "Mering procedure"), but was interestingly never advocated for pruritus of the scrotum or any other area. Lichenification of the affected skin may have been a protective factor, accounting for the relative success reported. Later publications by Friedrich recommended that intralesional triamcinolone (5–10 mg/cc) be tried initially and, most importantly, noted that subcutaneous alcohol injection was "of no value" to the patient with vulvar burning.[52,53] Nonlichenified skin is not as resistant to trauma and tissue slough is likely to occur; in some cases, postalcohol scarring is indistinguishable from atrophic lichen sclerosus.

MANAGEMENT PRINCIPLES

Chronic problems distress physicians most familiar with genital diseases (such as gynecologists), because they are resistant to "cure"; while physicians who are used to chronic conditions (dermatologists) may not be as confident of their diagnostic skills in the genital area. Mutual anxiety can cause poor doctor-patient communication and misunderstanding. The physician should directly address the patient's fears: "Is this contagious?" "Could this be cancer?" If either of these is a possibility, appropriate diagnostic tests should be performed if they have not already been.

Reluctance to discuss sexual implications of the disorder may further confuse the issue, and this too may come from the physician or the patient. Some patients seem almost eager to talk about sexual dysfunction; although this may make the physician uncomfortable, it may mean only that the patient feels at ease with the doctor. This is particularly true of women who have talked about their problems with friends and are now seeing a female physician. As with most cutaneous problems, symptoms vary considerably in severity from patient to patient. Women may be angry and are often tearful as they describe their frustration with previous treatments. Some do their own research, carrying copies of articles and books to the physician's office; groups like the ICA are very helpful in providing support, but some patients are too embarrassed to discuss their problem. Some patients think that stress makes them worse; others feel that they could handle stress if only they didn't have their chronic pain.

Painful intercourse can focus attention on the relationship between partners. If the situation is perceived to be genuine physical discomfort, mutual support is often remarkable; on the other hand, if either partner is thought to be psychologically "at fault," the problem is distinctly worsened. Fortunately, justification for the diagnosis of psychosomatic illness is becoming less common as more is learned about perineal pain syndromes. "Psychosomatic disease" is a diagnosis of exclusion—a function of the investigator's diligence (or lack of it) in recognizing and cataloging physical findings. Diseases of the genitalia are second only to those of the face in arousing anxiety. Patients with chronic perineal pain are no more psychologically unbalanced than those with atopic dermatitis or acne. Patients with psychiatric disease (obsessive-compulsive disorder, severe depression) present with a variety of somatic complaints, only one of which might be chronic mucosal burning.

Careful focus on appropriate diagnosis and therapy is essential to successful management; patients will improve in most cases. Regular follow-up appointments to review and emphasize progress encourage both the patient and physician to stay with adequate treatment trials. Symptomatic perineal or genital discomfort does not resolve rapidly, and several weeks or even months of therapy are not unusual. Episodic flares often occur for a few days, even during successful therapy. These gradually become less severe, last for a shorter period of time, and occur less often as the patient recovers. Physicians who can calmly explain management strategies for chronic symptomatic problems will usually be able to develop a pleasant working relationship with chronic pain patients, who appreciate genuine caring and concern for their problem.

REFERENCES

1. McKay M: Vulvodynia versus pruritus vulvae. *Clin Obstet Gynecol* 28:123, 1985.
2. Witkin SS: Immunology of recurrent vaginitis. *Am J Reprod Immunol Microbiol* 15:34, 1987.
3. McKay M: Vulvodynia: Diagnostic patterns. *Dermatol Clin* 10:423, 1992.
4. Turner ML, Marinoff SC: Pudendal neuralgia. *Am J Obstet Gynecol* 165:1233, 1991.
5. France RD: The future for antidepressants. Treatment of pain. *Psychopathology* (suppl 1) 20:99, 1987.
6. Stewart DE, Whelan CI, Fong IW, et al: Psychosocial aspects of chronic, clinically unconfirmed vulvovaginitis. *Obstet Gynecol* 76:852, 1990.
7. Wittkower E, Russell B: *Emotional Factors in Skin Disease.* London, Cassell. 1953, pp 74–83.
8. Cormia, FE: Basic concepts in the production and management of the psychosomatic dermatoses. *Br J Dermatol Syph* 63:83, 1951.
9. Jeffcoate TNA: Pruritus vulvae. *Br Med J* ii:1197, 1949.
10. Dureck CJ: Pruritus vulvae and repressed sexual urge. *Neurol Cutaneous Rev* 49:306, 1945.
11. Lynch FW: Pruritus vulvae as seen in dermatologic practice. *JAMA* 150:14, 1952.
12. Rosenbaum, M: Psychosomatic factors in pruritus. *Psychosom Med* 7:52, 1945.
13. Koblenzer, CS: Pruritus Ani, in *Psychocutaneous Disease*, Orlando, Grune & Stratton. 1987, pp 225.
14. Lynch PJ: Vulvodynia: A syndrome of unexplained vulvar pain, psychologic disability and sexual dysfunction. *J Reprod Med* 31:773, 1986.
15. Dodson MG, Friedrich EG Jr: Psychosomatic vulvovaginitis. *Obstet Gynecol* (suppl 1) 51:99, 1987.
16. McKay M: Subsets of vulvodynia. *J Reprod Med* 33:695, 1988.

17. Koblenzer, CS: Pruritus ani, in *Psychocutaneous Disease*, Orlando, Grune & Stratton. 1987, pp 220–221.
18. Verbov J: Pruritus ani and its management: A study and reappraisal. *Clin Exp Dermatol* 9:46, 1984.
19. Hanno R, Murphy P: Pruritus ani: classification and management. *Dermatol Clin* 5:811, 1987.
20. McKay M: Vulvodynia: A multifactorial problem. *Arch Dermatol* 125:256, 1989.
21. Burning vulva syndrome: report of the ISSVD task force. *J Reprod Med* 29:457, 1984.
22. Gilpin SF: Glossodynia *JAMA* 106:1722, 1936.
23. Ziskin DE, Moultan R: Glossodynia: a study of idiopathic oralingual pain. *J Am Dent Assoc* 33:1422, 1946.
24. Basker RM, Sturdee DW, Darenpert JC: Patients with burning mouths: A clinical investigation of causative factors, including the climacteric and diabetes. *Br Dent J* 145:9, 1978.
25. Zigarelli DJ: Burning mouth: An analysis of 57 patients. *Oral Surg Med Oral Pathol* 58:34, 1984.
26. Smith MJ, Hodson ME: High dose beclomethasone inhaler in the treatment of asthma. *Lancet* 1:265, 1983.
27. Cawson RA: Chronic oral candidosis, denture stomatitis, and chronic hyperplastic candidosis, in Winner HI, Hurley R (eds): *Symposium on Candida infections.* Edinburgh, Churchill Livingstone, 1966.
28. Powell FC: Glossodynia and other disorders of the tongue. *Dermatol Clin* 5:687, 1987.
29. Ray TL: Oral candidiasis. *Dermatol Clin* 5:651, 1987.
30. Bodner DR: The urethral syndrome. *Urol Clin North Am* 15:699, 1988.
31. Wilkins EGL, Payne SR, Pead PJ, et al: Interstitial cystitis and the urethral syndrome: A possible answer. *Br J Urol* 64:39, 1989.
32. Held P, Hanno PM, Wein AJ, et al. A study of women with painful bladder syndrome, NIH workshop on interstitial cystitis, 1987, *J Urol* 140:203–206, 1988.
33. The Interstitial Cystitis Association, ICA, PO Box 1553, Madison Square Station, New York, NY 10159.
34. Sobel J: Recurrent vulvovaginal candidiasis. A prospective study of the efficacy of maintenance ketoconazole therapy. *N Engl J Med* 315:1455, 1986.
35. Friedrich EG Jr: Vulvar vestibulitis syndrome. *J Reprod Med* 32:110, 1987.
36. McKay M, Frankman O, Horowitz BJ, et al: Vulvar vestibulitis and vestibular papillomatosis: Report of the ISSVD committee on vulvodynia. *J Reprod Med* 36:413, 1991.
37. Woodruff D, Friedrich EG Jr: The vestibule. *Clin Obstet Gynecol* 28:134, 1985.
38. Pyka RE, Wilkinson EJ, Friedrich EG Jr, et al: The histopathology of vulvar vestibulitis syndrome. *Int J Gynecol Pathol* 7:249, 1988.
39. Friedrich EG Jr: Therapeutic studies on vulvar vestibulitis. *J Reprod Med* 33:514, 1988.
40. McCormack WM: Two urogenital sinus syndromes: Interstitial cystitis and focal vulvitis. *J Reprod Med* 35:873, 1990.
41. McKay, M. Dysesthetic ("essential") vulvodynia: Successful treatment with amitriptyline. *J Reprod Med* 38:9, 1993.
42. McKay M: Vulvodynia and pruritus vulvae. *Semin Dermatol* 8:40, 1989.
43. McKay M: Pruritus vulvae and vulvodynia: Itching and burning, in Hurst JW (ed): *Medicine for the Practicing Physician,* 3d ed. Boston, Butterworth-Heinemann. 1992, Chap. 10–15, pp 678–680.
44. McKay M: Vulvar dermatoses. *Clin Obstet Gynecol* 34:614, 1991.
45. Chalmers RJG, Burton PA, Bennett RF, et al: Lichen sclerosus et atrophicus: A common and distinctive cause of phimosis in boys. *Arch Dermatol* 120:1025, 1984.
46. Dalziel KL, Millard R, Wojnarowska F: The treatment of vulval lichen sclerosus with a very potent topical steroid (clobetasol propionate 0.05%) cream. *Br J Dermatol* 124:461, 1991.
47. Ashman RB, Ott AK: Autoimmunity as a factor in recurrent vaginal candidosis and the minor vestibular gland syndrome. *J Reprod Med* 34:264, 1989.

48. Witkin SS: A controlled trial of nystatin for the candidiasis hypersensitivity syndrome. [letter to the editor] *N Engl J Med* 324:1593, 1991.
49. Friedrich EG Jr: Therapeutic studies on vulvar vestibulitis. *J Reprod Med* 33:514–518, 1988.
50. Rehder PA, Eliezer ET, Lane AT: Perianal cellulitis: Cutaneous group A streptococcal disease. *Arch Dermatol* 124:702, 1988.
51. Kokx NP, Comstock JA, Facklam RR: Streptococcal perianal disease in children. *Pediatrics* 30:659, 1987.
52. Clouser JK, Friedrich EG Jr: A new technique for alcohol injection in the vulva. *J Reprod Med* 31:971, 1986.
53. Kaufman RH, Friedrich EG Jr, Gardner HL: Non neoplastic epithelial disorders of the vulvar skin and mucosa, in *Benign Diseases of the Vulva and Vagina,* 3d ed. Chicago, Year Book. 1989, p 319.

TWELVE
NEUROGENIC PRURITUS AND STRANGE SKIN SENSATIONS

Jeffrey D. Bernhard

Itch is a sensation transmitted by nerves from the periphery to the central nervous system. It is therefore no surprise that any one of a number of diseases that affect the peripheral or central nervous systems may cause itching, paresthesias, sensations that are perceived as itching, or other strange skin sensations.[1] For the purposes of this discussion, itching is considered a primary sensation and not one of a number of "paresthesias." Because this area overlaps with clinical neurology, several basic neurologic terms are defined at the outset.

Paresthesia. "abnormal sensations such as tingling, prickling, burning, tightness, pulling, and drawing feelings, or a feeling of a band or girdle around the limb or trunk; occurs with disease of the peripheral nerves, roots, or posterior columns of the spinal cord."[2]

Dysesthesia. "1. impairment but not absence of the senses, especially of the sense of touch. 2. Painfulness or disagreeableness of any sensation not normally painful." The terms dysesthesia and paresthesia are now often used interchangeably.[3]

Hypesthesia. "impairment of sensation; lessened tactile sensibility."

Hyperesthesia. "increased sensitivity (usually cutaneous) to tactile, painful, thermal, and other stimuli."

Hyperalgesia. "excessive sensitivity to pain."

Hyperpathia. "an exaggerated or excessive perception of or response to any painful stimulus."

Allodynia. perception of an ordinarily nonpainful stimulus as painful.[4]

Alloknesis. perception of an ordinarily nonpruritic stimulus as itchy.[5]

The definitions of several of these terms overlap, which is not surprising as they share a common background. While complete sensory denervation abolishes all forms of sensation, nerve damage or partial sensory denervation can lead to paresthesias, pain, or other sensory phenomena described by the terms defined earlier. Itching and pruritic phenomena may occur in situations that ordinarily provoke paresthesias or pain. This must not be a common occurrence, however, as true itching is hardly ever described as a component of most neuropathic syndromes, and pruritus hardly ever has more than a few entries in the indexes of neurology textbooks. In some cases itch may be overshadowed by other complaints, in some cases it may not be noted, but in many it is probably absent.

STRANGE SKIN SENSATIONS AND PSYCHIATRIC DISEASE

Patients with psychiatric disorders may experience and complain of strange skin sensations as well. This subject is covered in detail in Chap. 25. Although psychiatric patients may have bizarre skin complaints, not all bizarre skin complaints are psychiatric in nature. It is also important to recognize that distinctions blur when the simple fact that psychiatric disorders can have organic causes is borne in mind. Nonetheless, we shall try to restrict this chapter's discussion to those situations in which itching or strange skin sensations occur on an organic, neurologic basis.

Because severe itching can have an extremely debilitating effect on its victims, because the complaint of strange skin sensations is often met with skepticism by physicians, and because both can be such a frustrating diagnostic challenge, it is not surprising that some patients become exasperated, desperate, and depressed. Care must be taken to avoid confusing effect and cause. Finally, as Shuster has argued most effectively, skin disease can cause mental disturbance and severe changes in self-image, perhaps more often than the converse.[6]

PERIPHERAL NEUROPATHY

Peripheral neuropathy may occur as a consequence of physical injury, chemical injury, systemic disease, and neurological disorders, as listed in Table 12-1.

More frequently than not, the predominant symptom of peripheral neuropathies is paresthesia rather than itching. The main complaints include

Table 12-1 Some causes of neuropathic syndromes

Category	Examples
Hereditary	Fabry's disease
Drugs/toxic substances	alcohol
	vincristine
	thallium
	solvents
	Ciguatera fish poisoning
Inflammatory	vasculitis
Systemic diseases	diabetes
	uremia
	neoplastic disease
	paraproteinemia
	myeloma
	malnutrition
Infectious	herpes zoster
	leprosy
	viruses
Injury, entrapment	reflex sympathetic dystrophy

Modified from Bernhard.[1]

pain, tingling, "pins and needles" sensations, stinging, or burning sensations more like pain than like itch. These symptoms often elicit the tendency to rub rather than scratch the part affected, or to avoid touching the affected part altogether. Other symptoms of peripheral neuropathy include numbness, prickling, crawling sensations, disturbance of sweating, and disturbance of temperature and touch sensation. Isolated peripheral neuropathies may affect single nerves, but metabolic neuropathies and those caused by systemic processes such as diabetes tend to present with classic, symmetric, acral, "stocking and glove" distribution. Patients with symptoms of this type or with other abnormalities of sensation often present to dermatologists, but have much (if not all!) to gain from neurological consultation as well. Similar symptoms can also be seen in psychiatric disorders such as dermatologic nondisease,[7] (see Chap. 25). Aside from several selected examples, the complex fields of pain[8,9,10] and of the myriad diseases affecting the nervous system are beyond the scope of this book; the reader is referred to standard neurology textbooks for further information.[3,11,12] Shelley and Shelley have also provided a detailed consideration of paresthesias.[13]

Several isolated peripheral sensory neuropathies are listed in Table 12-2; notalgia paresthetica is considered in detail because of its history and particular interest to dermatologists.

Table 12-2 Isolated peripheral sensory neuropathies[a]

Syndrome	Nerve(s)	Area involved/comment
Postherpetic neuralgia[14]	dorsal root ganglion of affected dermatome	In severe cases, adjacent motor and sensory roots may be affected. Although pain is usually more prominent, postherpetic pruritus can occur alone or in combination with pain.[15]
Notalgia paresthetica[16]	posterior rami of dorsal spinal nerves 2–6	Scapular or midscapular area of the back. See text for further discussion.
Meralgia paresthetica[17]	lateral femoral cutaneous nerve	Outer thigh, symptoms also include numbness, burning, and sometimes, pain.
Brachioradial pruritus[18]	cutaneous branch of radial nerve	Forearm near elbow.
Pruritus as sign of cervical rib[19]	possible variant of brachioradial pruritus	Patients with itching localized to left flexor aspect of elbow and proximal forearm, possibly related to cervical rib pressure on spinal nerves.
Incisura scapulae syndrome	suprascapular nerve	
Gonyalgia paresthetica	saphenous nerve	Knee
Cheiralgia paresthetica[20]	dorsal cutaneous branch of ulnar nerve	Dorsal medial aspect of hand; numbness and dysesthesia
Other	sural nerve, digital nerves, auriculotemporal nerve	

[a] Itching may be present, paresthesias may predominate.

NOTALGIA PARESTHETICA

Notalgia paresthetica (NP) is the name given to a form of localized itching that occurs on the upper midback or to one side or the other of the midscapular area. Patients may also complain of tingling, burning, formication, hyperalgesia, and even tenderness, but itching is usually the most prominent and often the only complaint. Localized neurologic findings may be present but are not required to make the diagnosis. Sensation to light touch, temperature, vibration, and two-point discrimination may be altered. Hypesthesia to pinprick may occur; sweating in the affected area may be reduced. Rarely, patients complain of localized sensory loss. Most often, at least early on, there is no visible abnormality of the skin, but the longer rubbing and scratching go on, the more likely it is that secondary changes such as hyperpigmentation and even lichenification will appear.

NP was first described as a neuritis affecting the posterior rami of spinal nerves T2 through T6, by Astwazaturow in 1934.[21] Wartenberg described a similar case in 1958.[22] In 1965, Comings and Comings reported a hereditary form of NP in which eight family members had what they called "hereditary localized pruritus."[23] Another kindred with hereditary NP was reported by Nunziata and colleagues.[24] In that kindred, NP was a phenotypic marker for medullary thyroid carcinoma. At least three additional kindreds with NP or NP-like findings in association with multiple endocrine neoplasia type 2A (Sipple's syndrome) have been described.[25,25a,25b] Some of these have been associated with lesions of cutaneous amyloidosis, which, in this setting, is probably the consequence of repeated rubbing, scratching, and damage to keratinocytes. After 1970, it became increasingly apparent that NP is not a rare disorder, and additional reports of small series of patients began to appear.[16,26–28] It also became clear that NP had probably also been given a variety of other names in isolated case reports over the years, and was probably the explanation for at least some cases of macular amyloidosis,[29] "puzzling posterior pigmented pruritic patch,[30] recurrent lichen simplex chronicus of the scapular area,[31] peculiar spotty pigmentation,[32] and puncta pruritica.[33] Some cases may be related to the presence of an occult Becker's nevus, which characteristically occurs in the same location as NP.[34] One case was related to saccharin ingestion.[35] One of the locations for PUVA-induced itching and skin pain[36] coincides with the location of NP. I have seen patients with what I would consider to be PUVA-induced notalgia paresthetica. The "unscratchable itch" described by poet Shel Silverstein is probably NP in most cases as well.

Massey and Pleet performed electromyography in nine patients with NP and found abnormalities indicative of paraspinal denervation localized to the T2 to T6 level in seven of the nine.[37] They suggest that spinal nerves arising at these levels may be damaged or entrapped, and note that these roots "emerge at right angles through the multifidus spinae muscle and may be exposed to harm from otherwise innocuous insults, such as back trauma . . ."[37] Weber and Poulos examined skin biopsies from 14 patients and found necrotic keratinocytes and melanin-laden dermal macrophages in all 14, but no evidence of amyloid deposition.[16] Using specialized immunohistochemical techniques, Springall and colleagues demonstrated that there is an increase in sensory epidermal innervation in the affected areas of skin in NP.[38] These changes could be a consequence of repeated rubbing and scratching, rather than the primary cause of NP, but are probably involved in perpetuating the localized itch–scratch cycle.

One of the most important reasons for making the diagnosis of NP is to spare the patient needless diagnostic tests. Another is that misdiagnosis can have unfortunate consequences. What appears to have been one case of NP was attributed to witchcraft.[39] The last is that it can be treated.

Treatment of notalgia paresthetica. In 1989, Wallengren reported that NP could be successfully treated by topical application of capsaicin 0.025 percent cream.[40,41] Most patients experience substantial itching, pain, or burning sensations during the first week of application, but thereafter both the side effects of capsaicin and the symptoms of NP subside. Remissions may last for many months, and relapses respond to retreatment. Layton and Cotterill treated three NP patients by topical application of the local anesthetic cream containing 2.5 percent lignocaine and 2.5 percent prilocaine (EMLA® cream).[42]

OTHER PARESTHESIAS OF PARTICULAR INTEREST TO DERMATOLOGISTS

Paresthesias or Dysesthesias Caused by Contactants

Skin contact with certain synthetic pyrethroids and other agents can cause paresthesia, with or without a rash. Surgeons and dentists are at risk of fingertip paresthesias from contact with methyl methacrylate monomer from acrylic bone cement. Acrylic monomer is such a strong solvent that it can penetrate rubber gloves, damage the skin, cause dermatitis, and lead to a peripheral neuritis from damage of nerve endings. The paresthesia may persist for weeks to months after the rash has subsided.[43] Synthetic pyrethroids[44] and strong solvents such as acetone, benzene, and turpentine can produce paresthesias as well.[45] One unusual case of fingertip hyperesthesia was caused by microfilaments of silica from hair curlers that became embedded in the skin of a hairdresser.[46]

Neuropathies Caused by Medication

Drugs that cause itching without a rash are discussed in Chap. 23. Medications can also cause a variety of neurotoxic reactions including seizures, encephalopathy, neuropsychiatric symptoms, and peripheral neuropathy in which acral paresthesias, numbness, and foot weakness may predominate. A variety of antibacterial agents in common use can be neurotoxic.[47] Antihistamines may cause paresthesias,[48] as can dapsone.[49] PUVA photochemotherapy can cause skin pain, sometimes in the form of notalgia paresthetica (see previous section).

The Pants Paresthesia Syndrome

The pants paresthesia syndrome consists of itching, tingling, burning, or formication of the inner aspects of the thighs. In some patients symptoms go further down the lower extremities, and in some men the scrotum is involved. It has been attributed to chemical contactants such as formaldehyde in clothing.[45,50] While many of its features point to chemical contactants as the initial cause and repetitive trigger for recurrent symptoms, the possibility of a localized neuropathy rather than repeated exposure to offending chemicals should be considered and may explain some of the symptoms better than repeated chemical exposure does. For example, some patients complain that certain materials or the "weight of the material itself" provoke symptoms. When the groin is involved, other causes such as subclinical tinea infection and erythrasma must be considered as well. I have seen several men with pants paresthesia syndrome in whom no infection or contactant could be implicated, who were not clinically depressed and who appeared entirely well adjusted, and whose symptoms had a neuropathic character despite the inability of neurologists and myself to confirm the diagnosis of a neuropathy. The fact that the administration of a tricyclic antidepressant may be helpful supports the neuropathy hypothesis. I suspect that time, more careful neurologic examination, or more refined diagnostic techniques could reveal that some cases have a neuroanatomic basis. Although the presentation is somewhat different, reflex sympathetic dystrophy can occur in the perineum, scrotum, and penis.[51] Reflex sympathetic dystrophy is discussed later.

PAINFUL SKIN

Reflex Sympathetic Dystrophy[52]

Reflex sympathetic dystrophy (RSD) is "a syndrome of burning pain, hyperesthesia, swelling, hyperhidrosis, and trophic changes in the skin and bone of an affected extremity."[53] The term RSD now encompasses a number of other disorders in which sympathetic hyperactivity is associated with persistent pain; these include causalgia, Sudek's atrophy of bone, algoneurodystrophy, shoulder–hand syndrome, and reflex neurovascular dystrophy. RSD is most frequently precipitated by peripheral nerve injury, but a wide variety of factors, including soft tissue injury, central nervous system lesions, cervical cord injury, shingles, and operative procedures have been associated with RSD. RSD has even been reported as a complication of skin diseases such as acrodermatitis continua.[54]

Because partial forms are more common than the full-blown syndrome, and because early recognition is the most critical factor in effective treatment for RSD, it is important that the diagnosis be considered by all physicians to whom patients with what may seem bizarre skin complaints may present. Because the complaints in RSD may seem bizarre and because its victims may appear tense and agitated (for just cause!) it is important not to dismiss the patient as neurotic. Diffuse burning pain, "tearing" sensations, and localized vasomotor instability are important clues.

RSD may progress through three stages which may last from weeks to years. In Stage I (Acute), burning or aching pain seemingly out of proportion to an antecedent injury is increased by dependency, physical contact, anxiety, or other emotional upset. Erythema, edema, dependent rubor, hyperthermia or hypothermia, and increased growth of hair and nails on the affected part may be present. Piloerection (a noradrenergic/sympathetic effect) is another important early sign. In Stage II (Dystrophic), sympathetic overactivity predominates. The skin becomes cool and hyperhidrotic, and may be indurated. Mottling, cyanosis, or a livedo pattern may be seen. In this phase hair loss occurs and the nails become brittle, ridged, and cracked. In Stage III RSD (Atrophic) irreversible tissue damage occurs and the pain spreads proximally. Anhidrosis rather than hyperhidrosis is seen, and the skin is cool, atrophic, thin, and shiny. The fingertips are tapered or wasted and fascia may thicken. By this time (or earlier) roentgenograms demonstrate osteoporosis and other changes such as ankylosis. Altered sensations and discomfort may spread beyond dermatomal limits to involve an entire quadrant of the body, or more. Webster and colleagues studied cutaneous changes in seven stage II and III RSD patients referred by neurologists for evaluation of associated skin problems.[55] Several patients had inflammatory papules and macules that tended to ulcerate. Two had reticulated hyperpigmentation. In this group, xerosis was more common than cutaneous atrophy. One patient with RSD of the foot, caused when the foot was run over by a car, developed pseudo-Kaposi's sarcoma in the affected area.[56]

A number of theories have been put forward to explain various aspects of RSD, but it is not clear that a single, unified theory to explain all of its manifestations exists. Reverberating circuits in the spinal cord, abnormal synapse formation at sites of injury followed by ephaptic transmission between efferent and afferent fibers, and abnormal firing of peripheral nerves that develop their own ectopic pacemakers, are among the suggested mechanisms. Spinal and supraspinal mechanisms must be involved; the consequent "centralization" of pain and the potential contribution of "memory traces" of pain, which might increase susceptibility to recurrent pain, may be among the factors that make RSD so difficult to treat.[53]

Many different treatments for RSD have been tried.[53] The most important factor is early recognition. Paravertebral sympathetic ganglion block is widely recommended; systemic corticosteroids and transcutaneous nerve stimulation may be helpful. Early physical therapy is important with any treatment modality.

Other Causes of Painful Skin

There are a number of settings in which diseases or lesions of the skin characteristically produce pain or give rise to tenderness on palpation. Skin lesions may cause pain from inflammation, from involvement of nerves, from destructive effects such as infection and ulceration, from space-occupying effects and impingement on nerves, and through miscellaneous effects such as fissure formation. Because they cannot all be considered in detail, a selection is provided in Table 12-3, and further information can be obtained from standard texts. Although many patients with psychogenic symptoms complain of "burning" sensations, not all patients who complain of burning sensations or other strange sensations of the skin have psychogenic problems! (See Chap. 25.)

NEUROGENIC PRURITUS

Unilateral or Isolated Itching After Strokes or Other Central Nervous System Lesions

Localized itching related to central nervous system lesions such as tumors,[71] abscesses,[72] strokes,[73,74] and multiple sclerosis[75,76] has been reported in a small number of cases. In multiple sclerosis the itching may be segmental, unilateral, or bilateral; may be accompanied by pain; and characteristically occurs in paroxysms. With strokes and mass lesions, the itching is characteristically contralateral and may be accompanied by other sensory abnormalities. Whether isolated cases of generalized pruritus described as "central pruritus"[77,78] are exceptional, or in fact due to something else is not known. Facial itching from spinal opiate administration almost certainly involves their action on central nervous system structures, perhaps an "itch center" in the brainstem or brain.[79] Unilateral facial itching has also been described as a presenting sign of brainstem glioma in two children with neurofibromatosis.[80]

Phantom Itch

Amputees and patients with severe nerve injuries can experience "phantom itching" analogous to phantom pain. It is probably of central origin.[81] Other otherwise inexplicable localized itches may be related to phantom mechanisms as well.[82]

Senile Pruritus (Essential Senile Pruritus)

Senile pruritus is distressing generalized itching in elderly people the cause of which is not known. It is a diagnosis of exclusion, and is discussed in

Table 12-3 Some additional causes of painful, burning, or tender skin

Infection
    deep pyogenic infections, furuncles, carbuncles
    Herpes zoster and post-herpetic neuralgia
    Herpes simplex infection
    some rickettsioses[57]
    syphilis, particularly tabes dorsalis
    Lyme disease (radicular burning pain)[58]
    influenza prodrome
    other viral infections causing peripheral neuropathy, e.g., HIV infection[59] + or − CMV
        infection[60]

Painful erythema
    acrodynia
    staph scalded skin syndrome
    toxic epidermal necrolysis
    Raynaud's phenomenon (including other color changes)
    erythromelalgia (in myeloproliferative disorders)[61]
    erythermalgia (primary idiopathic or secondary)[62,63]
    phototoxic reactions
    sunburn
    other photosensitivity reactions
    erythropoietic protoporphyria
    other porphyrias
    palmar-plantar erythrodysesthesia syndrome (painful acral erythema due to chemotherapy
        drugs)[64,65]

Painful swelling with or without erythema
    angioedema
    relapsing polychondritis

Painful erythematous papules or plaques
    some cases of psoriasis, particularly when eruptive or pustular
    psoriatic plaques subjected to UVB phototherapy in patients treated with hydroxyurea[66] or
        methotrexate
    many cases of parapsoriasis ("burning")
    some cases of dermatitis herpetiformis[67]
    chilblains
    thermal injury: frostbite & burns
    arthropod stings
    hives (urticaria) in urticarial vasculitis
    some cases of vasculitis with palpable purpura[68]
    nasociliary neuralgia caused by an acne papule[69]

Painful papules, nodules, or tumors
    erythema nodosum
    erythema nodosum like lesions in Sweet's syndrome
    nodulocystic acne
    any tumor that impinges on cutaneous nerves
    angiolipoma
    neuroma
    glomus tumor
    granular cell tumor

Table 12-3 Continued

Painful papules, nodules, or tumors (*continued*)
  eccrine spiradenoma
  leiomyoma
  chondrodermatitis nodularis helicis
  plantar warts
  clavi
  adiposus dolorosa (Dercum's disease)

Erosions
  in pemphigoid, pemphigus, other blistering disorders
  necrolytic migratory erythema (glucagonoma syndrome)

Cutaneous ulcerations
  most causes, with the notable exception of primary syphilis
  atrophie blanche
  pyoderma gangrenosum
  hypertensive ulcers
  Wegener's granulomatosis[70]
  other vasculitides
  reflex sympathetic dystrophy

Physical, chemical, and thermal injury produce a spectrum of changes ranging from
  erythema and swelling to ulceration

The itching or burning scalp—see Chap 3.

Miscellaneous
  Gardner–Diamond syndrome (painful bruising)
  lichen sclerosis et atrophicus
  balanitis xerotica obliterans
  scleroderma
  any cause of cutaneous calcinosis
  some cases of alopecia areata
  reflex sympathetic dystrophy, causalgia; see earlier
  Fabry's disease
  Shy–Drager syndrome
  Hansen's disease
  sinusitis
  fissures
  foreign bodies
  ingrown toenail
  psychogenic
    variants include vulvodynia, glossodynia, scrotodynia once other causes such as
    infection or nutritional disorder have been excluded

Chap. 3. One theory holds that it is a form of phantom itching related to age-related degenerative changes in the peripheral nervous system.[82]

Referred Itch, "Mitempfindungen"

Evans reported that about one out of four or five people "is conscious that scratching an irritation may produce an itch elsewhere."[83] According to

Evans, "scratch and referred itch are ipsilateral; scratching the spot of the referred itch does not cause the original spot to itch." Richter also described the experience he and his wife had with this phenomenon.[84] The mechanism of referred itch is not known, but Evans suggests that spread of excitation in the thalamus is a possibility.

Could Cholestatic Pruritus or Other Systemic Causes of Itching be Mediated in the Central Nervous System?

The observation that opiate antagonists can be effective in the treatment of cholestatic pruritus has led some investigators to suspect that abnormally produced endogenous opiates produce itching in this setting through their action in the central nervous system rather than in the skin.[85] Perhaps centrally active compounds that cause itching are produced or accumulate in other conditions, such as Hodgkin's disease and renal failure, as well.

Other Causes of "Strange" Skin Sensations

Although the majority of patients who complain of "strange" skin sensations have either itching, paresthesias, or painful skin secondary to any one of the many cutaneous, neurologic, or other systemic disorders listed earlier and discussed throughout this book, some articulate patients cannot describe their cutaneous symptom as anything other than "strange." The differential diagnosis is therefore rather broad. Some patients with "strange" skin sensations may have forms of tactile hallucinosis or other psychogenic phenomena.[86] Some have delusional parasitosis,[87] but, after having been disappointed by several physicians already, will not admit to their conviction that parasites are present unless carefully questioned by a physician they trust. Delusional parasitosis may be a manifestation of schizophrenia or the single manifestation of monosymptomatic hypochondriacal psychosis. It can also stem from a misattribution of causes when itching has actually been caused by fiberglass, a skin disease such as dermatitis herpetiformis, or an antecedent scabies infestation.[88] In one case, parasitophobia was the presenting symptom of vitamin B12 deficiency.[89] The distinctions between organic and psychogenic also begin to blur when one considers that many cases of delusional parasitosis respond to oral pimozide treatment.[90]

Lyell listed several causes of strange skin sensations,[87] to which I have added in Table 12-4. From personal experience of a phototoxic reaction to doxycycline, I can confirm that such sensations may be difficult to describe. My experience started with sudden, intense, prickling itching of the entire scalp (which, in strong denial, I attributed to bugs in the field I was watching a soccer game in), and then proceeded to a sensation that I could only describe as "wet prickling" on other sun-exposed areas. The latter prompted

Table 12-4 Other causes of strange skin sensations[a]

contact dermatitis
phototoxic drug reaction (e.g., doxycycline)
systemic disease (e.g., hepatic, renal)
vitamin B12 deficiency
senile pruritus
ciguatera fish poisoning (notable for sensation of
   temperature reversal and painful awareness of
   the teeth)[91]
scombroid fish poisoning[92,93]
pellagra
malnutrition
flushing syndromes
erythropoietic protoporphyria
drug addiction
alcoholism
peripheral neuritis
toxic states
medication reactions
organic brain disease
schizophrenia
dermatologic nondisease
monosymptomatic hypochondriacal psychosis
delusional parasitosis
aquagenic pruritus ("prickling" or "irritating"; see
   Chap. 3.)

   [a] "Strange" sensations may range from itching
to prickling, burning, crawling sensations, and various
paresthesias and dysesthesias.
      Note: modified from Lyell.[87]

me to ask my family if it was raining, much to their amusement on a bright, clear, and sunny summer afternoon.

REFERENCES

1. Bernhard JD: Itches, pains, and other strange skin sensations. *Current Challenges in Dermatology*, (monograph). New York, HP Publishing Co., Winter, 1991.
2. *Blakiston's Gould Medical Dictionary*, 4th ed. New York, McGraw-Hill, 1979.
3. Schaumburg HH, Berger AR, Thomas PK: *Disorders of Peripheral Nerves*, 2d ed. Philadelphia, Davis. 1992, p 8.
4. Asbury AK: Numbness, tingling, and other abnormalities of sensation, in Braunwald E, Isselbacher KJ, Petersdorf RG, et al, (eds): *Harrison's Principles of Internal Medicine*, 11th ed. New York, McGraw-Hill, 1987, p 99.

5. Simone DA, Alreja M, LaMotte RH: Psychophysical studies of the itch sensation and itchy skin ("alloknesis") produced by intracutaneous injection of histamine. *Somatosens Motor Res* 8:271–279, 1991.
6. Shuster S: Reason and the rash. Proc Roy Inst Gr Br 53:136–163, 1981.
7. Cotteril JA: Dermatologic non-disease: A common and potentially fatal disturbance of cutaneous body image. *Br J Dermatol* 104:611–619, 1981.
8. Fields HL: *Pain.* New York, McGraw-Hill, 1987.
9. Cooper BC, Lucente FE: *Management of Facial, Head and Neck Pain.* Philadelphia, Saunders, 1989.
10. Wall PD, Melzack R: *Textbook of Pain,* 2d ed. Edinburgh, Churchill Livingstone, 1989.
11. Dyck PJ, Thomas PK, Lambert EH, et al (eds): *Peripheral Neuropathy,* 2d ed. Philadelphia, Saunders, 1984.
12. Adams RD, Victor M: *Principles of Neurology,* 4th ed. New York, McGraw-Hill, 1989.
13. Shelley WB, Shelley ED: *Advanced Dermatologic Diagnosis.* Philadelphia, Saunders. 1992, pp 1035–1051.
14. Editorial: Postherpetic neuralgia. *Lancet* 336:537–538, 1990.
15. Liddell K: Post-herpetic pruritus. *BMJ* 4:165, 1974.
16. Weber PJ, Poulos EG: Notalgia paresthetica. Case reports and histologic appraisal. *J Am Acad Dermatol* 18:25–30, 1988.
17. Massey EW: Meralgia paresthetica. An unusual case. *JAMA* 237:1125–1126, 1977.
18. Massey EW, Massey JM: Forearm neuropathy and pruritus. *South Med J* 79:1259–1260, 1986.
19. Rongioletti F: Pruritus as presenting sign of cervical rib. *Lancet* 339:55, 1992.
20. Massey EW, Pleet AB: Handcuffs and cheiralgia paresthetica. *Neurology* 28:1312–1313, 1978.
21. Astwazaturow M: Über paresthetische neuralgien und eine besondere form derselben—notalgia paresthetica. *Dtsch Z Nervenheilkd* 133:188, 1934.
22. Wartenberg R: *Neuritis, Sensory Neuritis, and Neuralgia.* New York, Oxford University Press. 1958, pp 242–250.
23. Comings DE, Comings SN: Hereditary localized pruritus. *Arch Dermatol* 92:236–237, 1965.
24. Nunziata V, Giannattasio R, DiGiovanni G, et al: Hereditary localized pruritus in affected members of a kindred with multiple endocrine neoplasia type 2A (Sipple's syndrome). *Clin Endocrinol* 30:57–63, 1989.
25. Gagel RF, Levy ML, Donovan DT, et al: Multiple endocrine neoplasia type 2A associated with cutaneous lichen amyloidosis. *Ann Intern Med* 111:802–806, 1989.
25a. Ferrer JP, Halperin I, Conget Jl. Primary cutaneous amyloidosis and familial medullary thyroid carcinoma. *Clin Endocrinol* 34:435–439, 1991.
25b. Bugalho MJGM, Limbert E, Sobrinho LG, et al: A kindred with multiple endocrine neoplasia type 2A associated with pruritic skin lesions. *Cancer* 70:2664–2667, 1992.
26. Massey EW, Pleet AB: Localized pruritus—notalgia paresthetica. *Arch Dermatol* 115:982–983, 1979.
27. Streib EW, Sun SF: Notalgia paresthetica owing to compression neuropathy: Case presentation including electrodiagnostic studies. *Eur Neurol* 20:64–67, 1981.
28. Pleet AB, Massey EW: Notalgia paresthetica. *Neurology* 28:1310–1312, 1978.
29. Bernhard JD: Macular amyloidosis, notalgia paresthetica and pruritus: Three sides of the same coin? *Dermatologica* 183:53–56, 1991.
30. Marcusson JA, Lundh B, Siden A, et al: Notalgia paresthetica—puzzling posterior pigmented pruritic patch. *Acta Derm Venereol* (Stockh) 70:452–454, 1990.
31. Dean EA, Bernhard JD: Recurrence of lichen simplex chronicus after surgical excision. *Cutis* 40:157–158, 1987.
32. Gibbs RC, Frank S: A peculiar spotty pigmentation, report of five cases. *Int J Dermatol* 8:14–16, 1969.

33. Boyd AS, Zemtsov A, Neldner K: Puncta pruritica. *Int J Dermatol* 31:370, 1992.
34. Dobson RL: Pruritus confined to scapular and subscapular region? Occult Becker's nevus with mild folliculitis. *J Am Acad Dermatol* 10:296–297, 1989.
35. Fishman HC: Notalgia paresthetica. *J Am Acad Dermatol* 15:1304–1305, 1986.
36. Roelandts R, Stevens A: PUVA-induced itching and skin pain. *Photodermatol Photoimmunol Photomed* 7:141–142, 1990.
37. Massey EW, Pleet AB: Electromyographic evaluation of notalgia paresthetica. *Neurology* 31:642, 1981.
38. Springall DR, Karanth SS, Kirkham N, et al: Symptoms of notalgia paresthetical may be explained by increased dermal innervation. *J Invest Dermatol* 97:555–561, 1991.
39. Hillard JR, Rockwell JK: Dysesthesia, witchcraft, and conversion reaction: A case successfully treated with psychotherapy. *JAMA* 240:1742–1744, 1978.
40. Wallengren J: Treatment of notalgia paresthetica with capsaicin (Zostrix). *Skin Pharmacol* 2:229–230, 1989.
41. Wallengren J: Treatment of notalgia paresthetica with topical capsaicin. *J Am Acad Dermatol* 24:286–288, 1991.
42. Layton AM, Cotterill JA: Notalgia paresthetica—report of three cases and their treatment. *Clin Exp Dermatol* 16:197–198, 1991.
43. Fisher AA: Paresthesia of the fingers accompanying dermatitis due to methylmethacrylate bone cement. *Contact Derm* 5:56–57, 1979.
44. Knox JM, Tucker SB, Flannigan SA: Paresthesia from cutaneous exposure to a synthetic pyrethroid insecticide. *Arch Dermatol* 120:744–746, 1984.
45. Fisher AA: Dysesthesia and paresthesia caused by contactants. *Cutis* 33:442–460, 1984.
46. Shelley WB, Pillsbury DM: Fingertip hyperesthesia. Solitary sign of new occupational dermatosis due to silica hair curlers. *JAMA* 170:1779–1781, 1959.
47. Snavely SR, Hodges GR: The neurotoxicity of antibacterial agents. *Ann Int Med* 101:92–104, 1984.
48. Kaufman HS, Chang P, Chang G: Astemizole-induced paresthesia. *N Eng J Med* 323:684, 1984.
49. Koller WC, Gehlmann LK, Malkinson FD: Dapsone-induced peripheral neuropathy. *Arch Neurol* 34:644–646, 1977.
50. Fisher AA: Contact "pants paresthesia syndrome." *Contact Dermatitis* 9:92, 1983.
51. Olson WL: Perineal reflex sympathetic dystrophy treated with, bilateral lumbar sympathectomy. *Ann Int Med* 113:633–634, 1990.
52. Kozin F: Reflex sympathetic dystrophy syndrome. *Bull Rheum Dis* 36(3):1–8, 1986.
53. Schwartzman RJ, McLellan TL: Reflex sympathetic dystrophy. A review. *Arch Neurol* 44:555–561, 1987.
54. Stephens CJM, McGibbon DH: Algodystrophy (reflex sympathetic dystrophy) complicating unilateral acrodermatitis continua. *Clin Exp Dermatol* 14:445–447, 1989.
55. Webster GF, Schwartzman RJ, Jacopy RA, et al: Reflex sympathetic dystrophy. Occurrence of inflammatory skin lesions in patients with stages II and III disease. *Arch Dermatol* 127:1541–1544, 1991.
56. Shelton RM, Lewis CW: Reflex sympathetic dystrophy: A review. *J Am Acad Dermatol* 22:513–520, 1990.
57. Burnett JW: Rickettsioses: A review for the dermatologist. *J Am Acad Dermatol* 2:359–373, 1980.
58. Abele DC, Anders KH: The many faces and phases of borreliosis I. Lyme disease. *J Am Acad Dermatol* 23:167–186, 1990.
59. So Yt, Holtzman DM, Abrams DI, et al: Peripheral neuropathy associated with the acquired immunodeficiency syndrome: Prevalence and clinical features from a population based study. *Arch Neurol* 45:945–948, 1988.
60. D'Ivernois C, Dupon M, Catry-Thomas I, et al: Painful peripheral neuropathy and cytomegalovirus pneumonia in AIDS. *Lancet* 2:1329–1230, 1989.

61. Michiels JJ, Van Joost T: Erythromelalgia and thrombocythemia: A causal relation. *J Am Acad Dermatol* 22:107–111, 1990.
62. Michiels JJ, Van Joost T, Vuzevski VD: Idiopathic erythermalgia: A congenital disorder. *J Am Acad Dermatol* 21:1128–1130, 1989.
63. Michiels JJ, Erythromelalgia versus erythermalgia. *Lancet* 336:183–184, 1990.
64. Burke KC, Bernhard JD, Michelson A: Chemotherapy induced painful acral erythema in childhood: Burgdorf's reaction. *Am J Ped Heme Onc* 11:44–45, 1989.
65. Lokich JJ, Moore C: Chemotherapy-associated palmar-plantar erythrodysesthesia syndrome. *Ann Intern Med* 101:798–800, 1984.
66. Sparks MK, Moshell AN, Nigra TP: Hydroxyurea and pain in psoriatic plaques during ultraviolet-B radiation. *Arch Dermatol* 121:1107, 1985.
67. Leitao EA, Bernhard JD: Perimenstrual nonvesicular dermatitis herpetiformis. *J Am Acad Dermatol* 22:331–334, 1990.
68. Provost T: Presentation at American Academy of Dermatology, December, 1990.
69. Lambert WC, Okorodudu AO, Schwartz RA: Cutaneous nasociliary neuralgia. *Acta Derm Venereol* (Stockh) 65:257–258, 1985.
70. Bernhard JD, Mark EJ: Case records of the Massachusetts General Hospital. Case 17-1986. An 18-year-old man with cutaneous ulcers and bilateral pulmonary infiltrates, (Wegener's granulomatosis). *N Engl J Med* 314:1170–1184, 1986.
71. Andreev VC, Petkov I: Skin manifestations associated with tumors of the brain. *Br J Dermatol* 92:675–678, 1975.
72. Sullivan MJ, Drake ME: Unilateral pruritus and Nocardia brain abscess. *Neurology* 34:828–829, 1984.
73. King CA, Huff FJ, Jorizzo JL: Unilateral neurogenic pruritus: Paroxysmal itching associated with central nervous system lesions. *Ann Int Med* 97:222–223, 1982.
74. Massey EW: Unilateral neurogenic pruritus following stroke. *Stroke* 15:901–903, 1984.
75. Osterman PO: Paroxysmal itching in multiple sclerosis. *Br J Dermatol* 95:555–558, 1976.
76. Yamamoto M, Yabuki S, Hayabara T, et al: Paroxysmal itching in multiple sclerosis: A report of three cases. *J Neurol Neurosurg Psychiatry* 44:19–22, 1981.
77. Procacci P, Maresca M: Central pruritus. Case report. *Pain* 45:307–308, 1991.
78. Maheshwari MC: Neurogenic pruritus. *J Indian Med Assoc* 85:364–365, 1987.
79. Scott PV, Fischer HBJ: Spinal opiate analgesia and facial pruritus: A neural theory. *Postgrad Med J* 58:531–535, 1982.
80. Summers CG, MacDonald JT: Paroxysmal facial itch: A presenting sign of childhood brainstem glioma. *J Child Neurol* 3:189–192, 1988.
81. Melzack R: Phantom limbs. *Sci Am* 266:120–126, 1992.
82. Bernhard JD: Phantom itch, pseudophantom itch, and senile pruritus. *Int J Dermatol* 31:856–857, 1992.
83. Evans PR: Referred itch (mitempfindungen). *BMJ* 2:839–841, 1976.
84. Richter CP: Mysterious form of referred sensation in man. *Proc Nat Acad Sci USA* 74:4702–4705, 1977.
85. Bergasa N, Jones EA: Management of pruritus of cholestasis: Potential role of opiate antagonists. *Am J Gastroenterol* 86:1404–1412, 1991.
86. Musaph H: Psychogenic pruritus. *Sem Dermatol* 2:217–222, 1983.
87. Lyell A: Delusions of parasitosis. *Sem Dermatol* 2:189–195, 1983.
88. Schrut AH, Waldron WG: Psychiatric and entomological aspects of delusory parasitosis. *JAMA* 186:429–430, 1963.
89. Pope FM: Parasitophobia as the presenting symptom of vitamin B12 deficiency. *Practitioner* 204:421–422, 1970.
90. Munro A: Monosymptomatic hypochondriacal psychosis manifesting as delusions of parasitosis. A description of four cases successfully treated with pimozide. *Arch Dermatol* 114:940–943, 1978.

91. Lawrence DN, Enriquez MB, Lumish RM, et al: Ciguatera fish poisoning in Miami. *JAMA* 244:254, 1980.
92. Etkind P, Wilson ME, Gallagher K, et al: Bluefish-associate scombroid poisoning: An example of the expanding spectrum of food poisoning from seafood. *JAMA* 258:3409–3410, 1987.
93. Morrow JD, Margolies GR, Rowland J, et al: Evidence that histamine is the causative toxin of scombroid-fish poisoning. *N Engl J Med* 324:716–720, 1991.

UNSCRATCHABLE ITCH

There is a spot that you can't scratch
Right between your shoulder blades,
Like an egg that just won't hatch
Here you set and there it stays.
Turn and squirm and try to reach it,
Twist your neck and bend your back,
Hear your elbows creak and crack,
Stretch your fingers, now you bet it's
Going to reach—no that won't get it—
Hold your breath and stretch and pray,
Only just an inch away,
Worse than a sunbeam you can't catch
Is that one spot that
You can't scratch.

THIRTEEN
PRURITIC CURIOSITIES

Jeffrey D. Bernhard

"Many things which are false are transmitted from book to book and gain credit in the world."

Samuel Johnson*

Dermatologists seem to have an itch to name things, and even this itch has been given a name, logodaedalian pruritus.[1] Perhaps partly for that reason, and partly because itching is such a peculiar sensation, many curious itches have been reported as anecdotal observations or in small collections of patients. As the nature of medical experience goes, some itches that started out as isolated curiosities were gradually recognized with increasing frequency. Notalgia paresthetica, an itch usually localized to one side or the other of the mid-scapular area, is a case in point. It was first described in 1934. There were some scattered reports over the next few decades; then a gradual recognition that it was fairly common, and increasing acceptance of the notion that it is often, if not usually, the consequence of an isolated sensory neuropathy.[2] Now it can even be treated.[3] It has graduated from the ranks of "pruritic curiosities" and is discussed more fully in Chap. 12.

Based on a desire for completeness, on the possibility that other curiosities could follow a similar path of recognition and understanding, and partly for the sake of amusement, the following tabulation of itches is provided

* In: Boswell Life of Johnson. Chapman, RW, ed. London: Oxford University Press, 3d ed. 1976, p. 755.

with minimal comment and with the caveat that many stem from anecdotal reports on single patients. Some will turn out to be something else, some may be recognized in other patients, and some are destined to remain nothing more than curiosities.

Notalgia paresthetica. (Synonyms: hereditary localized pruritus, some cases of puncta pruritica, some cases of macular amyloidosis of the back.) An itch localized to one side or the other of the mid-scapular area of the back. Secondary changes caused by rubbing and scratching may develop. Probably an isolated sensory neuropathy. See Chap. 12.

Mitempfindungen.[4,5] (Synonym: referred itch). An itch that occurs more or less reproducibly at one spot when another spot is scratched. Neurologic basis presumed.

Brachioradial pruritus.[6,7,8,9] (Synonyms: solar pruritus of the elbow, brachioradial summer pruritus). Chronic, intermittent itching of the flexor surface of the elbows. Chronic solar damage may play a contributory role, and episodes are often precipitated by sunlight exposure. Some cases or variants may be related to the presence of a cervical rib.[10]

Polymorphic light eruption sine eruptione.[11] Probably a diminutive variant of or precursor to polymorphic light eruption. Itching of exposed skin after sunlight exposure, without a rash. Some cases may be variants of brachioradial pruritus. Important differential diagnoses: erythropoietic protoporphyria (EPP), photosensitive drug eruptions, and sunburn.

Aquagenic pruritus. (Synonym: bath pruritus). Itching provoked by contact with water. See full discussion in Chap. 3.

Atmoknesis.[12] (Synonym: aerogenic pruritus). Itching caused by, or that seems as though it is caused by, exposure to air on undressing. Particularly notable in many patients with atopic dermatitis and psoriasis.

Cold pruritus.[13] Probably a diminutive variant of cold urticaria. It would appear that analogous variants of most of the physical urticarias probably exist, and fall on a spectrum that ranges from itching alone to erythema to urticaria.[13a]

Pruritus prohibitus.[14] The itch that you can't scratch because your hands are full, because you are standing in front of an audience, or because you have scrubbed for surgery. Usually goes away by itself. The most famous case was Huckleberry Finn's:

> There was a place on my ankle that got to itching, but I dasn't scratch it; and then my ear began to itch; and next my back, right between my shoulders. Seemed like I'd die if I couldn't scratch. Well, I've noticed that thing plenty of times since. If you are with the quality, or at a funeral, or trying to go to sleep when you ain't sleepy—if you are anywheres where it won't do for you to scratch, why you will itch all over in upward of a thousand places . . . [15]

Puncta pruritica.[16,17] One or more intensely pruritic pinpoint spots in clinically normal skin. Some cases may actually be notalgia paresthetica.[18,19]

Peculiar persistent pruritic affection of the skin.[20] A momentary itch that "attacks only a small area, and is relieved by a single scratch or pinch." Described anecdotally in three paragraphs in 1977, proof that something that happens to everyone every day can be immortalized if named appropriately. On the other hand, "The beginning of wisdom is to call things by their right names," according to a Chinese proverb.

Recurrent lichen simplex chronicus.[21] Lichen simplex chronicus is common but curious nonetheless, especially when it recurs in the same location after surgical excision. The subject of the case cited here probably had notalgia paresthetica, and, it turns out, so did her mother (hereditary localized pruritus,[22] hereditary notalgia paresthetica). Lichen simplex chronicus[23]—the maddeningly itchy plaques of thickened skin with accentuated skin markings which practicing dermatologists see every day—often recurs after "successful" treatment on any part of the body. So, not every case can be notalgia paresthetica (which only occurs on the back), but some cases may be analogous to it.

Macular amyloidosis. The cutaneous and systemic amyloidoses produce a bewildering variety of skin lesions.[24,25] The classic presentation of macular amyloidosis is an itchy, hyperpigmented macule of the midback. The pigmentation may be brown or gray, and it may be "rippled." The amyloid in such cases is probably degenerated keratin (amyloid-K), deposited as the consequence of repeated rubbing and scratching. While not every case of macular amyloidosis is the consequence of notalgia paresthetica, many probably are.[26,27,28]

Post-herpetic pruritus.[29] Pain is more common but itching can occur.

Post-prandial pruritus in the dumping syndrome.[30] More than 20 years after a Bilroth II gastrectomy for a duodenal ulcer and a transthoracic vagotomy for recurrent ulceration, a 62-year-old man presented with symptoms of the dumping syndrome and with generalized itching that always occurred half an hour after meals. Treatment with oral pectin relieved both problems.

Prodromal itching in asthma.[31,32,33,34] Perhaps common. May appear in 40 to 70 percent of patients with asthma; usually the neck, chin, or back; before or at the beginning of an attack.

Orthostatic leg itching. Itching of the legs on standing in a patient with autonomic dysfunction.[35]

Piano player's practice pruritus. Can affect any part of the body; sometimes paroxysmal. Familiar to any parent who has ever convinced a child to practice the piano before the child was good and ready to do so. (As in many other itches, scratching is observed, itching is presumed.)

Nasal pruritus as atypical angina.[36] Reproducible itching of the bridge of the nose in a 60-year-old man associated with electrocardiographic evidence of angina. Naso-pruritic angina?

Nasal pruritus as a sign of advanced brain tumor.[37,38] Noted as a "ferocious" itching of the nostrils in a survey of patients with advanced brain tumors, particularly those with tumors infiltrating the base of the fourth ventricle. "Patients could be seen scratching for hours. Even when unconscious they scratched their nostrils and, if restrained, tried to rub their noses in the pillow." Particularly intriguing in light of the observation that the nose is a sight of predilection in itching of central origin in animal experiments.[39]

Nasal or facial pruritus as side-effect of opiate medication or abuse.[40] See Chap. 23.

Nasal pruritus in helminthoses. (e.g., in ascariasis)[41]

The nasal variant of pruritus prohibitus. Also described by Huckleberry Finn:

> ...My nose begun to itch. It itched till the tears come into my eyes. But I dasn't scratch. Then it begun to itch on the inside. Next I got to itching underneath. I didn't know how I was going to set still. The miserableness went on as much as six or seven minutes; but it seemed a sight longer than that. I was itching in eleven different places now . . . [15]

Nasal pruritus from flossing upper teeth.[42] If this also happens to you, please write to me.

Thinker's itch.[43] The itch that makes people scratch their heads when thinking or perplexed. For other causes of the itchy scalp, see Chap. 3, Table 3-6.

Red traffic light phenomenon.[44] Musaph "repeatedly" observed that drivers forced to stop at red traffic lights put their hands to their heads and scratch. He viewed this as a form of derived unconscious activity, "resolving an emotional conflict situation." I have repeatedly observed a nasal variant of this phenomenon.

Vulvovaginal pruritus cause by drug ingestion.[45] An 80-year-old woman developed vulvovaginal itching when treated with the angiotensin converting enzyme inhibitor, enalapril. My colleague, Dr. Lori Herman, and I have seen a very similar case in a much younger woman.

Anorectal pruritus after intravenous hydrocortisone.[46] Not the same as other cases of anorectal itching related to fecal soiling or passage of allergenic or irritant foods or spices. (See Chap. 11.)

Intercourse related pruritus. (Synonym: "spouse allergy") Can occur from allergy to sweat or semen,[47] or because of allergy to latex in condoms, or because of any irritant or allergenic substance, including systemic medication taken by partner, transmitted by connubial contact (see Chap. 3, section on "connubial contact dermatitis").

The itchy knee, eye, elbow, palm, or foot in superstition. An itchy knee, for example, is said to signify that its owner is about to kneel at a strange altar. See the section titled "Does scratching have a meaning?" in Chap. 6.

Localized uremic pruritus due to arteriovenous anastomosis.[48]

Judo-jogger's itch.[49] The itchy ankles and wrists one physician gets when jogging, but only if he has done a judo workout the day before.

Cardiac bypass pruritus.[50] An itch of the back with 2-minute to 2-hour episodes, usually beginning within 6 weeks of surgery and then gradually improving over 11 months or so.

Very unusual/anecdotal causes of generalized pruritus.
alcohol intolerance in neoplastic disease[51]
aquagenic pruritus after alcohol ingestion in sarcoidosis[52]
starvation (e.g., in anorexia nervosa)[53]
ciguatera fish poisoning
coffee[54]
banana[55]
other foods, such as mustard
see also Chap. 22

Mites and other bugs.[56] Discussed in several other chapters of this book, but so easy to overlook, so hard to find, and so varied in their presentation, that they deserve to be mentioned again here. Did you think of mites in the feather pillow?[57] Pigeon mites?[58] Carpet beetles?[59] Moths?[60] The cat?[61] See also Chap. 4 and 9.

Pearl Harbor itch (medusa sting) and other geographic itches.[62,63]

Stress-induced itching. See cholinergic and adrenergic pruritus in Chap. 18. See also psychogenic pruritus in Chap. 25.

Telepathic pruritus.[64] The delusion that someone is making you itch by mental telepathy.

"Epidemic" delusional or "hysterical" itching.[65,66] In one epidemic, 57 of 159 students at a rural elementary school developed itching and an irregular, macular, erythematous rash with excoriations only at sites accessible to the hands, and only during school hours.[67]

Pruritus idiosyncratica. Many people seem to have "their own little itch" that recurs intermittently at the same site and that doesn't fall easily into any other category. No visible skin changes can be detected, and most people will not bother to mention it (unless their dermatologist is already running late). It may be one heel or the other, a spot on the foot, or anywhere else. Other causes of localized itching should be considered before this diagnosis is made. Dr. Kenneth Appelbaum collaborated with me in naming it.

Undefined episodic mediator release syndromes. In one well-documented case, a 29-year-old woman developed episodic attacks of flushing along with severe skin, bone, and abdominal pain, as well as an organic psychosis. The skin pain was "burning." Generalized pruritus developed about 7 years after the onset of illness. The syndrome was similar to those induced by hallucinogenic drugs such as lysergide and mescaline. Mast cell disease and carcinoid syndrome were excluded. The clinical response to opiate antagonists suggested the possibilty that the syndrome was related to episodic release of an endogenous opiate.[68] Since the original description of this patient, several patients with similar complaints have been evaluated by the authors but none have had the same syndrome. One of those referred for evaluation had temporal lobe epilepsy. The original patient is now doing well under treatment with the oral opiate antagonist, nalmefene.[69]

Paresthesias and other strange skin sensations. See Chap.12.

Neurogenic itches. See Chap. 12.

Psychogenic itches. See Chap. 25.

Metaphysical urticaria. Not easy to define but sometimes seen in dermatologists struggling with a case of dermatitis nonrecollecta.[70] Also, and originally, a very helpful mnemonic for the causes of chronic urticaria.[71]

"How these curiosities would be quite forgott, did not such idle fellowes as I am putt them downe."

John Aubrey
Brief Lives, 'Venetia Digby'[72]

REFERENCES

1. Bernhard JD: Editorial comment, in Sober AJ, Fitzpatrick TB (eds): *1991 Year Book of Dermatology.* St. Louis, Mosby Year Book, 1991, p 431.
2. Weber PJ, Poulos EG: Notalgia paresthetica. Case reports and histologic appraisal. *J Am Acad Dermatol* 18:25–30, 1988.
3. Wallengren J: Treatment of notalgia paresthetica with topical capsaicin. *J Am Acad Dermatol* 24:286–288, 1991.
4. Evans PR: Referred itch (mitempfindungen). *BMJ* 2:839–841, 1976.
5. Richter CP: Mysterious form of referred sensation in man. *Proc Nat Acad Sci USA* 74:4702–4705, 1977.
6. Waisman M: Solar pruritus of the elbows (brachioradial summer pruritus). *Arch Dermatol* 98:481, 1968.
7. Heyl T: Brachioradial pruritus. *Arch Dermatol* 119:115, 1983.
8. Kestenbaum T, Kalivas J: Solar pruritus. *Arch Dermatol* 115:1368, 1979.
9. Walcyk PJ, Elpern DJ: Brachioradial pruritus: A tropical dermopathy. *Br J Dermatol* 115:177–180, 1986.
10. Rongioletti F: Pruritus as presenting sign of cervical rib. *Lancet* 339:55, 1992.

11. Dover JS, Hawk JLM: Polymorphic light eruption sine eruptione. *Br J Dermatol* 118:73–76, 1988.
12. Bernhard JD: Nonrashes 5. Atmoknesis. Pruritus provoked by contact with air. *Cutis* 44:143–144, 1989.
13. Shelley WB, Shelley ED: Diary of a practice. *Cutis* 46:471, 1990.
13a. Bernhard JD: A theorem of pruritus and urticarial diminution. *J Am Acad Dermatol* 28:800,1993.
14. Bernhard JD: Nonrashes 3. Pruritus prohibitus. *Cutis* 29:358–359, 1982.
15. Twain M: *The Adventures of Huckleberry Finn.* Avon, The Heritage Press, 1968, p 17.
16. Toomey N: Itchy points (puncta pruritica). *Arch Dermatol* 5:744–747, 1922.
17. Crissey JT: Puncta pruritica. *Int J Dermatol* 30:722–724, 1991.
18. Boyd AS, Zemtsov A, Neldner KH; Puncta pruritica. *Int J Dermatol* 31:370, 1992.
19. Crissey JT: Puncta pruritica. *Int J Dermatol* 31:166, 1992.
20. Schamberg IL: Peculiar persistent pruritic affection of the skin. *Arch Dermatol* 113:986, 1977.
21. Dean EA, Bernhard JD: Recurrence of lichen simplex chronicus after surgical excision. *Cutis* 40:157–158, 1987.
22. Comings DE, Comings SN: Hereditary localized pruritus. *Arch Dermatol* 92:236–237, 1965.
23. Shaffner B: Lichen simplex chronicus and its variants. *Arch Dermatol* 64:340–351, 1951.
24. Breathnach SM: Amyloid and amyloidosis. *J Am Acad Dermatol* 18:1–16, 1988.
25. Wang W-J: Clinical features of cutaneous amyloidosis. *Clin Dermatol* 8:13–19, 1990.
26. Bernhard JD: Macular amyloidosis, notalgia paresthetica and pruritus: Three sides of the same coin? *Dermatologica* 183:53, 1991.
27. Wong C-K, Lin C-S: Friction amyloidosis. *Int J Dermatol* 27:302–307, 1988.
28. Hashimoto K, Ito K, Kumakiri M, et al: Nylon brush macular amyloidosis *Arch Dermatol* 123:633–637, 1987.
29. Liddell K; Post-herpetic pruritus. *BMJ* 4:165, 1974.
30. Harries AD, Tredree R, Heatley RV, et al: Pruritus as a manifestation of the dumping syndrome. *Br J Dermatol* 107:707–709, 1982.
31. Salter HH: *Asthma: Its pathology and treatment.* Philadelphia, Blanchard & Lee, 1864, p 62.
32. David TJ, Wybrew M, Hennessen U: Prodromal itching in childhood asthma. *Lancet* 2:154–155, 1984.
33. Wright DJM: Prodromal itching in asthma. *Lancet* 2:822, 1984.
34. Derbes VJ: Prodromal itching in asthma. *Lancet* 2:822, 1984.
35. Hines S, Houston M, Robertson D: The clinical spectrum of autonomic dysfunction. *Am J Med* 70:1091–1096, 1981.
36. Reichstein RP, Stein WG: Nasal pruritus as atypical angina? *N Engl J Med* 309:667, 1983.
37. Wartenberg R: Pruritus nasi bei hirntumoren. *Klin Wochenschr* 11:461, 1932.
38. Andreev VC, Petkov I: Skin manifestations associated with tumors of the brain. *Br J Dermatol* 92:675–678, 1975.
39. Rothman S: Physiology of itching. *Physiol Rev* 21:357–381, 1941.
40. Scott PV, Fischer HBJ: Intraspinal opiates and itching: A new reflex? *BMJ* 284:1015–1016, 1982.
41. Canizares O: Helminthic deseases I. Nematodes—cutaneous manifestations of intestinal parasites, in Canizares O, Harmon R (eds): *Clinical Tropical Dermatology,* 2d ed. Boston, Blackwell Scientific Publications, 1992, pp 324–334.
42. Sotos JG: *Zebra cards. An Aid to Obscure Diagnosis.* Nose, NO-003. Philadelphia, American College of Physicians, 1989.
43. Bernhard JD: Does thinking itch? *Lancet* 1:589, 1985.
44. Musaph H: Psychogenic pruritus. *Sem Dermatol* 2:217–222, 1983.
45. Heckerling PS: Enalapril and vulvovaginal pruritis (sic). *Ann Int Med* 112:879–880, 1990.

46. Novak E, Gilbertson TJ, Seckman CE, et al: Anorectal pruritus after intravenous hydrocortisone sodium succinate and sodium phosphate. *Clin Pharmacol Ther* 20:109–112, 1976.
47. Freeman S: Woman allergic to husband's sweat and semen. *Contact Dermatitis* 14:110–112, 1986.
48. Monk BE, Sarkany I: Localized uraemic pruritus due to arteriovenous anastomosis. *Br J Dermatol* Suppl 19 105:92–94, 1981.
49. Sullivan SN: Judo-jogger's itch. *N Engl J Med* 300:866, 1979.
50. Carmichael AJ, Weston C, Marks R, et al: Cardiac bypass pruritus: A new itch. *Br J Dermatol* Suppl 38 125:13, 1991.
51. Brewin TB: Alcohol intolerance in neoplastic disease. *BMJ* 2:437–441, 1966.
52. Sharma OP, Balchum OJ: Alcohol-induced pain and itching on hot shower in sarcoidosis. An unusual association. *Am Rev Respir Dis* 106:763–766, 1972.
53. Gupta MA, Gupta AK, Voorhees JJ: Starvation-associated pruritus: A clinical feature of eating disorders. *J Am Acad Dermatol* 27:118–120, 1992.
54. Bureau Y, Barriere E: Une etiologie trop meconnue des prurits: l'intoxication par le cafe. *Bull Soc Francaise Dermatol Syphil* 68:484, 1961.
55. Lyell A: The itching patient: A review of the causes of pruritus. *Scott Med J* 17:334–347, 1972.
56. Blankenship ML: Mite dermatitis other than scabies. *Dermatol Clin* 8:265–275, 1990.
57. Aylesworth R, Baldridge D: Dermatophagoides scheremetewskyi and feather pillow dermatitis. *Minn Med* 66:43, 1983.
58. Regan AM, Metersky ML, Craven DE: Nosocomial dermatitis and pruritus caused by pigeon mite infestation. *Arch Intern Med* 147:2185–2187, 1987.
59. Ahmed AR, Moy R, Barr AR, et al: Carpet beetle dermatitis. *J Am Acad Dermatol* 5:428–432, 1981.
60. Dinehart SM, Archer ME, Wolf JE Jr, et al. Caripito itch: Dermatitis from contact with Hylesia moths. *J Am Acad Derm* 13:743–747, 1985.
61. Lee BW: Cheyletiella dermatitis: A report of fourteen cases. *Cutis* 47:111–114, 1991.
62. Lin AN, Imaeda S: A dermatologic gazetteer. *Int J Dermatol* 29:468–471, 1990.
63. Stewart WD: Geographic dermatology. *Int J Dermatol* 29:477–478, 1990.
64. Bernhard JD, Gardner MR: Nonrashes 6. Telepathic pruritus. *Cutis* 45:59, 1990.
65. Anderson FE: The mystery of itching telephonists. *Australas J Dermatol* 27:64–66, 1986.
66. Berg M: Facial skin complaints and work at visual display units. Epidemiological, clinical and histopathological studies. *Acta Derm Venereol* (Stockh) Suppl 150, 1989.
67. Robinson P, Szewczyk M, Haddy L, et al: Outbreak of itching and rash. Epidemic hysteria in an elementary school. *Arch Intern Med* 144:1959–1962, 1984.
68. Goldstein DJ, Keiser HR: A case of flushing and organic psychosis: Reversal by opiate antagonists. *Ann Intern Med* 98:30–34, 1983.
69. Keiser HR: Personal telephone communication. September 22, 1992.
70. Shelley WB, Shelley ED: *Advanced Dermatologic Diagnosis*. Philadelphia, Saunders, 1992, p 626.
71. Torrelo A, Allegue F, Harto A: Metaphysical urticaria. *Arch Dermatol* 128:999, 1992.
72. Aubrey J: *Brief Lives*. Edited from the original manuscripts and with an introduction by Oliver Lawson Dick. London: Secker and Warburg, 1949, p 101.

FOURTEEN

SEVEN MEMORABLE ITCHES

Thomas B. Fitzpatrick

Persistent severe pruritus, like pain, is a symptom that dominates and controls all other facets of life. It may, in fact, be more maddening than pain inasmuch as pain can usually be ameliorated by analgesics but there is as yet no effective therapy for pruritus. Pruritus leads to sleepless nights; a state of permanent fatigue ensues that precludes work, and confounds and compounds family relationships.

My approach to the patient with generalized pruritus is similar to my approach to the patient with factitious dermatosis—generalized pruritus and factitious dermatosis are both diagnoses of exclusion: all possible organic causes must first be excluded. The work-up of these patients that I use is presented in Table 14-1.

The following seven patients did not have any clinical findings (i.e., *specific* skin lesions) that could readily provide a clue to the etiology of their pruritus; routine laboratory tests were negative but in some instances the diagnosis became evident with special laboratory tests (e.g., liver function tests, thyroid tests, chest X-ray) or imaging.

The pruritus in each of these patients was memorable for me because they were so miserable. We were careful to look for evidence of xerosis, a very frequent cause of generalized pruritus in older patients, who live in heated rooms with low-humidity, especially in winter in northern latitudes; oil-in-water baths followed by emollients did not have any effect on the severity of the pruritus, nor did it reduce the frequency of attacks. As will be discovered, the cryptic etiology of the pruritus was found in some but not all of the patients.

Table 14-1 Approach to the diagnosis of generalized pruritus without diagnostic skin lesions*

Initial visit

1. Detailed history of pruritus:
   are there any skin lesions that precede the itching?
   severity: does the itching keep the patient awake?
2. History of weight loss, fatigue, fever, malaise.
3. Has there been a recent emotional stress situation?
4. History of oral or parenteral medication which can be a cause of generalized pruritus without a rash. (See Chap. 23.)
5. Examine carefully for subtle primary skin disorders as a cause of the pruritus: xerosis or asteatosis, scabies, pediculosis (nits?).
6. Give the patient bath oil, followed by an emollient ointment. No soap; the bath is therapeutic, not for cleansing the skin; shower to clean.
7. Follow-up appointment in 2 weeks.

Subsequent visit(s)

If symptomatic treatment given on the first visit does not provide relief, proceed as follows:
1. Detailed review of systems.
2. General physical examination including *all* the lymph nodes; rectal examination and stool guaiac in adult patient. Refer patient for pelvic examination, pap smear.
3. Obtain chest roentgenogram.
4. Laboratory tests: complete blood count (CBC), erythrocyte sedimentation rate, fasting blood sugar, renal function tests, liver function tests, hepatitis antigens, thyroid tests, stool for parasites.
5. Consider skin biopsy.
6. If the diagnosis has not been established at this point, the patient should be referred to an internist for a complete work-up including further imaging (scans, ultrasound, etc.) if indicated.

*See also Chaps. 5 and 24.

A WEALTHY, NERVOUS, MIDDLE-AGED WIDOW WITH MANY FAMILY PROBLEMS: ALL ATTEMPTS FAILED TO CONTROL HER GENERALIZED PRURITUS

This patient was vexing to all the physicians whom she had seen, as they had not been able to control her generalized pruritus. There were serious problems at home and these were regarded by all to be the major cause of the pruritus. Laboratory tests were negative. Because of her long periods of sleepless nights and out of mere frustration we put her in the hospital for rest and sedation. During the hospital stay one of the medical consultants suggested a liver biopsy despite the negative liver function tests, including the alkaline phosphatase. Much to our surprise, she was discovered, on liver biopsy, to have biliary cirrhosis—the cause of her pruritus, despite the normal value of alkaline phosphatase. At the time, the antimitochondrial antibody test was not available; no treatment helped.

AN AGITATED 38-YEAR-OLD DIVORCE LAWYER WITH GENERALIZED INTRACTABLE PRURITUS

This patient was so nervous that he could barely sit on the examining table. He had a very successful law practice and was overwhelmed with professional work. We attributed his generalized pruritus to the stress of his practice. Several screening tests were performed to search for causes of the pruritus and one showed very high T4 levels. The generalized pruritus was the presenting symptom of thyrotoxicosis, and with treatment of this, the pruritus completely disappeared.

A CONSERVATIVELY DRESSED FINANCIER WITH ITCHING FOR 6 MONTHS LOCALIZED TO THE ANTERIOR CHEST AND UPPER AND LOWER ABDOMEN

This patient, aged 53 years, was an investment counsellor, conservatively dressed in a three-piece suit. There was a history of itching for 6 months, but this was strictly localized to the skin from the hairy presternal region to the pubic area. There were no skin lesions. Heat increased the itching and it was much worse after he went to bed. His wife did not have any itching. The attacks of pruritus were episodic, periods of weeks would go by with only mild pruritus. The patient was not taking any medication. A peculiar feature was the strict limitation of the pruritus to a quadrilateral area from the sternum to the pubic symphysis; there was intense itching around the navel.

I then sat down and with a head magnifier slowly surveyed the skin that itched so intensely. On examination, the presternal area contained tiny dark crusts that looked like dried blood and could be scraped off. On close examination of the pubic hair, on the hairs around the navel and in the presternal area there were nits. The diagnosis was pubic lice. I had never seen this disorder involve the hair on the upper chest or around the navel. There were no nits on the eyelashes. After he was informed that he had pubic lice he told of his contact with a female teacher 6 months previously at a convention in Los Angeles. He was concerned about AIDS and syphilis but both of these tests were negative. Apparently he did not have any contact with his wife for the 6-month period.

THE SPEECHLESS STROKE PATIENT WITH INTRACTABLE GENERALIZED PRURITUS

This 75-year-old patient could not speak and constantly pointed to scratch marks on his skin. He was a prominent merchant who had had a cerebrovascular accident 2 years previously that left him paralyzed on the left side and without any speech.

The pruritus began at the time the stroke occurred. He had developed some lichenification from constant scratching, and by the use of corticosteroids and plastic wrap we were able to slightly improve his pruritus. Nevertheless, his wife related tales of his scratching for hours without stopping, night and day. We were completely helpless in giving him relief from his pruritus.

We never discovered the etiology of this patient's intractable pruritus and wondered whether he could have had an infarct in an area of the central nervous system that could result in "spontaneous activity in diencephalic or cerebral structures mediating pruritus" as was reported by King, Huff, and Jorizzo.[1]

THE MANAGING EDITOR OF A LARGE NEWSPAPER WITH INTRACTABLE PRURITUS THAT FAILED TO RESPOND TO ORAL PREDNISONE

I received a call from the managing editor of a large metropolitan newspaper who had a 6-month history of pruritus that was not controlled by any medication that had been given him by his internist. He had not seen a dermatologist. He had been given oral prednisone but this did not help at all. This patient was a friend of my family and I felt it necessary to ask him to make a trip to Boston. When he arrived I discovered that he had pubic lice! The nits were difficult to detect except by careful inspection.

SUDDEN ONSET OF SEVERE INTRACTABLE GENERALIZED PRURITUS WHILE 60-YEAR-OLD MAN WAS WALKING HIS DOG

This patient, apparently healthy, took his dog for their customary walk in the city one evening. In a matter of a few minutes he noted intense pruritus on the chest area and later when he returned home there was a generalized pruritus but no rash was evident. He could not get to sleep at all that night and the next day he consulted a dermatologist who gave him a topical antipruritic containing camphor and menthol, some oatmeal baths, and an antihistamine. After a second night of no sleep he was sent to us and we decided to obtain laboratory tests and a chest X-ray. We found a large hilar mass; subsequent studies led to a diagnosis of Hodgkin's disease. Following treatment, the pruritus disappeared.

A PHLEGMATIC PRIEST
WHO ITCHED MADLY FOR WEEKS

A big (6′3″) 55-year-old Irish-American Catholic priest was beside himself with intense generalized pruritus. He had been seen by a dermatologist and a biopsy had been obtained of a 4.0-mm shiny reddish brown nodule on his buttocks—this was one of only three similar nodules of 4.0 to 7.0 mm on the buttock. This was read as mycosis fungoides by a highly qualified dermatopathologist. The patient was sent to me for a second opinion. I could not believe that these few papules could be mycosis fungoides—possibly lymphomatoid papulosis but not mycosis fungoides. I was, moreover, perplexed by the *generalized* pruritus that accompanied these few lesions, localized to the buttock area. In another biopsy of one of these nodules we were able to detect portions of the scabies mite in the stratum corneum. The message here is: In a patient with severe generalized itching and in whom the clinical presentation is consistent with scabies but in whom all attempts to demonstrate the organism have failed, obtain a biopsy.[2]

REFERENCES

1. King CA, Huff J, Jorizzo JL: Unilateral neurogenic pruritus: Paroxysmal itching associated with central nervous system lesions. *Ann Intern Med* 97:222–223, 1982.
2. Head ES, Macdonald EM, Ewert A, et al: Sarcoptes scabei in histopathologic sections of skin in human scabies. *Arch Dermatol* 126:1475–1477, 1990.

SYSTEMIC ASPECTS OF PRURITUS

CHAPTER FIFTEEN

RENAL ITCH

Andrew J. Carmichael

INTRODUCTION

Intolerable itching, without primary skin manifestations, associated with chronic uremia, was originally described by Rosenstein[1] over a century ago. The first investigative work in the field was performed by Chargin and Keil in 1932.[2] In the ensuing half century great advances have been made in medicine, resulting in prolongation of life. Part of the expense of this progress has been increased morbidity, exemplified by the management of chronic renal failure (CRF) and the ability to treat patients with dialysis.

As the number of patients in dialysis programs continues to expand, without a corresponding increase in the rate of transplantation, the population in CRF grows (Fig. 15-1). Thus, effective treatment of the attendant complications, such as anemia, hyperparathyroidism, hypertension, peripheral neuropathy, and pruritus becomes ever more important. Fortunately, many of these complications are now amenable to therapy. For example, erythropoietin is now available for the treatment of the anemia.[3] In sad contrast, the last 50 years has seen little progress in our understanding of either the mechanism, or the management of renal itch.[4,5]

Why should there be such inertia in renal itch? There is the unspoken suspicion that the itch is viewed by the nephrologist as unimportant. The dermatologist, confronted every day by unexplained itch, recites the difficulty of its quantification and takes refuge in a diagnosis—"uremic pruritus"— which in reality is merely a descriptive label, masking poor understanding.

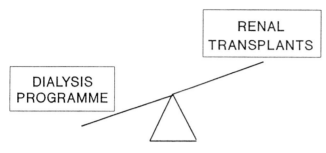

Figure 15-1 The problem.

DEFINITION

"Renal itch" is localized or generalized itch, occurring in a patient with CRF, where there is no primary cutaneous disease and no other systemic or psychological dysfunction that might cause pruritus. It is unfortunate that the term uremic pruritus is used synonymously by some authors for this condition, as the implication that the itch results from a raised serum urea is untrue.

EPIDEMIOLOGY

Renal itch is a feature of chronic, not acute, kidney failure. The epidemiology of renal itch is extremely unreliable because of the difficulty in defining this most subjective of symptoms, the limited number of patients in most of the series, and the retrospective nature of some of the information.[6]

The wide range of figures quoted for the prevalence of renal pruritus in those on dialysis, 41 to 86 percent,[7,8] epitomizes the problem. The occurrence of renal itch is not associated with sex, age, race, duration of dialysis, or etiology of the renal failure.[6,8,9]

In the majority of those affected, the itch is paroxysmal and may be localized (56%) or generalized (44%).[6] Patients on continuous ambulatory peritoneal dialysis (CAPD) are less affected by itch than those on hemodialysis.[7] Whether this reflects the different personality types allocated to these modes of dialysis, the boredom factor associated with hemodialysis, or the differences in the filtration properties of the membranes in the two types of dialysis is unresolved.

The incidence of pruritus increases with deterioration of renal function. Nielsen and colleagues[10] reported pruritus in less than 30 percent of pre-dialysis patients (mean serum creatinine level 580μmol/l), whereas 70 percent of dialysis patients with terminal renal failure suffered with itch. The impact of dialysis on pruritus is slight. Young and colleagues[9] recorded amelioration of pruritus in only 11 percent of patients within 6 months of starting dialysis.

Renal itch has been shown to be an independent marker of mortality at 3 years for patients on hemodialysis.[11]

ETIOLOGY

The etiology of renal itch is unknown. In order to try and chart a logical path through the many hypotheses put forward, this discussion will initially consider stimuli, then facilitatory factors, alteration of itch receptors and afferent nerve fibers, and finally central modulation (Fig. 15-2).

Stimuli

Histamine, as one of the few known endogenous chemicals capable of inducing itch, deserves thorough investigation. Suspicion of its potential role was heightened by Neiman and colleague's chance observation[12] that uremic patients undergoing hemodialysis show proliferation of mast cells in spleen, bone-marrow, bowel wall, and skin. Subsequent work,[13] however, has demonstrated that dermal mast cell proliferation appears to be a response to extracorporeal circulation of blood. No mast cell proliferation was seen in those not on hemodialysis with renal itch and no difference was noted in the number of mast cells between those with and those free from pruritus in

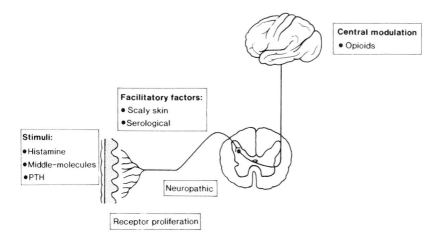

Figure 15-2 Possible etiological factors in renal itch.

end stage renal failure. Further evidence which argues against endogenous histamine as the cause of renal itch, is the demonstration of a lowered histamine itch threshold and the ability to rapidly develop tachyphylaxis to histamine in uremic patients.[14] However, the debate remains unresolved, with two groups[15,16] having detected raised circulating histamine levels in patients on hemodialysis, most marked in those suffering with itch.

There is an hypothesis that renal itch results from the accumulation of poorly dialyzed compounds—so called "middle molecules"—that cross dialysis membranes more slowly than smaller molecules such as creatinine. With further developments in dialysis membranes, removal of such middle molecules may become a possibility, thereby clarifying their role in the pruritus.

Parathyroid gland activity is commonly increased in chronic renal failure. In 1968 two reports[17,18] appeared suggesting that parathyroid hormone (PTH) may have a permissive role in renal itch. This hypothesis has not stood the test of time. When levels of circulating PTH have been measured no correlation with itch has been demonstrated.[10,19] Immunohistochemical studies have failed to demonstrate the presence of PTH peripherally in the skin and intradermal injection of PTH failed to produce itch.[20] There is, therefore, no evidence that PTH acts as a peripheral mediator of renal itch and only anecdotal suggestions that it has a role at all.

Facilitatory Factors

Itch threshold in CRF is lowered, perhaps reflecting an "itch-friendly" environment in the skin. Dry skin is the most frequent dermatological feature of CRF.[7] The frequency of pruritus is significantly higher in those with clinically diagnosed xerosis.[8,10] When this dry or xerotic skin has been objectively investigated, its hydration is not reduced[21]—scaliness in CRF has been misinterpreted as dryness. Why the skin is scaly in CRF and why it should itch are unanswered. One could hypothesize a unifying role for vitamin A, which is elevated in the epidermis in chronic renal failure[22] and is associated with scaly skin.

The contribution of circulating factors to the milieu has been investigated from a number of points of view. Serological parameters, when ranked with the degree of itch, have shown a significant correlation with the concentration of magnesium and phosphate.[19] This observation is interesting in view of a previous report of resolution of renal pruritus on a low magnesium dialysate.[23] However, subsequent use of a magnesium-free dialysate failed to show a role for magnesium, despite adequate lowering of the serum magnesium.[24] The positive association with phosphate has not been the experience of other workers[7] and the suspicion that phosphate acts as a marker of the adequacy of dialysis has not been confirmed by analysis of the clearances on dialysis.[25] There is anecdotal evidence of a role for aluminum overload in prurigo nodularis in patients on maintenance hemodialysis. Treatment of three such patients with the chelating agent desferrioxamine resulted in resolution of the itch within 1 month.[26]

Receptors

The receptors responsible for itch have not been clearly defined. Of interest is controversial work[27] that showed increased neuron-specific enolase activity extending into the epidermis in those with CRF. These findings require confirmation, in view of the contradictory data from Fantini and colleagues.[28] It is also difficult to explain the abruptness of the response to transplantation if receptor proliferation plays a major role.

Afferent Nerve Fibers

Peripheral neuropathy affects 65 percent of patients about to begin dialysis[29] and is the other main complication of CRF, equally defying a mechanism and treatment.[30] Clinically it may present with paresthesia or dysesthesia although not "restless legs".[31] It is interesting to conjecture that the itch could be a manifestation of the neuropathy.

Central Modulation

Given the poor definition of the ascending pathway of itch, one can speculate widely on central modulation of its perception. In broad terms it could be that dialysis results in the accumulation of a substance capable of facilitating itch transmission in the spinal cord, or having a stimulatory effect on the perception of itch. A favorite candidate for this putative pruritogen must be the opioids. A decade ago several groups produced work indicating opioids have a pruritogenic effect.[32,33] More recently Thornton and Losowsky[34] have shown opioid accumulation in those with hepatic impairment and that therapy with an opiate antagonist resulted in marked improvement of associated hepatic pruritus. Opioids accumulate in renal failure,[35–37] are unrelated to the duration of dialysis and are unaltered by hemodialysis.[36] Renal itch shares all these features and raises the important possibility of opioids having a pivotal role in renal itch, as they appear to in hepatic pruritus.

THERAPEUTICS

The number of treatments that have been tried in uremic pruritus bears witness to the challenge it offers dermatologists. In our enthusiasm to find a solution to this most troublesome problem, we must not overlook the altered physiology, pharmacokinetics, and overwhelming hospital dependency of those affected with CRF.

Antihistamines

There can be few instances of pruritus in which antihistamines have not been tried, despite the very limited role of histamine in producing pathological itch—a reflection of dermatological impotence in treating itch. When antihistamines have been given in renal itch, the response has been at best marginal.[6] An isolated report relates improvement in five patients on hemodialysis treated with the putative mast cell stabilizing agent ketotifen.[16] More recently De Marchi and colleagues[38] observed a reduction of itch and histamine levels in a small group of patients with chronic renal insufficiency, who had received erythropoietin. This response of the renal itch to erythropoietin has not been confirmed by a subsequent larger study in dialysis patients.[39]

Correction of the Milieu

Emollients are another of the staffs of dermatology. When patients with renal pruritus have been surveyed, only 17 percent derived benefit from this mode of therapy.[6]

Correcting hypermagnesemia[23] cannot be recommended, as it was not successful in the short term when examined according to a double-blind protocol, and caused hyperparathyroidism.[24]

Despite the impressive small series reporting dramatic improvement of itch following parathyroidectomy,[17,18] subsequent work has failed to define a role for parathyroid hormone in renal itch.[20]

Detoxification

The implication that CRF results in the accumulation of a pruritogen is reinforced by evidence that a number of detoxificants have shown a beneficial effect in renal itch. The metabolic load can be reduced by prescribing a low-protein amino-acid supplemented diet. Although apparently successful in improving renal itch,[40] further loss of choice, in an already severely restricted life style, makes long-term compliance most unlikely.

Alternatively, various systemic therapies, thought to work by chelating an unidentified pruritogen, have been described. Oral activated charcoal is inexpensive, has a favorable side-effect profile, and showed impressive results in a double-blind cross-over trial.[41] Cholestyramine has had more varied success,[42,43] is less acceptable to patients, and care should be taken to monitor for acidemia in those not on dialysis.[44] Twice daily intravenous heparin, a recognized detoxifying agent, has shown benefit in a small open trial,[45] but the literature has since been silent on the role of this agent. Practically, the risk in allowing patients to give themselves intravenous heparin injections condemns this treatment option.

To augment the diminished glomerular function, stimulation of the sweat glands with saunas has shown benefit,[46] perhaps by encouraging excretion of a pruritogen. At a practical level, the concept of a sauna "en suite" to dialysis units is a little surreal and the unquantifiable insensible water loss could cause major complications with fluid balance.

Altered Nerve Conduction

Lidocaine is a membrane-stabilizing antiarrhythmic, metabolized in the liver, with a normal plasma half-life in patients in renal failure. An impressive response of renal itch to parenteral lidocaine was achieved in a double-blind trial by Tapia and colleagues.[47] Why the benefit lasted 24 hours, given the drug's short half-life, is unexplained. The potential side effects of this therapy were also significant, highlighted by two patients who developed acute hypotension, one progressing to a grand mal convulsion. As maintenance therapy, daily intravenous lidocaine is impractical, but mechanistically the response is interesting. It lends support to the neuropathic hypothesis and suggests that an orally active, membrane-stabilizing antiarrhythmic, with a longer half-life, less liable to produce acute toxicity, might be a useful drug in the management of renal itch. Mexiletine is such a drug and is metabolized in the liver.

Topical capsaicin depletes and prevents the reaccumulation of substance P in peripheral nerves. Breneman and colleagues[48] reported benefit with this agent in a few patients with renal itch.

Central Modulation

A controlled trial of a modified acupuncture technique, electrical needle stimulation (ENS), has been beneficial,[49] presumably through modulation of the transmission of itch afferents, and is an area of investigation with potential.

The capacity for sedative antihistamines to be effective in itch has been clearly shown to be due to decreased central perception but represents a very blunt means of decreasing itch sensation. Undoubtedly, occasions arise in which the need to suppress renal itch warrants this crude tool. Prescribers should ensure that the sedative chosen is not renally excreted and thereby risk inducing toxicity.

Phototherapy

The role of phototherapy in renal pruritus must be assessed by double-blind trials, in view of the potential for placebo response.[50,51] UVB has generally,[52–54] although not uniformly,[55] been shown to be therapeutic (see Chap. 28). However, the need for the patient to attend another department on a regular basis and be subjected to further machine dependence should not be underestimated. Equally, the potentially carcinogenic effect of the ultraviolet radiation in a group of patients prospectively known to be at great risk of epidermal dysplasia, once they receive their transplantation and begin life-long immunosuppression,[56] requires serious consideration.

MANAGEMENT

Faced by a patient with generalized pruritus and renal failure, how should the dermatologist proceed? Table 15-1 provides a summary.

Of primary importance is confirmation of the diagnosis. Significant renal failure must be identified, and its chronicity established. The latter can be difficult, in view of the silent nature of the presentation of CRF. Indicators include: a history of several months of nocturia, lassitude, and fluid overload; investigations at presentation showing a normochromic normocytic anemia and hyperphosphatemia; and best, but not always available, reviewing previous levels of urea and creatinine over several months. Other causes for pruritus should be excluded through a combination of history, examination, and screening investigations. There are no primary manifestations of renal pruritus, although the skin may show signs of scratching, with excoriations and lichenification, as well as features of CRF, such as scaling, hyperpigmentation, and "half and half" nails.

When the diagnosis of renal itch is confirmed, it is important to establish the severity of the problem, through enquiry of its interference with the patient's life style and semiquantitative assessment using visual analog scales. Excoriations provide more objective evidence for assessment and can be most relevant, as severe secondary skin infection may act as a contraindication to transplantation, in view of the subsequent risk with immunosuppression. For patients whose life has been taken over by itching there will be no

Table 15-1 Summary of management of renal itch

- Establish diagnosis of chronic renal failure.
- Exclude primary dermatosis and systemic or psychological causes for itch.
- Quantify severity of the problem.
- Trial of:
  - (a) Oral activated charcoal 6 g daily.
  - (b) Cholestyramine 5 g b.d.
  - (c) Ultraviolet radiation (short course).
- Encourage transplant program.

debate on the need for treatment—indeed they will demand help. For others the decision will be less straightforward.

Currently two oral medications can be recommended. Both are economical and convenient, but need to be taken on a long-term basis. Oral activated charcoal, at a dose of 6 g once a day in capsule form, is preferable, as it is acceptable to patients, is safe, and showed an excellent response in the only double-blind cross-over study reported.[41] Cholestyramine at a dose of 5 g twice a day can also be successful,[42] but its unpalatable nature and high incidence of gastrointestinal side effects raises serious doubts over long-term compliance. It should be used with extreme caution in those not on dialysis because of the risk of acidosis.[44]

If these oral therapies prove ineffective one can consider the use of ultraviolet radiation. This treatment carries two major drawbacks: further machine and hospital dependence and the potential risk of future nonmelanoma skin cancer. The latter reason may make this treatment inadvisable for long-term use in certain patients.

Ultimately, although some of these measures may help, only renal transplantation will guarantee a complete cure of the pruritus. Dermatologists must make every effort to encourage the transplant program to try and redress the current imbalance between those starting dialysis and those being transplanted.

THE FUTURE

The etiology and mechanism underlying renal itch requires definition. Three areas particularly worthy of further attention in CRF are: cutaneous innervation; vitamin A and opioid kinetics; and dynamics.

Stahle-Backdahl[27] has demonstrated an increased epidermal activity of neuron-specific enolase in dialysis patients. These findings must be confirmed and their relevance explored. Itch as a manifestation of peripheral neuropathy requires consideration by quantification and correlation.

The commonly observed scaliness of the skin in CRF is unexplained, but there is evidence associating it with the pruritus.[10] Vitamin A metabolism is altered in uremia, resulting in excess epidermal retinol.[22] Theoretically, the chelating agents activated charcoal and cholestyramine might partially correct this excess. Equally, ultraviolet light has been shown to decrease epidermal retinol.[57] The hypothesis that altered vitamin A status has a central role in both the scaliness and itch of CRF needs further investigation.

Opioids are thought to have a facilitatory effect on pruritus centrally.[32–34] Opioid metabolism is partially renal-dependent.[35] Measurement of opioid levels in renal failure and their correlation with itch is needed. Therapeutically, the role of opioid antagonists deserves investigation.

CONCLUSION

Renal itch is a common problem in those with CRF, contributing significantly to the morbidity of many on long-term dialysis. With the number of patients awaiting transplantation increasing, the relevance grows.

The mechanism responsible for renal itch is undefined. Treatment is often difficult, but oral activated charcoal, cholystyramine, and possibly UVB are worth considering for those well motivated by severe pruritus. The definitive treatment is transplantation.

The cause for renal itch requires further investigation. Avenues worthy of exploration include cutaneous innervation, and vitamin A and opioid kinetics and dynamics in CRF. It is the responsibility of dermatologists to take up the challenge offered by renal itch to help resolve one of the outstanding sources of morbidity for those on dialysis.

ACKNOWLEDGMENTS

I am grateful to Dr. A. Y. Finlay for his constructive criticism of this chapter.

REFERENCES

1. Thursfeld H: *Tr Med-Chir Soc Edinburgh* 83:221, 1990.
2. Chargin L, Keil H: Skin diseases in nonsurgical renal disease. *Arch Dermatol Syph* 26:314, 1932.
3. Eschbach JW, Egrie JC, Downing MR, et al: Correction of the anemia of end-stage renal disease with recombinant human erythropoietin. *N Engl J Med* 316:73, 1987.
4. Rosen T: Uremic pruritus: A review. *Cutis* 23:790, 1979.
5. Ponticelli C, Bencini PL: Uremic pruritus: A review. *Nephron* 60:1, 1992.
6. Gilchrest BA, Stern RS, Steinman TI, et al: Clinical features of pruritus among patients undergoing maintenance hemodialysis. *Arch Dermatol* 118:154, 1982.
7. Bencini PL, Montagnino G, Citterio A, et al: Cutaneous abnormalities in uremic patients. *Nephron* 40:316, 1985.
8. Young AW, Sweeney EW, David DS et al: Dermatological evaluation of pruritus in patients on hemodialysis. *N Y State J Med* 73:2670, 1973.
9. Stahle-Backdahl M, Hagermark O, Lins L-E: Pruritus in patients on maintenance hemodialysis. *Acta Med Scand* 224:55, 1988.
10. Nielsen T, Hemmeloff Andersen KE, Kristiansen J: Pruritus and xerosis in patients with chronic renal failure. *Dan Med Bull* 27:269, 1980.
11. Carmichael AJ, McHugh MI, Martin AM: Renal itch as an indicator of poor outcome. *Lancet* 337:1225, 1991.
12. Neiman RS, Bischel MD, Lukes RJ: Uraemia and mast-cell proliferation. *Lancet* i:959, 1972.
13. Matsumoto M, Ichimaru K, Horie A: Pruritus and mast cell proliferation of the skin in end stage renal failure. *Clin Nephrol* 23:285, 1985.
14. Stahle-Backdahl M, Hagermark O, Lins L-E: The sensitivity of uremic and normal human skin to histamine. *Acta Derm Venereol* (Stockh) 68:230, 1988.

15. Stockenhuber F, Kurz RW, Sertl K, et al: Increased plasma histamine levels in uraemic pruritus. *Clin Sci* 79:477, 1990.
16. Francos GC, Kauh YC, Gittlen SD, et al: Elevated plasma histamine in chronic uremia. Effects of ketotifen on pruritus. *Int J Dermatol* 30:884,1991.
17. Hampers CL, Katz AI, Wilson RE, et al: Disappearance of "uremic" itching after subtotal parathyroidectomy. *N Engl J Med* 279:695, 1968.
18. Massry SG, Popovtzer MM, Coburn JW, et al: Intractable pruritus as a manifestation of secondary hyperparathyroidism in uremia. Disappearance of itching after subtotal parathyroidectomy. *N Engl J Med* 279:697, 1968.
19. Carmichael AJ, McHugh MM, Martin AM, et al: Serological markers of renal itch in patients receiving long term haemodiaysis. *BMJ* 296:1575, 1988.
20. Stahle-Backdahl M, Hagermark O, Lins L-E, et al: Experimental and immunohistochemical studies on the possible role of parathyroid hormone in uraemic pruritus. *J Intern Med* 225:411, 1989.
21. Stahle-Backdahl M: Stratum corneum hydration in patients undergoing maintenance hemodiaysis. *Acta Derm Venereol* (Stockh)68:531, 1988.
22. Vahlquist A, Berne B, Berne C: Skin content and plasma transport of vitamin A and beta-carotene in chronic renal failure. *Eur J Clin Invest* 12:63, 1982.
23. Graf H, Kovarik J, Stummvoll HK, et al: Disappearance of uraemic pruritus after lowering dialysate magnesium concentration. *BMJ* ii:1478, 1979.
24. Carmichael AJ, Dickinson F, McHugh MI, et al: Magnesium free dialysis for uraemic pruritus. *BMJ* 297:1584, 1988.
25. Carmichael AJ, McHugh MI, Martin AM: Itch unrelated to adequacy of haemodialysis. *Br J Dermatol* 126:95, 1992.
26. Brown MA, George CRP, Dunstan CR, et al: Prurigo nodularis and aluminum overload in maintenance haemodialysis. *Lancet* 340:48, 1992.
27. Stahle-Backdahl M: Uremic pruritus. Clinical and experimental studies. *Acta Derm Venereol* (Stockh) 69(Suppl 145):28, 1989.
28. Fantini F, Baraldi A, Sevignani C, et al: Cutaneous innervation in chronic renal failure patients. An immunohistochemical study. *Acta Derm Venereol*(Stockh) 72:102, 1992.
29. Robson JS: Uraemic neuropathy, some aspects of neurology. Robertson RF (ed): Edinburgh, Royal College of Physicians, 74, 1968.
30. Nielsen VK: The peripheral nerve function in chronic renal failure. Intercorrelation of clinical symptoms and signs and clinical grading of neuropathy. *Acta Med Scand* 190:113, 1971.
31. Raskin NH, Fishman RA: Neurological disorders in renal failure. *N Engl J Med* 294:204, 1976.
32. Bernstein JE, Swift R: Relief of intractable pruritus with naloxone. *Arch Dermatol* 115:1366, 1979.
33. Summerfield JA: Naloxone modulates the perception of itch in man. *Br J Clin Pharmac* 10:180, 1980.
34. Thornton JR, Losowsky MS: Opioid peptides and primary biliary cirrhosis. *BMJ* 297:1501, 1988.
35. Thornton JR, Losowsky MS: A role for the kidney and liver in plasma beta-endorphin elimination? *Clin Sci* 74:(Suppl 18) 51, 1988.
36. Hwang J-C, Hsu K-T, Tsai H-C, et al: Serum endorphin levels in uremic patients under maintenance hemodialysis. *J Formosan Med Assoc* 88:360, 1989.
37. Yamakado M, Tagawa H, Kiyose H, et al: Plasma β-endorphin in patients on maintenance hemodialysis. *Nippon Jinzo Gakkai Shi* 31:963, 1989.
38. De Marchi S, Cecchin E, Villatta D, et al: Relief of pruritus and decrease in plasma histamine concentrations during erythropoietin therapy in patients with uremia. *N Engl J Med* 326:969, 1992.

39. Balaskas EV, Uldall RP. Erythropoietin treatment does not improve uremic pruritus. *Perit Dial Int* 12:330, 1992.
40. Boulton-Jones JM, Sissons JGP, Harrison ER: Itching in renal failure. *Lancet* i:355, 1974.
41. Pederson JA, Matter BJ, Czerwinski AW, et al: Relief of idiopathic generalised pruritus in dialysis patients treated with activated oral charcoal. *Ann Intern Med* 93:446, 1980.
42. Silverberg DS, Iaina A, Reisin E, et al: Cholestyramine in uraemic pruritus. *BMJ* i:752, 1977.
43. Van Leusen R, Kutsch Lojenga JC, Th Ruben A: Is cholestyramine helpful in uraemic pruritus? *BMJ* i:918, 1978.
44. Wrong OM: Cholestyramine in uraemic pruritus. *BMJ* i:1662, 1977.
45. Yatzidis H, Digenis P, Tountas C: Heparin treatment of uremic itching. *JAMA* 222:1183, 1972.
46. Snyder D, Merrill JP: Sauna baths in the treatment of chronic renal failure. *Trans Amer Soc Artif Int Organs* 12:188, 1966.
47. Tapia L, Cheigh JS, David DS, et al: Pruritus in dialysis patients treated with parenteral lidocaine. *N Engl J Med* 296:261, 1977.
48. Breneman DL, Cardone JS, Blumsack RF, et al: Topical capsaicin for treatment of hemodialysis-related pruritus. *J Am Acad Dermatol* 26:91, 1992.
49. Duo LJ: Electrical needle therapy of uremic pruritus. *Nephron* 47:179, 1987.
50. Taylor R, Taylor AEM, Diffey BL, et al: A placebo-controlled trial of UVA phototherapy for the treatment of uraemic pruritus. *Nephron* 33:14, 1983.
51. Spiro JG, Scott S, MacMillan J, et al: Treatment of uremic pruritus with blue light. *Photodermatol Photoimmunol Photomed* 2:319, 1985.
52. Saltzer EI: Relief from uremic pruritus: A therapeutic approach. *Cutis* 16:298, 1975.
53. Gilchrest BA, Rowe JW, Brown RS, et al: Relief of uremic pruritus with ultraviolet phototherapy. *N Engl J Med* 297:136, 1977.
54. Shultz BC, Roenigk HH: Uremic pruritus treated with ultraviolet light. *JAMA* 243:1836, 1980.
55. Simpson NB, Davison AM: Ultraviolet phototherapy for uraemic pruritus. *Lancet* i:781, 1981.
56. Shuttleworth D, Marks R, Griffin PJA, et al: Epidermal dysplasia and cyclosporine therapy in renal transplant patients: A comparison with azathioprine. *Br J Dermatol* 120:551, 1989.
57. Berne B, Vahlquist A, Fischer T, et al: UV treatment of uraemic pruritus reduces the vitamin A content of the skin. *Eur J Clin Invest* 14:203, 1984.

SIXTEEN

CHOLESTATIC PRURITUS

C.N. Ghent

DEFINITION

Cholestatic Pruritus

Various disciplines within medicine define cholestasis differently. Pathologists define it by the presence of identifiable bile stasis, that is, discrete plugs within bile canaliculi, interlobular ducts, or neocholangioles, or diffusely within hepatocytes on microscopic examination of liver tissue.[1] This definition of cholestasis does not correlate well with the presence of absence of cholestatic pruritus—many patients with severe histologic cholestasis will have no pruritus, and conversely patients with certain disorders will itch for months or years before histologic cholestasis develops. Furthermore, this definition presupposes that liver tissue has been obtained for examination. For the physician faced with a patient complaining of generalized pruritus, this definition of cholestasis is not particularly useful.

Clinical physicians and physiologists define cholestasis as a decrease from normal in the production and/or flow of bile.[2] As there are no noninvasive, readily available tests to determine the rate of bile production and flow in human subjects, this definition also lacks clinical utility. It is by inference that one can assume that patients with conjugated hyperbilirubinemia have cholestasis. However, bilirubin is only a minor component of bile, and absence of hyperbilirubinemia does not exclude cholestasis as the cause of itching.

Practically, in the liver clinic, a history of generalized pruritus is usually considered prima facie evidence of cholestasis as a component of the liver disorder being investigated. In the dermatology clinic, cholestasis in the patient with generalized pruritus often may be diagnosed only indirectly by physical signs or laboratory tests pointing to hepatobiliary abnormalities or a specific diagnosis. In many situations, cholestatic pruritus is a difficult condition to define and, therefore, difficult to diagnose with confidence without also diagnosing a precise underlying hepatobiliary disorder.

EPIDEMIOLOGY AND CLINICAL FEATURES

Few studies document the incidence or prevalence of cholestatic pruritus overall.[3] Unless questioning about itch is routine, its incidence and prevalence in chronic liver disease will be underestimated, as patients fail to report it. Nevertheless, certain hepatobiliary diseases are commonly accompanied by pruritus whereas others are not. A partial list of these is shown in Table 16-1.

Pruritus is often an early symptom in chronic cholestasis, developing years before any other manifestations of liver disease. A high index of suspicion of cholestasis is necessary in all patients presenting with generalized

Table 16-1 Association of liver diseases with pruritus

Commonly associated	Not commonly associated
Primary·biliary cirrhosis	Alcoholic cirrhosis
Primary sclerosing cholangitis	Hemochromatosis
Obstructive choledocholithiasis	Wilson's disease
Chronic pancreatitis with obstruction of common bile duct	Chronic hepatitis B
Carcinoma of head of pancreas	Autoimmune chronic active hepatitis
Carcinoma of bile ducts	Cholestasis of sepsis
Drug-induced cholestasis	
Estrogens	
Phenothiazines	
Allopurinol	
Erythromycin	
Nitrofurantoins	
Chronic rejection of liver transplant	
Acute viral hepatitis	
Chronic hepatitis C	
Cholestasis of pregnancy	
Familial estrogen-induced cholestasis	
Alagilles syndrome	
Biliary atresia	
Byler's disease	
Porphyria cutanea tarda[a]	

[a] Accompanied by rash.

pruritus. The pruritus is typically worst on the hands and feet and around tight-fitting clothing and is often most pronounced at night. It may be intermittent and mild and so insidious in onset that patients will ignore it or more commonly, attribute it to "dry skin." As patients seldom make the mental connection between liver disease and itch, this symptom may be overlooked even in those with known chronic liver disease unless they are carefully questioned about it.

The physical findings are rarely specific but may give clues to cholestasis as the cause of generalized pruritus. Jaundice is an obvious potent clue but is often absent. Peripheral stigmata of chronic liver disease such as spider nevi, white nails, Dupuytren's contractures, and gynecomastia in males are usually absent in the course of chronic cholestatic liver disease. A very useful sign is the presence of xanthelasma strongly suggesting hypercholesterolemia which is a feature of chronic cholestasis in many patients. Abdominal examination may provide further clues if palpable splenomegaly, abnormal venous collaterals, or ascites is present. These findings suggest complicating portal hypertension. The size and consistency of a palpable liver edge may confirm the presence of chronic liver disease, but these features are subjective and very dependent on the experience of the examiner.

Primary Biliary Cirrhosis

The incidence, natural history, and prognosis of this disorder has been extensively studied.[4–10] Itch is associated with this disease at some point during its course in approximately 80 percent of patients and is the major presenting complaint in about 60 percent. This disease is notable for its long anicteric phase, with the insidious onset of nonspecific fatigue and pruritus and its associations with other autoimmune diseases. Ninety percent of patients with this disease are female. Any woman presenting to a dermatologist or family physician with persistent fatigue and generalized pruritus should be suspected of having this disease. From extrapolation of incidence and prevalence studies in Great Britain[11,12] and in Ontario, Canada,[13] the incidence appears to be about 3 per million per year with a prevalence of approximately 20 per million. There is no marked racial, geographic, or familial clustering.

Primary Sclerosing Cholangitis

Primary sclerosing cholangitis is a somewhat rarer disease than primary biliary cirrhosis.[14] It begins at any age, affects both sexes equally and is associated with chronic inflammatory bowel disease in 30 to 80 percent of subjects.[15] This disease is much more likely to be accompanied by fluctuating jaundice, pyrexia, abdominal pain, and intermittent pruritus than is primary biliary cirrhosis, although the onset in both is typically insidious. It is also more variable in its course than primary biliary cirrhosis and recent reports have emphasized the better prognosis than was previously reported, with median survival from the time of diagnosis exceeding 10 years.[16,17] Primary sclerosing cholangitis is mainly a radiologic diagnosis based on endoscopic retrograde (ERCP) or percutaneous transhepatic cholangiography (Fig. 16-1). In contrast, primary biliary cirrhosis is diagnosed by liver biopsy and positive serologic tests for mitochondrial antibodies.

Detailed discussion of the epidemiology of the other disease entities in Table 16-1 is beyond the scope of this chapter but a few generalities are worthy of mention. All of those diseases associated with acute obstruction of the extrahepatic ducts are usually accompanied by jaundice of short duration and an abrupt onset of pruritus. The jaundiced alcohol abuser who complains of pruritus should be suspected of having biliary obstruction, usually due to chronic calcific pancreatitis. Pruritus is the clue in these patients that jaundice is not due to alcoholic liver disease alone. Pruritus is also a common accompaniment of acute viral hepatitis but usually only transiently during the prodromal phase. Particularly in acute hepatitis B, itching, arthralgias, and urticarial rashes may herald the onset and then disappear when

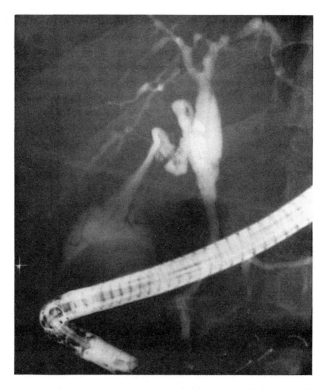

Figure 1 Endoscopic retrograde cholangiogram appearance of sclerosing cholangitis. Note multiple areas of irregular narrowing in intrahepatic bile ducts (arrows). The patient had chronic hepatitis B; the clue to coexisting sclerosing cholangitis was persistent pruritus.

icteric hepatitis develops. Chronic hepatitis C is more commonly associated with persistent pruritus than is chronic hepatitis B, and the pathologic correlate is more pronounced bile duct injury.[18] Drug-induced hepatitis, especially that due to sensitivity to phenothiazines or estrogens (pill cholestasis) is often accompanied by pruritus. Porphyria cutanea tarda is unique in this list in that it is the only liver disease with pruritus associated with a skin rash, and it is problematic whether to consider the pruritus an effect of the cholestasis, or a primary dermatologic problem.

ETIOLOGY AND PATHOGENESIS

The nature of the substance or substances which mediate pruritus of cholestasis and the mechanism of action on neurogenic pathways mediating itch sensation are unknown. There are several major theories about the mediators and mechanisms,[19–24] enumerated in chronologic order in Table 16-2. Each has proponents and challengers. It should be obvious that these, particularly the last three, are not mutually exclusive theories but rather variations on a theme.

The association of itch with jaundice is believed to have been first commented on by Areateus the Cappadocian over 1800 years ago.[19] This astute clinician distinguished two types of icterus, one of which he believed to arise from the spleen and the other from liver. It is difficult to determine what modern day diseases he was referring to, but he concluded that in both types of jaundice "the whole body is itchy . . . the bilious particles being prickly." It is a humbling reflection on modern scientific medicine that this perceptive observation could be considered as the state-of-the-art with respect to cholestatic pruritus. Although we believe that the phenomenon is somehow due to "bilious particles being prickly," we have not yet identified precisely which bilious particles are prickly, or why.

The second theory proposes that bile salts which accumulate in cholestatic plasma and skin are directly pruritogenic.[20] This theory is no longer tenable.[21,22,24,25]

The hypothesis that pruritus is caused by accumulation of an intermediate in bile salt synthetic pathways[21] (as I have proposed) remains highly

Table 16-2 Theories of the mechanism of cholestatic pruritus

1. "Bilious particles . . . being prickly"[19]
2. Retained bile salts acting on the skin[20]
3. Accumulation of a pruritogenic intermediate in bile salt synthetic pathways[21]
4. Bile salt toxicity to hepatocyte membranes, with release of an unidentified pruritogen[22]
5. Histamine-mediated itch from activation of mast cells by unidentified activators[23]
6. Centrally acting pruritogenic endogenous opiates accumulating as a result of hepatocyte secretory failure[24]

theoretical and has little support. Although alternative pathways of bile salt biosynthesis may be activated in cholestatic syndromes, a consistent association between pruritus and any intermediate has not been demonstrated.

I have proposed that pruritus of cholestasis is due to hepatocyte injury from high concentrations of retained hydrophobic bile salts, with release of a secondary pruritogen.[22] While there is abundant evidence of hepatocyte membrane injury from retained bile salts in cholestasis,[26,27] the link to pruritus and the nature of the proposed secondary mediator remains speculative. Relief of pruritus by rifampin[28-31] and by ursodeoxycholic acid[32] support this theory, as both agents probably decrease intrahepatic concentrations of hydrophobic bile salts. However, it is possible that the putative mediator released by the toxic bile salts comes not from hepatocytes but from mast cells, Ito cells, or other cells lining hepatic sinusoids. This theory is compatible with histamine or endogenous opiates as the mediators. Rifampin may act by altering hydroxylation and conjugation reactions in bile salt metabolism rather than by inhibition of hepatic uptake of bile salts.[33]

The theory that histamine is a mediator of pruritus of cholestasis has received renewed interest, and there is convincing evidence that among patients with cholestasis those with pruritus have higher venous plasma histamine concentrations than do controls without pruritus.[23] The presence of itch and not the nature of the underlying disease is the discriminating factor. The source of this histamine is unknown and histaminase levels do not differ in pruritic and nonpruritic subjects. Furthermore, the almost universal failure of antihistamine treatment to control pruritus of cholestasis in clinical trials[34] is a major unexplained feature challenging this theory.

The mediation of pruritus of cholestasis by endogenous opiates is suggested by the finding in one study that the specific narcotic antagonist naloxone relieves itch of cholestasis.[35] It has been long appreciated that pruritus is a major side effect of morphine, particularly when given by the epidural route, suggesting a relationship between opiate receptor activity and itch. However, naloxone does not alter the augmentation of histamine-induced itch by methionine enkephalin, beta endorphin, or morphine.[36] This suggests itch sensation is neuronally separate from pain, and that the effect of naloxone in cholestatic pruritus may not involve opiate receptors. The origin and nature of the mediator affected by naloxone also thus remains speculative. The relief of cholestatic pruritus by subhypnotic doses of propofol,[37] which also relieves itching due to spinal morphine administration, strongly suggests that endogenous opiates, perhaps released from the liver, may mediate itch by a central mechanism. Equating pruritus with quantitation of scratching activity[38] is conceptually flawed (by this definition of pruritus, handcuffs would provide a sure cure). However, this technology is useful in research, and has led to identification of a serum factor which may be a mediator of itch of cholestasis.[39]

LABORATORY FEATURES

Laboratory tests can be conveniently divided into nonspecific tests which can be used to screen for cholestasis as the cause of pruritus and those which confirm a specific diagnosis of the cholestatic disorder (Tables 16-3 and 16-4). For screening purposes, the hallmark of cholestasis is an elevation of serum alkaline phosphatase. Rarely, asymptomatic patients have been diagnosed as having primary biliary cirrhosis on the basis of liver biopsy and abnormal serology with a normal serum alkaline phosphatase level, but by the time itch develops, almost all patients with cholestasis will have an elevation of this enzyme.

For those rare patients who may have an elevation of serum alkaline phosphatase from bone disease, a confirmatory test for hepatobiliary alkaline phosphatase may be necessary. Tests based on substrate specificity of alkaline phosphatase or serum tests for other enzymes released from the canalicular membrane, such as gammaglutamyl transpepdidase are available in most laboratories. However, they contribute little to diagnostic specificity in most cases.

Serum cholesterol is nonspecifically elevated in cholestasis due to the presence of an abnormal cholesterol-rich lipoprotein, LP-X.[40] Lipoprotein quantitation in these patients is difficult, often inaccurate, and not diagnostically useful.

Accurate tests to quantitate bilirubin fractions in serum will occasionally show elevation of the conjugated fraction of serum bilirubin before there is elevation of the total bilirubin. However, there may be completely normal levels of all fractions of serum bilirubin in early cholestasis with pruritus.

Laboratory, radiologic, and histologic methods of confirming the diagnosis of specific common cholestatic disorders are listed in Table 16-4. For illustrative purposes, an example of the typical radiologic appearances of sclerosing cholangitis is shown in Figure 16-1.

DIFFERENTIAL DIAGNOSIS

There is usually little difficulty in attributing itch to cholestasis in a patient with an elevated serum alkaline phosphatase. Normal alkaline phosphatase

Table 16-3 Screening for cholestasis

1. Serum alkaline phosphatase
2. Fasting serum cholesterol
3. Serum bilirubin, total and conjugated

Table 16-4 Tests for specific cholestatic disorders

Disorder	Test	Expected result
Primary biliary cirrhosis	Antimitochondrial antibody (AMA)	Strong positive
	Immunoglobulins	Elevated IgM
	Liver biopsy	Bile duct destruction
Primary sclerosing cholangitis	Cholangiogram (ERCP)	Strictures
Chronic hepatitis C	Serum anti-HCV	Positive
Choledocholithiasis	Cholangiogram (ERCP)	Filling defects in common bile duct
Drug hepatitis/cholestasis	Drug withdrawal	Prompt improvement

levels are age dependent, with higher levels in children. In occasional patients with more than one disease associated with pruritus, it may not be easy to determine which is the cause of the itch and a therapeutic trial may be the only way to do so. Control of coexistent hyperglycemia or thyrotoxicosis in a patient with primary biliary cirrhosis may relieve the itch and establish that in spite of having primary biliary cirrhosis, the itch is not related to that. Patients with atopy or atopic dermatitis often have little dermatitis and much itch (see Chap. 3). If these people develop a chronic cholestatic disorder, the cause of the pruritus is very difficult to establish. In one such patient only failure of response to treatment for cholestatic pruritus and subsequent response to treatment for atopic dermatitis identified the cause of the itch.[28] Table 16-5 offers a partial differential diagnosis for cholestatic pruritus.

TREATMENT

The general principles of treatment are outlined in Chap. 26. Only those aspects of the treatment unique to cholestatic pruritus will be discussed.

The goal of treatment is to relieve the itch by curing the disease if possible.

Table 16-5 Differential diagnosis of cholestatic pruritus

Hematologic neoplasm
    Polycythemia rubra vera
    Hodgkins disease
    Non-Hodgkins lymphoma
Chronic renal failure
Thyrotoxicosis
Hyperglycemia
Occult internal malignancy

Table 16-6 Standard treatment modalities for cholestatic liver diseases

Disorder	Treatment
Choledocholithiasis	Surgical or endoscopic stone removal
Iatrogenic biliary stricture	Surgical reconstruction
Drug hepatitis/cholestasis	Drug withdrawal
Chronic Hepatitis C	Interferon[a]
Carcinoma of pancreas/bile ducts	Surgical resection or bypass
Porphyria cutanea tarda	Phlebotomy
Primary biliary cirrhosis	Ursodeoxycholic acid[a]
Primary sclerosing cholangitis	Ursodeoxycholic acid[a]
End-stage liver failure of any cause	Liver transplantation

[a] Experimental

This should be the objective in the disorders listed in Table 16-6. The treatment of some of these disorders remains controversial, particularly the treatment of chronic hepatitis C with interferon and treatment of primary biliary cirrhosis and sclerosing cholangitis, the two most common cholestatic disorders in adulthood, with ursodeoxycholic acid. The latter treatment is under intense investigation in several controlled trials at this time and has been reported to relieve pruritus in primary biliary cirrhosis.[32] It is believed to exert this effect by replacing hydrophobic bile salts in the enterohepatic circulation (Fig. 16-2) with the relatively hydrophilic ursodeoxycholic acid.

Symptomatic or palliative treatment is a stepwise process, often necessitating frequent review and revision. While there is no consensus as to the logical steps in this process, the author suggests a sequence as presented in Table 16-7.

Cholestyramine is the first agent to be prescribed. This anion exchange resin is believed to work by interrupting the enterohepatic circulation of bile salts by anion exchange in the small bowel[20] (Fig. 16-2) When biliary obstruction is complete, no bile salts enter the small bowel and this agent then cannot be expected to relieve pruritus. It does control itch very well in the majority of patients with partial biliary obstruction.[20] Short-term side effects include a bitter taste, nausea, vomiting, abdominal fullness, and constipation. The oral intake can be made more acceptable by mixing the cholestyramine with an ice cold beverage or using it in cooking. Patients should be told to expect the relief of itch at the earliest 3 or 4 days after commencing treatment. Thereafter, the dose can be titrated slowly over days or weeks to the minimum which will control pruritus. Cholestipol may be substituted but its efficacy has not been documented.

With the administration of any medication, potential and actual long-term side effects must be considered. Bile salt-sequestering resins may

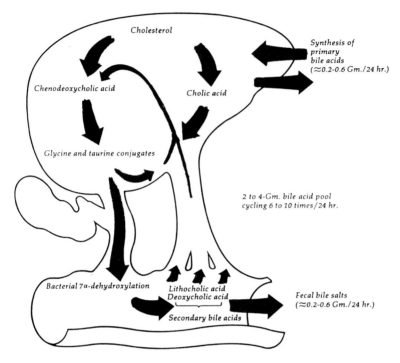

Cholesterol

Synthesis of
primary
bile acids
($\approx$0.2-0.6 Gm./24 hr.)

Chenodeoxycholic acid

Cholic acid

Glycine and taurine conjugates

2 to 4-Gm. bile acid pool
cycling 6 to 10 times/24 hr.

Bacterial 7α-dehydroxylation

Lithocholic acid
Deoxycholic acid

Secondary bile acids

Fecal bile salts
($\approx$0.2-0.6 Gm./24 hr.)

Figure 2 The enterohepatic circulation of bile salts. Primary bile salts (mainly conjugates of cholic acid and chenodeoxycholic acid) are synthesized in the liver. Active ileal absorption and hepatic extraction results in less than 5 percent per day fecal excretion (mainly deconjugated and dehydroxylated deoxycholic and lithocholic acid).

produce serious long-term metabolic effects. As these agents exchange a chloride ion for any other available anion in the gut, the absorption of many other drugs given concomitantly may be impeded, and their effects decreased or negated. The exchange of bicarbonate ion for chloride ion with absorption of the latter produces a mild hyperchloremic metabolic acidosis,

Table 16-7 Palliative or symptomatic treatment of cholestatic pruritus

Cholestyramine	4 gm	1 p.o. Q.I.D.
Rifampin	150 mg	1 p.o. Q.I.D.
Terfenadine	60 mg	1 p.o. B.I.D.
Phototherapy[a]	See Chap. 28	
Plasmapheresis[a]		
External biliary drainage[a]		
Liver transplantation		

[a] Experimental

which may accelerate bone mineral loss. The decrease in intraluminal bile salts may produce or worsen malabsorption of fats and fat soluble vitamins, especially vitamins A and K. This leads to night blindness, coagulopathy and worsening malnutrition. Effects on vitamin D metabolism are not as well delineated as osteoporosis and not osteomalacia is the major component of hepatic osteodystrophy.[41]

Rifampin administration has been shown to relieve pruritus in chronic cholestasis.[28–31] Because this is a new treatment, long-term effects have not been studied. The theoretical side effects of induction of hepatic mixed function oxidases with this agent in chronic liver disease include alterations in metabolism of a wide variety of drugs and xenobiotics. I have successfully used this treatment in five patients with primary biliary cirrhosis and otherwise intractable pruritus for up to 5 years with no obvious side effects. Other inducers of mixed function oxidases are less effective than rifampin[29] and have the disadvantage that they may cause drowsiness.

Of all the antihistamines available, only one, terfenidine, has been evaluated for its effect on pruritus of cholestasis.[34] A modest effect was documented. All antihistamine treatment should be regarded as adjunctive rather than first line therapy in cholestatic pruritus. The metabolism of hydroxyzine is markedly altered in chronic cholestasis[42] and treatment with this agent should be carefully monitored for efficacy and side effects.

Phototherapy[43] (see Chap. 28), plasmapheresis[44] and external biliary drainage[45] have all been reported to relieve intractable pruritus of cholestasis but these reports have not been verified. Therefore, these modalities of treatment must be considered experimental. The concept of partial interruption of the enterohepatic circulation by a permanent cholecystostomy is appealing, and this may be an appropriate treatment for truly refractory itch in early primary biliary cirrhosis, in childhood cholestatic syndromes[45] or as palliation in advanced distal biliary obstruction.

Anabolic steroids relieve pruritus but worsen cholestasis.[46] The patient's itch may disappear but he or she is likely to turn bright yellow. The aggravated cholestasis may diminish the patient's life expectancy. This treatment is not recommended.

Orthotopic liver transplantation is the treatment of choice for chronic cholestatic liver disease when life threatening complications ensue.[47] Although it seems unwarranted to subject a patient with less advanced disease to the 10 to 30 percent mortality rate and the need for life long antirejection therapy accompanying this procedure, truly intractable pruritus may be disabling. Such patients, if well informed and realistic, may reasonably choose to accept the risks involved in transplantation to improve their quality of life. Severe pruritus resistant to therapy has been accepted by the National Institutes of Health Consensus Conference on Liver Transplantation as a valid indication for the procedure.[48] Because of the improvements in antipruritic therapy over the last decade, the need to resort to liver transplantation to treat pruritus should be rare.

REFERENCES

1. Desmet VJ: Cholestasis: Extrahepatic obstruction and secondary biliary cirrhosis, in MacSween RNM, Anthony PP, Scheuer PJ (eds): *Pathology of the Liver* 2d ed. New York, Churchill Livingstone. 1987, Chap 12, pp 364–423.
2. Scharschmidt BF: Bile formation and cholestasis, in Zakim D, Boyer TD (eds): *Hepatology* 2d ed. Philadelphia, Saunders. 1990, Chap 12, pp 303–340.
3. McPhedran NT, Henderson RD: Pruritus and Jaundice. *Can Med Assoc J* 92:1258–1260, 1965.
4. Shapiro JM, Smith H, Schaffner F: Serum bilirubin: A prognostic factor in primary biliary cirrhosis. *Gut* 20:137–140, 1979.
5. Roll J, Boyer JL, Barry D, et al: The prognostic importance of clinical and histologic features in asymptomatic and symptomatic primary biliary cirrhosis. *N Engl J Med* 308:1–7, 1983.
6. Christensen E, Neuberger J, Crow J, et al: Beneficial effect of azathioprine and prediction of prognosis in primary biliary cirrhosis: Final result of an international trial. *Gastroenterology* 89:1084–1091, 1985.
7. Dickson ER, Grambsch PM, Fleming TR, et al: Prognosis in primary biliary cirrhosis: Model for decision making. *Hepatology* 10:1–7, 1989.
8. Grambsch PM, Dickson ER, Kaplan M, et al: Extramural cross-validation of the Mayo primary biliary cirrhosis survival model establishes its generalizability. *Hepatology* 10:846–850, 1989.
9. Rydning A, Schrumpf E, Abdelnoor M, et al: Factors of prognostic importance in primary biliary cirrhosis. *Scand J Gastroenterol* 24:119–126, 1990.
10. Goudie BM, Burt AD, Macfarlane GJ, et al: Risk factors and prognosis in primary biliary cirrhosis. *Am J Gastroenterol* 84:713–716, 1989.
11. Hamlyn AN, Sherlock S: The epidemiology of PBC: A survey of mortality in England and Wales. *Gut* 15:473–479, 1974.
12. Long GR, Scheuer PJ, Sherlock S: Presentation and course of asymptomatic primary biliary cirrhosis. *Gastroenterology* 72:1204–1207, 1977.
13. Witt-Sullivan H, Heathcoate J, Cauch K, et al: The demography of primary biliary cirrhosis in Ontario, Canada. *Hepatology* 12:98–105, 1990.
14. Chapman RWG, Marbough BA, Rhodes JM, et al: Primary sclerosing cholangitis: A review of the clinical features, cholangiography, and hepatic histology. *Gut* 21:870–877, 1980.
15. Weisner RH, LaRusso NF, Ludwig J, et al: Comparison of the clinicopathologic features of primary sclerosing cholangitis and primary biliary cirrhosis. *Gastroenterology* 88:108–114, 1985.
16. Helzberg JH, Peterson JM, Boyer JL: Improved survival with primary sclerosing cholangitis. *Gastroenterology* 92:1869–1875, 1987.
17. Weisner RH, Grambach PM, Ludwig J, et al: Primary sclerosing cholangitis: Natural history, prognostic factors, and survival analysis. *Hepatology* 10:430–435, 1989.
18. Lefkowitch JH, Schiff ER, Davis GL, et al: Pathological diagnosis of chronic hepatitis C: A multicenter comparative study with chronic hepatitis B. *Gastroenterology* 104:595–603, 1993.
19. Aretaeus, the Cappadocian (circa 160 A.D.): *The Extant Works of Aretaeus the Cappadocian.* Edited by F. Adams, London, Sydenham Society, 1856.
20. Carey JB Jr: Lowering of serum bile acid concentrations and relief of pruritus in jaundiced patients fed bile acid sequestering resin. *J Lab Clin Med* 56:797–798, 1960.
21. Ghent CN, Bloomer JR: Itch in liver disease: Facts and speculations. *Yale J Biol Med,* 52:77–82, 1979.
22. Ghent CN: Pruritus of cholestasis is related to effects of bile salts on the liver, not the skin. *Am J Gastroenterol* 82:117–118, 1987.
23. Gittlen SD, Schulman ES, Maddrey WC: Raised histamine concentrations in chronic cholestatic liver disease. *Gut* 31:96–99, 1990.

24. Jones EA, Bergasa NV: The pruritus of cholestasis: From bile acids to opiate agonists. *Hepatology* 11:884–887, 1990.
25. Ghent CN, Bloomer JR, Klatskin G: Elevations in skin tissue levels of bile acids in human cholestasis: Relationship to serum levels and to pruritus. *Gastroenterology* 3:1125–1130, 1978.
26. DeBroc ME, Roels F, Nouwen EJ, et al: Liver plasma membrane: The source of high molecular weight alkaline phosphatase in human serum. *Hepatology* 5:118–128, 1985.
27. Layden TJ, Boyer JL: Taurolithocholate-induced cholestasis. Taurocholate, but not dehydrocholate, reverses cholestasis and bile canalicular membrane injury. *Gastroenterology* 73:120–128, 1977.
28. Ghent CN, Carruthers SG: Treatment of pruritus in primary biliary cirrhosis with rifampin: Results of a double-blinded crossover randomized trial. *Gastroenterology* 94:488–493, 1988.
29. Bachs L, Pares A, Montserrat E, et al: Comparison of rifampicin with phenobarbitone for treatment of pruritus in biliary cirrhosis. *Lancet* I:574–578, 1989.
30. Cynamon HA, Andres JM, Iafrate RP: Rifampin relieves pruritus in children with cholestatic liver disease. *Gastroenterology* 98:1013–1016, 1990.
31. Podesta A, Lopez P, Terg R, et al: Treatment of pruritus in primary biliary cirrhosis with rifampin. *Dig Dis Sci* 36:216–220, 1991.
32. Matsuzaki Y, Tanaka N, Osuga T, et al: Improvement of biliary enzyme levels by administration of ursodeoxycholic acid in primary biliary cirrhosis. *Am J Gastroenterol* 85:15–23, 1990.
33. Wietholtz H, Marschall H-U, Reuschenbach R, et al: The influence of rifampicin on urinary bile acid gluconide excretion. *Hepatology* 12:896, 1990.
34. Duncan JS, Kennedy HJ, Triger DR: Treatment of pruritus due to chronic obstructive liver disease. *BMJ* 289:22, 1984.
35. Bergasa NV, Talbot TL, Alling DW, et al: A controlled trial of naloxone infusions for the pruritus of cholestasis. *Gastroenterology* 102:544–549, 1992.
36. Fjellner B, Hagermark O: Potentiation of the histamine-induced itch and flare responses in human skin by the enkephalin analogue FK-33-824, beta-endorphin and morphine. *Arch Dermatol Res* 274:29–37, 1982.
37. Borgeat A, Wilder-Smith OHG, Mentha G: Subhypnotic doses of propofol relieve pruritus associated with liver disease. *Gastroenterology* 104:244–247, 1993.
38. Bergasa NV, Talbot T, Schmit J, et al: Objective quantitation of pruritus in patients with cholestatic liver disease. *Hepatology* 10:639, 1989.
39. Bergasa NV, Thomas DA, Vergalla J, et al: Serum extracts from cholestatic patients induce naloxone-reversible centrally mediated facial scratching in monkeys. *Hepatology* 16:152D, 1992.
40. Cooper AD: Hepatic lipoprotein and cholesterol metabolism, in Zakim D, Boyer TD (eds): *Hepatology* 2d ed. Philadelphia, Saunders, 1990. Chap 5, pp 96–123.
41. Stellon AJ, Webb A, Compston J, et al: Lack of osteomalacia in chronic cholestatic liver disease. *Bone* 7:181, 1986.
42. Dimond FE, Watson WT, Chen XY, et al: The pharmacokinetics and pharmacodynamics of hydroxyzine in patients with primary biliary cirrhosis. *J Clin Pharmacol* 29:809–815, 1989.
43. Hanid MA, Levi AJ: Phototherapy for pruritus in primary biliary cirrhosis. *Lancet* 2:530, 1980.
44. Lauterberg BH, Taswell HF, Pineda AA, et al: Treatment of pruritus of cholestasis by plasma perfusion through USP-charcoal-coated glass beads. *Lancet* 2:53–55, 1980.
45. Whitington PF, Whitington GL: Partial external biliary diversion of bile for the treatment of intractable pruritus associated with intrahepatic cholestasis. *Gastroenterology* 95:130–136, 1988.

46. Walt RP: Effect of Stanozolol on itching in primary biliary cirrhosis. *BMJ* 296:607, 1988.
47. Maddrey, W, VanThiel DH: Liver Transplantation: An overview. *Hepatology* 8:948–959, 1988.
48. Salens LB, Roth HP, Crout JR, et al: National Institutes of Health Concensus Development Conference Statement: Liver Transplantation. *Hepatology* 4:1075–1105, 1984.

SEVENTEEN
IRON DEFICIENCY AND OTHER HEMATOLOGICAL CAUSES OF GENERALIZED PRURITUS

S.J. Adams

Pruritus has long been recognized as a presenting or concomitant symptom of many hematological, myeloproliferative and neoplastic diseases.[1] The most notable of these are listed in Table 17-1 and discussed in the following sections.

THE LEUKEMIAS AND MYELOPROLIFERATIVE DISEASE

Pruritus is an uncommon manifestation of chronic leukemia. It is said to be more often encountered in the lymphatic than the granulocytic form.[2] Greenwood and Barker[3] in a survey of patients with B cell chronic lymphocytic leukemia and their dermatological manifestations describe 6 patients, one with leukemia cutis, the others with "nonspecific" rashes, but they do not mention generalized pruritus as a manifestation of the disease. Generalized pruritus is well recognized in Hodgkin's disease. Bluefarb[1] states that itching occurs in nearly 30 percent of patients with the disease: Indeed it may be the presenting complaint in a significant proportion of sufferers. The irritation is intense and resistant to all therapy save that of treatment of the lymphoma. Sometimes, sufferers complain of an associated burning sensation. Feiner and colleagues[4] and Goggi and colleagues[5] found that pruritus in Hodgkin's disease was associated with a poor prognosis—it is argued that it should therefore be considered a "B" symptom.[5] The pruritus may antedate further manifestations of Hodgkin's disease by several months. Itching in Hodgkin's disease is discussed more fully in Chap. 21. Beare[6], in his study of 43 cases of generalized pruritus describes one patient with a malignant lymphoma of

Table 17-1 Hematologic and myeloproliferative disorders associated with pruritus*

Leukemias
Hodgkin's disease and non-Hodgkin's lymphomas
Paraproteinemia (myelomatosis)
Polycythemia rubra vera
Iron deficiency with or without a microcytic hypochromic anemia
Myelodysplastic syndrome
Hypereosinophilic syndrome
Essential thrombocythemia

*See also Chap. 21.

undescribed cellular type. Certainly, other non-Hodgkin's lymphomas may present in a similar manner. Other myeloproliferative disorders described in this context are myelomatosis[7] and paraproteinemia.[8]

POLYCYTHEMIA RUBRA VERA

Pruritus is a well recognized manifestation of polycythemia rubra vera. It occurs most commonly following a hot bath, the triggering factor seeming to be a drop in temperature. Fjellner and Hägermark[9] found that this symptom occurred in 70 percent of their patients suffering from polycythemia rubra vera. Winkelmann and colleagues[10] found that the symptom was present in 60% of patients. Post bathing pruritus or aquagenic pruritus is, however, not specific for polycythaemia rubra vera. It may occur in other myeloproliferative disorders and in Hodgkin's disease,[11] and the hypereosinophilic syndrome.[12] McGrath and Greaves[13] described an association between aquagenic pruritus and the myelodysplastic syndrome. In a retrospective study of 268 patients with essential thrombocythemia, 6 patients experienced pruritus and 3 noted post-bath pruritus.[14]

Idiopathic aquagenic pruritus, described in more detail in Chap. 3, was first described by Shelley in 1979[15] and subsequently by Greaves and colleagues.[16] Typically presenting with a complaint of a prickling skin discomfort, it occurs in susceptible individuals within minutes of contact with water at any temperature. The symptoms may be associated with significant emotional liability.[17] Within the context of hematological disease, aquagenic pruritus may antedate the diagnosis of polycythemia vera by a number of years.[17,18] As such, the regular assessment of such individuals' hematological status is mandatory.

Some degree of iron deficiency is universal in polycythemia rubra vera[20] and there are several reports in the literature of the resolution of polycythemia rubra vera-associated itching with oral iron.[21–23] Rector and colleagues[24] document the appearance of symptoms in response to venesection. Tucker and colleagues[25] were unable to induce generalized pruritus in their study of 21 normal males undergoing serial venesection and suggest that iron deficiency per se does not, therefore, cause pruritus. There may be an underlying tendency to histamine release in the polycythemia vera group. Also the volunteers in Tucker's group were of a younger age group than the polycythemia vera patients. As chronic iron treatment for individuals with polycythemia rubra vera may result in a progressive increase in red cell mass, the indiscriminate long-term use of oral iron for this condition is not advocated.

IRON DEFICIENCY

An association between iron deficiency anemia and generalized pruritus has long been recognized by dermatologists[21,26,27] although this association was and is still not widely recognized by general physicians.[28] Sneddon and Garretts[21] noted that the pruritus of iron deficiency anemia responded to iron therapy, the symptoms resolving on restoration of a normal hemoglobin and/or serum iron levels. These authors describe 9 of their 20 patients who were iron deficient but not anemic. Fielding and colleagues[29] described iron deficiency sine (without) anemia. Nine of Sneddon and Garretts series of iron deficient patients were not anemic and Vickers in his personal series of 87 patients[22] (72 female, 15 male) with generalized pruritus comments on this association. Of interest is the presence of malignancy in 14 of the 15 males. Vickers does not state the age at which the symptoms presented nor the hemoglobin levels but states that these patients were iron deficient sine anemia and comments that a low serum iron with pruritus may be indicative of sinister pathology in men.[30]

In a personal series,[31] the author studied a group of 50 patients presenting with a symptom of generalized pruritus. They were compared with a nonitchy age- and sex-matched study group. The age and sex is documented in Table 17-2.

Investigations included hemoglobin, full blood count, serum ferritin, serum iron and total binding capacity, urea and electrolytes, liver function tests, thyroid function tests, chest x-ray, autoantibodies, fecal occult bloods and urinalysis.

Table 17-2 Patients suffering from generalized pruritus

Sex	Number	Mean age (years)	Range (years)
Women	20	62.3	24–98
Men	30	62.7	32–91

In 22 patients, no specific disease was identified and they were regarded as suffering from idiopathic pruritus. Twenty of the 50 patients were iron deficient as indicated by an assessment of their iron stores (serum ferritin). Twelve of this group had a low serum iron. Table 17-3 describes the iron deficient patients. Table 17-4 demonstrates the relationship of serum ferritin to hemoglobin. Only 1 of the iron deficient female patients was anemic: She was a girl with thalassemia trait who had a hemoglobin of 9.7 g/dl. All other iron deficient patients were well hemoglobinized with no demonstrable microcytosis, so supporting Vickers'[22] assertion that the pruritus is iron, not hemoglobin related.

The breakdown of the findings in this iron deficient group is fascinating: Table 17-5 demonstrates the sex-related findings.

The female iron deficient group represents a miscellaneous group. In the male group, the origins of the iron deficiency is more cohesive. It was associated principally with alcohol-related disease (diet, ulcers, gastritis, and post-gastrectomy induced iron deficiency). However, four men were found to have previously unrecognized carcinoma. I shall document two such individuals:

Case 1 A 63-year-old man who presented with a 6-month history of severe generalized pruritus. He was found to have a normal hemoglobin (15.3 g/dl) but low serum ferritin (7 ug/l). Fecal occult bloods were positive and gastroscopy and biopsy demonstrated a gastric adenocarcinoma. Although he remained pruritic after surgery, his symptoms resolved when his serum ferritin was restored to normality.

Case 2 (not included in this series) A 67-year-old man with a year's history of generalized pruritus. He had recently noticed some nasal stuffiness. He was found to be iron deficient sine anemia. Fecal occult bloods were positive. A nasopharyngeal carcinoma was detected. He is still pruritic post surgery.

In the author's series, none of the men suffering from malignancy required costly or invasive investigation to determine the presence of a sinister

Table 17-3 Age and sex of patients suffering from iron deficiency*

Sex	Number	Mean age (years)	Range (years)
Women	6	59.7	24–98
Men	14	64.7	30–91

*Low iron stores as indicated by serum ferritin.

Table 17-4 Hematological parameters in patients with generalized pruritus and low ferritin compared to controls

Women		Generalized pruritus	Control
Mean Hb	(NR 11.5–16)	12.8 g/dl	12.6 g/dl
Mean MCV	(NR 78–98)	87.2 fl	87.0 fl
Mean Ferritin	(NR 9–142)	6.1 μg/l p < 0.001	82 μg/l
Men		Generalized pruritus	Control
Mean Hb	(NR 13–18)	14.2 g/dl	13.7 g/dl
Mean MCV	(NR 78–98)	87.4 fl	87.0 fl
Mean Ferritin	(NR 41–480)	15 μg/l p < 0.001	270 μg/l

This table shows the normal hemoglobin and MCV in the group with generalized pruritus despite low iron stores as manifested by the low ferritin levels.

Note: Hb = hemoglobin
MCV = mean corpuscular volume

abnormality, and it would appear that simple screening procedures such as serum ferritin, fecal occult blood, and urinalysis would be sufficient to expose the organ system involved in individuals with generalized pruritus, malignant disease, and iron deficiency sine anemia. I would agree with Vickers that generalized pruritus with iron deficiency, particularly in the elderly male, is a sinister sign.

Although I have principally described iron deficiency-associated pruritus presenting in a generalized manner, localized pruritus, especially in the perianal or vulval regions, may also present in iron deficient individuals or indeed in a patient suffering from pruritus associated with any of the hematological or myeloproliferative diseases. Staubli[32] describes five episodes of iron deficiency anemia associated with localized pruritus in four women. In a recent

Table 17-5 Reasons for iron deficiency in patients with generalized pruritus

Women	Menorrhagia	1		
	"Old age"	1		
	Filiariasis	1		
	Diet	1		
	Hiatus hernia	1		
	Thalassemia	1		
Men	Diet	4 (1 vegan)		
	Alcohol	1		
	Ulcer post gastrectomy	3		
	Hemorrhoids	1		
	Carcinoma	4—Bladder	1	
		Stomach	2	
		Large Bowel	1	
	Unknown	1		

series of women suffering from lichen simplex vulvae, 44 individuals presented to a clinic for vulvar disease from their primary, referring physician, with a diagnosis of "pruritus vulvae." Nineteen of the 44 women were suffering from lichen simplex vulvae. Of these, 50 percent had a low serum ferritin. Seventy percent responded to oral iron supplementation, although in combination with moderately potent topical corticosteroids, an emollient wash cream and nocturnal sedation.[33]

PATHOPHYSIOLOGY OF PRURITUS ASSOCIATED WITH HEMATOLOGIC DISEASE

On the whole, the pathophysiology of the itch precipitated in such diseases is unclear. Jackson and colleagues[34] measured mast cell numbers, circulating basophils and whole blood histamine in 13 patients with polycythemia vera and found that itching, which was present in nine patients, correlated well with numbers of skin mast cells but not with circulating basophils or whole blood histamine. They attributed aspirin's effect on pruritus to interference with the effect of mast cell prostaglandins and felt that local PG-mediated vascular responses may trigger mast cell degranulation.

Fjellner and Hägermark[9] suggested that in polycythemia vera, serotonin and prostaglandin E2 were important as inflammatory mediators. McGrath and Greaves[13] suggest within the context of aquagenic pruritus and the myelodysplastic syndrome that functionally and structurally abnormal platelets may release inflammatory mediators as part of the response to water.

Iron deficiency may lead to psychological[35,36] and to epithelial changes that may result in a predisposition to itch. As iron is a critical component of many enzymes, it is also not difficult to imagine that alterations in their function could lead to itching through a variety of metabolic paths.

TREATMENT

Pruritus associated with hematological or myeloproliferative disease is usually only responsive to treatment of the underlying disorder. Salem and colleagues,[23] Sneddon and Garretts,[21] and Vickers[22] describe the response of iron deficient patients with polycythemia rubra vera to oral iron therapy but this is not to be recommended in the long term because of its disadvantageous effect on red cell mass. Aspirin has been reportedly useful in the treatment of polycythemia vera although bleeding is a potentially serious complication.[9,34] Cholestyramine, said to act by binding pruritogenic substances in the gut thereby reducing bile salt concentration, has been reported by Chanarin and Szur[37] to be helpful in the treatment of severe, intractable pruritus in polycythemia rubra vera.

Photochemotherapy has been reported to be useful in the treatment of pruritus associated with polycythemia vera[38,39] (see Chap. 28). Cimetidine has been reportedly helpful in the treatment of pruritus associated with polycythemia vera[40] and Hodgkin's disease.[41] Others describe a similar response to pruritus associated with polycythemia rubra vera to cimetidine.[42] However, in a pilot study of 12 patients with polycythemia rubra vera who complained of pruritus, no benefit from treatment with cimetidine was observed although these authors comment that it was possible that the dose was insufficient to produce H_2 receptor antagonism.[43]

Pruritus precipitated by iron deficiency responds to iron, which should be continued until the iron stores—as assessed by serum ferritin—are back to normal. In the case of localized pruritus proceeding to lichenification, the administration of a moderately potent topical corticosteroid and a nocturnal antihistamine may be helpful in addition to dietary supplementation with oral iron if required.

REFERENCES

1. Bluefarb SM: *Cutaneous Manifestations of Malignant Lymphomas*. Springfield, Il, Charles C Thomas 1959.
2. Cunliffe WJ, Savin JA: The skin and the nervous system, in *Textbook of Dermatology*, Rook A, Wilkinson DS, Ebling FJG, Champion RH, Burton JL (eds). Blackwell Scientific Publications 4th Ed, 1986, p 2251.
3. Greenwood RA, Barker DJ, Tring FC, et al: Clinical and immunological characterisation of cutaneous lesions in chronic lymphocytic leukaemia. *Br J Dermatol* 113:447–453, 1985.
4. Feiner AS, Mahmood T, Wallner SF: Prognostic importance of pruritus in Hodgkin's disease. *JAMA* 240:2738–2745, 1978.
5. Gobbi PG, Attardo-Parrinello G, Lattanzio G, et al: Severe pruritus should be a B-symptom in Hodgkin's disease. *Cancer* 57:1934–1936, 1983.
6. Beare JM: Generalised pruritus, a study of 43 cases. *Clinical Exp Derm* 1:343, 1976.
7. Erskine JG, et al: Pruritus as a presentation of myelomatosis. *BMJ* 1:687, 1977.
8. Zelicovici A, Lahav M, Cahane P, et al. Pruritus as a possible early sign of paraproteinaemia. *Isr J Med Sci* 5:1079–1081, 1969.
9. Fjellner B, Hägermark Ö: Pruritus in polycythaemia: treatment with aspirin and possibility of platelet involvement. *Acta Dermatovener* (Stockh) 59:505–512, 1979.
10. Winkelmann RK, Muller SA: Pruritus. *Ann Rev Med* 15:53, 1964.
11. Herndon JH: Itching: The pathophysiology of pruritus. *Int J Dermatol* 14:465, 1975.
12. Newton JA, Singh AK, Greaves MW, et al: Aquagenic pruritus associated with the idiopathic hypereosinophilic syndrome. *Br J Dermatol* 122:103, 1990.
13. McGrath JA, Greaves MW: Aquagenic pruritus and the myelodysplastic syndrome. *Br J Dermatol* 123:414, 1990.
14. Itin PH, Winkelmann RK: Cutaneous manifestions in patients with essential thrombocythemia. *J Am Acad Dermatol* 24:59, 1991.
15. Shelley WB: Questions and answers. *J Am Med Assoc* 212:1385, 1970.
16. Greaves MW, Black AK, Eady RAJ, et al: Aquagenic pruritus. *BMJ* 282:2008, 1981.
17. Steinman HK, Greaves MW: Aquagenic pruritus. *J Am Acad Dermatol* 13:91, 1985.
18. Archer CB, Camp RDR, Greaves MW: Polycythaemia vera can present with aquagenic pruritus. *Lancet* 1:1451, 1988.

19. Reid CDL: Pruritus preceding the development of polycythaemia vera. *Lancet* ii:964, 1988.

20. Berlin NI: Diagnosis and classification of the polycythaemias. *Seminar Haematol* 12:339, 1975.

21. Sneddon IB, Garretts M: The significance of low serum iron levels in the causation of itching, in Jadassohn W, Schinnen CG (eds): Proceedings of XIII International Congress of Dermatology. Vol 2. Berlin, Springer Verlag, 1061–1063, 1968.

22. Vickers CFH: Nutrition and the skin: Iron deficiency in dermatology. Proceedings of 10th Symposium in Advanced Medicine, London, Royal College of Physicians, 1974, pp 311–316.

23. Salem HT, Van der Weyden MB, Young IF, et al: Pruritus and severe iron deficiency in polycythaemia vera. *BMJ* 285:91, 1982.

24. Rector WJ, Fortuin NJ, Conley CL: Non-haematologic effects of chronic iron deficiency. A study of patients with polycythaemia vera treated soley with venesections. *Medicine* (Baltimore) 1982, 61(6):382–389, 1982.

25. Tucker WF, Briggs C, Challoner T: Absence of pruritus in iron deficiency following venesection. *Clin Exp Dermatol* 9:186, 1984.

26. Sneddon IB, Church RE: *Practical Dermatology*, 2nd ed. London, Edward Arrow, 125, 1991.

27. Rook A, Wilkinson DS, Ebling F: *Textbook of Dermatology*. Blackwell Scientific Publications 2 ed, 1972.

28. Lewiecki MC, Rahman F: Pruritus, a manifestation of iron deficiency. *JAMA* 236(20):2319, 1976.

29. Fielding J, O'Shaughnessy MC, Brunstrom GM: Iron deficiency without anaemia. *Lancet* ii:9, 1965.

30. Vickers CFH: Iron deficiency and the skin. *Br J Dermatol* Suppl 10, 1974.

31. Adams SJ: Iron deficiency, serum ferritin, generalised pruritus and systemic disease—a case controlled study. *Br J Dermatol* Suppl 34, 121:15, 1989.

32. Staubli M: Pruritus—a little known iron deficiency symptom. *Schweltz Med Wochenschr* 111(38):1394, 1981.

33. Adams SJ: A study of lichen simplex chronicus vulvae. In press.

34. Jackson N, Burt D, Crocker J, et al. Skin mast cell in polycythaemia vera: Relationship to the pathogenesis and treatment of pruritus. *Br J Dermatol* 116:121, 1987.

35. Chisholm M: Tissue changes associated with iron deficiency. *Clin Haematol* 2:303, 1973.

36. Dallman PR: Tissue effects of iron deficiency, in Jacobs A, Worwood M (eds): *Iron in Biochemistry and Medicine*. London, Academic Press 437–475, 1974.

37. Chanarin I, Szur L: Relief of intractable pruritus in polycythaemia rubra vera with cholestyramine. *Br J Haematol* 29:669, 1975.

38. Swerlick RA: Photochemotherapy treatment of pruritus associated with polycythaemia vera. *J Am Acad Dermatol* 13:675–677, 1985.

39. Morison WL, Nesbitt JA: Oral psoralen photochemotherapy (PUVA) for pruritus associated with polycythemia vera and myelofibrosis. *Am J Hematol* 42:409–410, 1993.

40. Easton P, Galbraith PR: Cimetidine treatment of pruritus in polycythaemia vera. Letter, *N Engl J Med* 299:1134, 1978.

41. Aymard JP, et al: Cimetidine for pruritus in Hodgkin's disease. *BMJ* 157, 1980.

42. Weick JK, Donovan PB, Najean Y, et al. The use of cimetidine for the treatment of pruritus in polycythemia vera. *Arch Intern Med* 142:241–242, 1982.

43. Scott GL, Horton RJ: Pruritus, cimetidine and polycythemia. Letter to the Editor *N Engl J Med* 300:434, 1979.

EIGHTEEN

ENDOCRINE AND METABOLIC ITCHES

Jeffrey D. Bernhard

The association of itching with several endocrine and metabolic disorders is clear cut; in several others, such as gout, the association is anecdotal at best (see Table 18-1). In diabetes, the nature of the itch and the nature of the association are somewhat controversial. Several disorders that have endocrine or metabolic features are discussed elsewhere in this text (see Table 18-2).

HYPERTHYROIDISM

Pruritus in patients with thyrotoxicosis was first described by Sir William Osler.[1] It may affect as many as 4 to 11 percent of patients and may be the presenting complaint.[2–5] In my own experience, hyperthyroidism has been the leader *among systemic causes* of generalized pruritus in patients who present themselves to my clinic with the chief complaint of itching. It is said that itching is more common among patients with Graves' disease or in patients with long-standing, untreated hyperthyroidism. Scratch papules, prurigo papules, excoriations, and secondary eczematous changes may be present. A case of thyrotoxicosis presenting as generalized pruritic exfoliative dermatitis and fever has also been reported.[6] The skin may appear entirely normal, although it is often noted to be warm, smooth, and "fine."[7]

The cause of itching in hyperthyroidism is not known but there are several reasonable theories, especially when one considers the wide range of effects that thyroid hormone has on the skin.[8] Thyroid hormone influences the differentiation and maturation of skin, its oxygen consumption, protein

Table 18-1 Endocrine and
metabolic disorders associated
with itching discussed in this
chapter

Hyperthyroidism
Hypothroidism
Carcinoid syndrome
Mastocytosis
Diabetes (localized; generalized)
Cholinergic pruritus
Adrenergic pruritus
Gout (doubtful; anecdotal)
Hypercalcemia
Autoimmune progesterone dermatitis
Sipple's syndrome (MEN 2a)

synthesis, thickness, hair formation, and sebum secretion. Theories on how excessive thyroid hormone may lead to itching range from activation of kinins from increased tissue metabolism to a reduction in the itch threshold due to warmth and vasodilatation. In one study, patients with hyperthyroidism and pruritus had elevated levels of serum chenodeoxycholic acid (CDC); when their hyperthyroidism was treated the itching resolved and the CDC levels returned toward normal.[9] Whether alterations in serum and biliary bile acid composition will turn out to be the cause of itching in hyperthyroidism, or only a marker for it, remains to be seen. The potential link to biliary cirrhosis is intriguing to say the least.

Urticaria and pruritus or urticaria alone can also be seen in hyperthyroidism.[10] Chronic urticaria and angioedema (CUA) can be the presenting sign of underlying thyroid autoimmunity, even in patients who appear clinically euthyroid. In a remarkable study, Leznoff and colleagues detected thy-

Table 18-2 Disorders with
endocrine or metabolic features
and itching discussed in other
chapters of this text

Disorder	Chapter
Notalgia paresthetica	12
Uremic pruritus	15
Cholestatic pruritus	16
Iron deficiency	17
Pregnancy	19
Paraneoplastic pruritus	21

roid autoimmunity in 12.1 percent of 140 consecutive cases of chronic urticaria; 8 of the 17 had goiter or thyroid dysfunction.[11] Each of the 17 also had angioedema. The urticaria and angioedema improved in some, but not all of the patients when they were treated with levothyroxine, but the nature of the link between CUA and thyroid autoimmunity remains unclear.

HYPOTHYROIDISM

According to the classic picture, the skin in hypothyroidism is cold, dry, pale, rough, and scaly. There is a diffuse waxy pallor, sweating is decreased, and the epidermis may be thinned but hyperkeratotic. Skin "dryness" is seen in 80 to 90 percent of cases of hypothyroidism.[8] Asteatotic eczema is noted in some cases as well. It is not at all surprising that itching would accompany such changes in the skin of hypothyroid patients, and some textbooks indicate that the skin in hypothyroid patients may itch; what is surprising is the relative paucity of recent reports of this phenomenon in the medical literature. In the 1950s, Goldblatt administered thyroid extract to patients with pruritus and excoriation at a state psychiatric hospital and to 32 private patients with similar findings.[12] Scratching ceased in many cases and from this Goldblatt concluded that "factitial dermatitis is probably the result of scratching in response to a deficiency of thyroid hormone." As this trial was not blinded or controlled, it provides tenuous support for the widely held notion that hypothyroidism is a direct cause of itching. Experienced thyroidologists have not registered itching as a frequent complication of hypothyroidism.[13]

CARCINOID SYNDROME

Carcinoid syndrome routinely appears on lists of systemic causes of generalized pruritus without a rash and, nowadays, itching is often mentioned as one of the symptoms in textbook descriptions of the carcinoid syndrome. Case reports of this phenomenon are actually rare. Mengel reported the case of a 57-year-old man who complained of severe pruritus, erythema of the upper half of the body, flushing, abdominal fullness, and watery diarrhea for 6 weeks.[14] In addition to a violaceous hue over the face and shoulders, a dusky gray appearance over the rest of his body, and deep red telangiectatic lesions over facial prominences, he also developed peculiar orange blotches spontaneously or when he rubbed or scratched. In another single case report, a 41-year-old woman developed severe pruritus during a carcinoid crisis also manifested by peripheral vascular collapse, flushing, chest pain, paresthesias, and hyperesthesias.[15] Intravenous administration of the antiserotonin compound, cyproheptadine, led to immediate relief.

DIABETES

There is no question that itching of the genital and perianal areas, as well as a number of nonpruritic skin disorders, may be associated with diabetes.[16] In a substantial number of cases this may be due to the predisposition to candidiasis or dermatophyte infection in those areas among diabetics. Generalized pruritus also occurs, but is not as common. In 1927, Greenwood surveyed 500 diabetic patients and found that 16 had generalized pruritus and 17 had localized itching, principally of the vulva.[17] He also found that the skin was "dry" in 26 percent of cases. Forty percent had dermatophytosis of the feet. In 1986, Neilly and colleagues reported a study of 300 diabetic hospital outpatients and 100 nondiabetic hospital outpatient controls.[18] Among the diabetics, they found that 13 had generalized pruritus. Of these, two had iron deficiency anemia, one had ichthyosis, one psoriasis, and one eczema. Thus eight (2.7%) had generalized pruritus for which there was no other explanation, compared to only 1 percent of the controls. Twenty-nine of the diabetic women had pruritus vulvae, compared to only three in the control group; of the 21 examined, seven had detectable yeast infection and two had beta streptococcal infection. Also 7.7 percent of the diabetics and 10 percent of the controls had other, nondefined, "localized itches." Neither Greenwood nor Neilly comments on whether itching of any sort was the initial presenting complaint in any of their patients. Given the minimal expense of blood glucose determination, however, the now common practice of measuring it as part of the evaluation of generalized pruritus does not seem unreasonable. Cases of generalized itching as a presentation of diabetes are reported from time to time.[19]

Anecdotal reports also indicate that diabetes may lead to isolated, "unrelenting" pruritus of the scalp, the only physical sign of which may be excoriation, and that "complete relief" may be achieved when the diabetes is brought under control.[20] According to Steven K. Shama, a dermatologist associated with the Joslin Diabetes Center and the New England Deaconess Hospital (with which Greenwood was affiliated as well), a number of diabetic patients complain of an itchy scalp.[21] According to Shama, physical examination reveals widely spaced inflammatory papules and some crusts, mostly, but not entirely, around hair follicles. Although most patients are not sure if the papules or the itch appears first, Shama feels that their response to topical corticosteroids indicates that they are inflammatory in nature.

If diabetes does cause generalized pruritus, the mechanism remains unknown. Metabolic abnormalities, including those that may be associated with diabetic renal failure, could account for some cases.[22] Autonomic dysfunction, by itself or because of related anhydrosis or oligohydrosis, could be another mechanism. Diabetic neuropathy is more characteristically associated with pain, burning, or prickling sensations, although pruritic sensations may be described as well.[23] Idiopathic autonomic dysfunction is a cause of one of the most rare pruritic curiosities, orthostatic leg itching.[24] There are at least two other ways in which diabetes may account for the complaint of generalized pruritus. One is that a localized focus of intense itching, as in anogenital pruritus, may lower the threshold for perception of itching elsewhere on the skin.[25] The other is that some patients will complain of "itching all over" to avoid the embarrassment of admitting to localized, anogenital pruritus.

MASTOCYTOSIS[26,27]

There are systemic and cutaneous forms of mastocytosis in which pharmacologically active mediators released by mast cells present in excessive numbers and/or abnormal locations cause a variety of systemic or local cutaneous symptoms, among which itching is often prominent. In solitary mastocytomas, macular, papular, or nodular skin-colored to tannish-pink lesions become redder and urticate on gentle stroking (Darier's sign). In urticaria pigmentosa, similar papules may be present, but the classic presentation includes many (10 to more than 100) skin-colored to cafe-au-lait-colored macules that exhibit Darier's sign on stroking. Flushing may be precipitated by rubbing the skin, by ingestion of mast cell degranulating agents, or after ingestion of alcohol. In infants the lesions may become bullous. In telangiectasia macularis eruptiva perstans (TMEP) the characteristic lesions are widespread telangiectatic macules that may be slightly tan to tan and that usually urticate on stroking as well. In diffuse cutaneous mastocytosis, yellow, thickened, doughy skin that resembles leather results from massive infiltration of mast cells. It may occur in an erythrodermic form. Bullae may occur spontaneously or after trauma. In systemic mastocytosis the liver, spleen, and bone marrow may be infiltrated by mast cells but as many as half of the patients may not have any skin findings. In all forms of mastocytosis, symptomatic (i.e., pruritic) dermographism may occur. Systemic mastocytosis may occur as mast cell leukemia or in association with a number of hematologic disorders. An aggressive variant, which may occur with or without urticaria pigmentosa, is called lymphadenopathic mastocytosis with eosinophilia. Although paresthesias and pruritus may occur in systemic mastocytosis they are actually not that common; flushing, sometimes with syncope, is more common. A 1991 supplement to the *Journal of Investigative Dermatology* included 14 excellent papers on mastocytosis, and reviewed every aspect from classification[28] to treatment.[29]

The diagnosis of mastocytosis can be challenging when classic skin lesions are not present.[30] The differential diagnosis of flushing, in particular, includes neurogenic flushing, autonomic epilepsy, autonomic neuropathy, carcinoid syndrome, insulinoma, and pheochromocytoma. Pathologic examination of involved skin (with special stains for mast cells) is straightforward; evidence of mast cell infiltration may also be sought in clinically normal looking skin or in the bone marrow. Measurement of urinary histamine levels, urinary histamine metabolites,[31] or other mast cell mediators such as tryptase[32] may be helpful. Cases of cutaneous mastocytosis without clinically obvious skin lesions, presenting as generalized pruritus or as dermographism, and diagnosed by skin biopsy, have been reported.[33,34]

CHOLINERGIC PRURITUS

Cholinergic pruritus represents one end of a spectrum ranging from itching without visible skin changes to cholinergic erythema to cholinergic urticaria.[35] Nomland reported three cases in 1944,[36] but there were no further reports until 1989; how rare it may be is not known. In the case reported by Berth-Jones and Graham-Brown, a 19-year-old man presented with a 3-year history of increasingly severe pruritus triggered by physical exertion, warm surroundings, anxiety, and hot food.[35] Initially the symptoms could be relieved by going to a cool place for a few minutes. As time went on and the severity of his symptoms increased, a mild erythema and then two small papules typical of cholinergic urticaria were noted. In the cases reported by Nomland, exercise, emotional stress, and heat were precipitating factors.[36] Like cholinergic erythema,[37] cholinergic pruritus would appear to be a diminutive variant of cholinergic urticaria. The patient reported by Berth-Jones and Graham-Brown had a low plasma level of alpha-1-antichymotrypsin and responded to treatment with danazol.

ADRENERGIC PRURITUS

In 1985, Shelley and Shelley described adrenergic urticaria, a new form of stress-induced hives.[38] In contrast to cholinergic urticaria, where the characteristic lesion is a small urticarial papule in the center of a large erythematous flare, the distinctive lesion of adrenergic urticaria is the "halo hive:" a small papule at the center of a small blanched halo. In addition, the acetylcholine skin test is positive in the former, negative in the latter. Intradermal injection of noradrenaline reproduces typical halo hives. Propranalol was effective in both of the cases reported by Shelley and Shelley.

Given the existence of cholinergic urticaria and its relative, cholinergic pruritus, followed by the report of adrenergic urticaria, it was inevitable that the symmetry of itches provoked by stress would be completed, and it was when Haustein reported a patient with adrenergic pruritus in 1990.[39] In that case, a 34-year-old woman developed generalized itching within 1 hour after episodes of emotional stress. The episodes lasted for 2 to 3 hours and no wheals, flares, or other rash was observed. Intradermal injection of adrenalin reproduced the symptoms and could be blocked by local administration of either propranalol or the alpha-blocker, tolazoline. Propranalol 25 mg by mouth twice daily was helpful in reducing further attacks.

How many patients with so-called psychogenic pruritus may actually have emotionally triggered or stress-related adrenergic or cholinergic pruritus remains to be seen. As noted by Shelley and Shelley, other agents that reduce autonomic discharge may also provide relief in the various forms of "autonomic urticaria," and, we presume, in "autonomic pruritus."[38] Finally, adrenergic pruritus may play a role in the itching of atopic dermatitis.[40]

PREGNANCY AND PERIMENSTRUAL PRURITUS

The itches and pruritic dermatoses of pregnancy are covered in Chap. 19. Premenstrual pruritus related to recurrent cholestasis has been observed,[41] and itching as a consequence of cholestasis induced by oral-contraceptive hormonal treatment is well recognized. A variety of other pruritic skin disorders may vary with the menstrual cycle.[42] Autoimmune progesterone dermatitis may take many forms: pompholyx, eczematous eruptions, erythema multiforme, and urticaria.[43,44] A well-documented case of recurrent premenstrual urticaria related to estrogen sensitivity has also been reported.[45]

MULTIPLE ENDOCRINE NEOPLASIA TYPE 2A (SIPPLE'S SYNDROME) AND NOTALGIA PARESTHETICA

Notalgia paresthetica (NP) is a localized itch of the midupper back or scapular area. Most cases are probably the consequence of an isolated sensory neuropathy. Repeated rubbing and scratching can lead to secondary change such as hyperpigmentation. Nunziata and colleagues from the University of Naples described a kindred in which NP is present only in family members who also have multiple endocrine neoplasia (MEN) 2A (Sipple's syndrome: medullary thyroid carcinoma and phaeochromocytoma).[46] In affected family members, NP appeared in childhood, before biochemical or clinical presentation of thyroid tumor. Three children of the last generation, aged 4 to 11 years, who have NP have undergone testing. Thyroid C-cell hyperplasia was detected in the 11-year-old. The authors conclude that, "In this MEN 2A kindred the presence of such a characteristic hereditary itch in affected members may be considered as a phenotypic marker giving advance warning of medullary thyroid carcinoma." As it is unlikely that NP in this family was caused by a circulating hormone, it seems likely that affected family members also inherited a separate anatomic abnormality predisposing them to NP. Notalgia paresthetica is discussed further in Chap. 12.

ANECDOTAL OR QUESTIONABLE ASSOCIATIONS

Gout

In 1961 Winkelmann pointed out that, "On the basis of clinical observation, many diseases have been said to be associated with pruritus," and that, despite the absence of evidence, "the myth of such relationships persists as part of medical folklore."[47] Winkelmann points out that itching in gout is an example of such folklore, and that although itchy patients with polycythemia may have hyperuricemia, "no modern treatise on the gouty patient includes description of pruritus as a primary symptom."

Hypercalcemia and Hypocalcemia

Hyperparathyroidism

Textbooks mention pruritus as a symptom of calcemia in primary hyper-parathyroidism, but I have not been able to locate primary citations.[48,49] Microscopic deposits of calcium in the dermis are thought to be the cause. The association of secondary hyperparathyroidism and itching in renal failure[50] is discussed in Chap. 15. In one case of intractable pruritus as the presenting symptom of carcinoma of the bronchus, an elevated parathyroid hormone level was detected and the authors suggested that ectopic PTH secretion could be the cause of pruritus associated with neoplasia.[51]

Hypoparathyroidism

In hypoparathyroidism the skin may be dry and scaly. An itchy exfoliative dermatitis has been described in several patients with idiopathic hypopara-thyroidism or other causes of hypocalcemia, and it is noteworthy that other clinical signs of hypocalcemia may not be dramatic.[52,53] Mucocutaneous candidiasis occurs in some cases of primary hypoparathyroidism and can cause itching, particularly in intertriginous areas.

REFERENCES

1. Osler W: *Principles and Practice of Medicine,* 5th ed. New York, Appleton. 1904, p 839.
2. Eliakim M, Rachmilewitz M: Pruritus: A neglected symptom in thyrotoxicosis. *Israel Med J* 18:262, 1959.
3. Barrow MV, Bird ED: Pruritus in hyperthyroidism. *Arch Dermatol* 93:237–238, 1966.
4. Rothfield B: Pruritus as a symptom in hyperthyroidism. *JAMA* 205:122, 1968.
5. Barnes HM, Sarkany I, Calnan CD: Pruritus and thyrotoxicosis. *Trans St. Johns Hosp Dermatol Soc* 60:59–62, 1974. [This journal is now known as *Clin Exp Dermatol.*]
6. Zemtsov A, Elks M, Shehata B: Thyrotoxicosis presenting as generalized pruritic exfoliative dermatitis and fever. *Dermatology* 184:157, 1992.

7. Braverman LE: Personal communication. December 21, 1986.
8. Bijlmer-Iest JC, van Vloten WA: Thyroid and the skin, in Vermeer BJ, Wuepper KD, van Vloten WA, et al (eds): *Metabolic Disorders and Nutrition Correlated with Skin. Curr Probl Dermatol.* Basel: Karger, 1991, vol 20, pp 34–44.
9. Kinsey MD, Donowitz M, Wartofsky L, et al: The correlation between pruritus and elevated serum chenodeoxycholic acid (CDC) levels in hyperthyroidism. Abstract. *Gastroenterology* 70:A-44/902, 1976.
10. Isaacs NJ, Ertel NH: Urticaria and pruritus: Uncommon manifestations of hyperthyroidism. *J Allerg Clin Immunol* 48:73–81, 1971.
11. Leznoff A, Josse RG, Denburg J, et al: Association of chronic urticaria and angioedema with thyroid autoimmunity. *Arch Dermatol* 119:636–640, 1983.
12. Goldblatt S: Hypothyroid pruritus. On the etiology and treatment of certain cases of neurotic excoriations. *Acta Derm Venereol* (Stockh) 35:167–173, 1955.
13. Braverman LE: Written personal communication. August 17, 1992.
14. Mengel CE: Cutaneous manifestations of the malignant carcinoid syndrome. Severe pruritus and orange blotches. *Ann Intern Med* 58:989–993, 1963.
15. Kahil ME, Brown H, Fred HL: The carcinoid crisis. *Arch Intern Med* 114:26–28, 1964.
16. Huntley AC: The cutaneous manifestations of diabetes mellitus. *J Am Acad Dermatol* 7:427–455, 1982.
17. Greenwood AM: A study of the skin in five hundred cases of diabetes. *JAMA* 89:774–776, 1927.
18. Neilly JB, Martin A, Simpson N, et al: Pruritus in diabetes mellitus: Investigation of prevalence and correlation with diabetes control. *Diabetes Care* 9:273–275, 1986.
19. Ghattas G, Clermont G: A new case of diabetes presenting with pruritus. *Union Med Can* 121:225–226, 1992.
20. Scribner M: Diabetes and pruritus of the scalp. (letter). *JAMA* 237:1559, 1977.
21. Shama SK: Personal communication. February 1, 1991.
22. Knick B: Juckreiz bei diabetes. *Much med Wschr* 123:1197–1199, 1981.
23. Dyck PJ: New understanding and treatment of diabetic neuropathy. *N Engl J Med* 326:1287–1288, 1992.
24. Hines S, Houston M, Robertson D: The clinical spectrum of autonomic dysfunction. *Am J Med* 70:1091–1096, 1981.
25. Edwards AE, Shellow WVR, Wright ET, et al: Pruritic skin disease, psychological stress, and the itch sensation. *Arch Dermatol* 112:339–343, 1976.
26. Soter NA: The skin in mastocytosis. *J Invest Dermatol* 96:32s–39s, 1991.
27. Austen KF: Systemic mastocytosis. *N Engl J Med* 326:639–640, 1992.
28. Metcalfe DD: Classification and diagnosis of mastocytosis: Current status. *J Invest Dermatol* 96:2s–4s, 1991.
29. Metcalfe DD: The treatment of mastocytosis: An overview. *J Invest Dermatol* 96:55s–59s, 1991.
30. Kuter I, Harris NL: Case records of the Massachusetts General Hospital, Case 7-1992, (systemic mastocytosis). *N Engl J Med* 326:472–481, 1992.
31. Keyzer JJ, deMonchy JGR, vanDoormaal JJ, et al: Improved diagnosis of mastocytosis by measurement of urinary histamine metabolites. *N Engl J Med* 309:1603–1605, 1983.
32. Schwartz LB, Metcalfe DD, Miller JS, et al: Tryptase levels as indicator of mast-cell activation in systemic anaphylaxis and mastocytosis. *N Engl J Med* 316:1622–1626, 1987.
33. Ruiz-Maldonado R, Tamayo L, Ridaura C: Diffuse dermographic mastocytosis without visible skin lesions. *Int J Dermatol* 14:126–129, 1975.
34. Kendall ME, Fields JP, King LE: Cutaneous mastocytosis without clinically obvious skin lesions. *J Am Acad Dermatol* 10:903–905, 1984.
35. Berth-Jones J, Graham-Brown RAC: Cholinergic pruritus, erythema and urticaria: A disease spectrum responding to danazol. *Br J Dermatol* 121:235–237, 1989.

36. Nomland R: Cholinogenic urticaria and cholinogenic itching. *Arch Dermatol Syph* 50:247–250, 1944.
37. Murphy GM, Kobza Black A, Greaves MW: Persisting cholinergic erythema: A variant of cholinergic urticaria. *Br J Dermatol* 109:343–348, 1983.
38. Shelley WB, Shelley ED: Adrenergic urticaria: A new form of stress-induced hives. *Lancet* 2:1031–1033, 1985.
39. Haustein U-F: Adrenergic urticaria and adrenergic pruritus. *Acta Derm Venereol* (Stockh) 70:82–84, 1990.
40. Shelley WB, Shelley ED: Diary of a practice. *Cutis* 46:198, 1990.
41. Dahl M: Premenstrual pruritus due to recurrent cholestasis. *Trans St Johns Hosp Dermatol Soc* 56:11, 1970.
42. Leitao E, Bernhard JD: Perimenstrual non-vesicular dermatitis herpetiformis. *J Am Acad Dermatol* 22:1079–1081, 1990.
43. Stephens CJM, Black MM: Autoimmune progesterone dermatitis. *Br J Dermatol* (suppl 34)121:64, 1989.
44. Miura T, Matsuda M, Yanbe H, et al: Two cases of autoimmune progesterone dermatitis. Immunohistochemical and serological studies. *Acta Derm Venereol* (Stockh) 69:308–310, 1989.
45. Mayou SC, Charles-Holmes R, Kenney A, et al: A premenstrual urticarial eruption treated with bilateral oophorectomy and hysterectomy. *Clin Exp Dermatol* 13:114–116, 1988.
46. Nunziata V, Giannattasio R, DiGiovanni G, et al: Hereditary localized pruritus in affected members of a kindred with multiple endocrine neoplasia type 2A (Sipple's syndrome). *Clin Endocrinol* 30:57–63, 1989.
47. Winkelmann RK: Dermatologic clinics. 1. Comments on pruritus related to systemic disease. *Proc Staff Meetings Mayo Clinic* 36:187–196, 1961.
48. Aurbach GD, Marx SJ, Spiegel AM: Parathyroid hormone, calcitonin, and calciferols, in Wilson JD, Foster DW (eds): *Williams Textbook of Endocrinology*, 7th ed. Philadelphia, Saunders. 1985, p 1173.
49. Freinkel RK, ·Freinkel N: Cutaneous manifestations of endocrine disorders, in Fitzpatrick TB, Eisen AZ, Wolff K, et al (eds): *Dermatology in General Medicine*, 3d ed. New York, McGraw-Hill. 1987, p 2066.
50. Massry SG, Popoutzer MM, Coburn JW, et al: Intractable pruritus as a manifestation of secondary hyperparathyroidism in uraemia, disappearance of itching after subtotal parathyroidectomy. *N Engl J Med* 279:697–700, 1968.
51. Thomas S, Harrington CI: Intractable pruritus as the presenting symptom of carcinoma of the bronchus: A case report and review of the literature. *Clin Exp Dermatol* 8:459–461, 1983.
52. Dent CE, Garretts M: Skin changes in hypocalcemia. *Lancet* 1:142–146, 1960.
53. Hirano K, Ishibashi A, Yoshino Y: Cutaneous manifestations in idiopathic hypoparathyroidism. *Arch Dermatol* 109:242–244, 1974.

NINETEEN
PRURITUS IN PREGNANCY

J. K. Shornick

INTRODUCTION

"Pruritus of pregnancy" is a potentially massive subject, as the pregnant woman may be subject to the entire repertoire of the dermatologists' trade. The preexisting skin diseases that may be aggravated by pregnancy have recently been reviewed,[1] and will not be discussed here. The more limited subject of those pruritic entities unique to pregnancy is the subject of this chapter.

The group of pregnancy-related diseases has engendered tremendous confusion. Many diseases of similar or identical clinical appearances have been given different names by different authors, usually without benefit of complete histopathologic or laboratory investigations. Information that was originally anecdotal has then been perpetuated in texts. Table 19-1 presents a summarized view of a typical classification scheme incorporating reviews published as recently as 1982.[2] But the classification of diseases is a dynamic process, subject to evolution, and fortunately the last several years has seen this list condense. The student of history will note, for example, that impetigo herpetiformis has been accepted as pustular psoriasis, perhaps induced by the relative hypocalcemia that pregnancy creates. Other entities may also be dropped from the list. Prurigo annularis was reported in 1941:[2a] No histology or laboratory information accompanied the text, and no subsequent report has been noted. Similarly, history has not reproduced autoimmune progesterone dermatitis of pregnancy, which was reported a single time in 1973.[2b] Spangler and colleagues's papular dermatosis of pregnancy[3] has caused particular confusion, being widely reproduced in standard references, yet seldom seen.

Table 19-1 Old classification of the dermatoses of pregnancy

Herpes gestationis
Pruritic urticarial papules and plaques of pregnancy
Intrahepatic cholestasis of pregnancy
Prurigo gestationis (Besnier)
Toxaemic rash of pregnancy (Bourne)
Prurigo of pregnancy (Nurse)
  early onset form
  late onset form
Papular dermatosis of pregnancy (Spangler)
Pruritic folliculitis of pregnancy
Linear IgM disease of pregnancy
Autoimmune progesterone dermatosis of pregnancy
Impetigo herpetiformis
Prurigo annularis

Much of the confusion regarding classification can be dispelled by an appreciation for the historical context in which the various terminologies arose, and by careful reading of the original articles. In 1904, Besnier and colleagues[4] first used the term "prurigo gestationis" to include all patients with pregnancy-related dermatoses, other than those with herpes gestationis. Costello[5] referred to these patients as "prurigo gestationis of Besnier" and estimated an incidence of 2 percent of all pregnancies. He suggested symptomatic treatment only, and, curiously, advocated injections of serum from healthy, pregnant women as a source of estrogens.

In 1962 Bourne[6] first characterized a subset of patients with intensely pruritic, symmetrical papules or urticarial plaques that tended to appear during the later part of the third trimester. Initial lesions typically developed within the abdominal striae of short women who had experienced excessive weight gain during pregnancy. They generally suffered recurrences during subsequent gestations, and had a tendency to develop fetal distress. Bourne coined the term "toxaemic rash of pregnancy" to describe this entity. Unfortunately, he offered no histology or laboratory information.

Spangler and colleagues (also 1962)[3] attempted to identify another subset of patients with distinctive clinical and biochemical abnormalities, which they referred to as "papular dermatitis of pregnancy." They reported 12 women seen over 3 years with intensely pruritic, generalized, excoriated papules in areas both easy and difficult to reach. First onset was generally during the second or third trimester, and all patients suffered recurrences during subsequent gestations. Three to eight new lesions developed per day in no particular pattern and all patients were unresponsive to topical therapies. The hallmark of papular dermatitis was purported to be the biochemical abnormalities, including an elevated urinary human chorionic gonadotropin, decreased plasma hydrocortisone, and decreased serum half-life of hydrocortisone. In 2 of 12 patients in whom estrogen levels were measured, the levels were found to be in the low–normal range. Liver function tests and histopathology were not reported, and immunofluorescence was not yet available. Spangler and colleagues[3] reported 37 pregnancies with 10 stillbirths or abortions prior to referral and treatment, yielding a fetal wastage of 37 percent. Only one fetal death was seen in the treated group, emphasizing the need for early diagnosis and treatment.

Nurse (1968)[7] cited all of the above literature, but ignored it, dividing all patients with (non-HG) pregnancy rashes into "early" and "late" forms. The late, papular, and urticarial form clearly overlapped with Bourne's "toxaemic rash of pregnancy," and has since been described as pruritic urticarial papules and plaques of pregnancy[8] (see following), but the early onset form has remained enigmatic. Nurse characterized the clinical features of these early onset patients as discrete, excoriated, grouped papules, predominantly on extensor surfaces, and estimated the incidence of this disorder at 1 in 200 pregnancies. By Nurse's description, lesions developed during the second or third trimester and persisted for up to 3 months postpartum. Recurrences during subsequent gestations were uncommon, and there were no maternal or fetal risks. Unfortunately, Nurse failed to perform histopathology or the biochemical tests described by Spangler, and his observations were also made before the advent of immunofluorescence.

Nurse's "early onset" patients and Spangler's "papular dermatitis" patients were undoubtedly the same group, viewed from different perspectives. Certainly, their clinical descriptions were nearly identical. As neither group reported liver function studies or histopathology and Nurse failed to exclude the biochemical abnormalities of papular dermatitis, one can only separate the two by their differences in fetal risks. Spangler's paper has been roundly criticized on this score, however. Of the 11 deaths in his group, only 3 were associated with the clinical features of papular dermatitis, the rest occurred prior to the first occurrence of skin disease. To include fetal deaths that were not associated with cutaneous disease clearly and grossly exaggerated risks. Second, Spangler made no attempt to distinguish spontaneous abortions in the first trimester from fatalities later on. As first trimester abortions are common in normal women, it is not clear that the fetal death rate in Spangler's group was, in fact, elevated. Finally, history has offered little encouragement that papular dermatitis is real. Only two groups have reported papular dermatitis since Spangler's own cases were reported.[9,10]

Pruritic folliculitis of pregnancy[11] was added to the group of pregnancy specific diseases in 1981. Yet all of the patients in this report were thought to have papular dermatitis clinically. They were defined as different based solely on their shared histologic features. None had biochemical investigations. Until *all* patients with the shared clinical features of early onset prurigo are thoroughly evaluated, it seems prudent to consider them together.

Table 19-2 Rational classification of the pruritic entities of pregnancy

Classification	Synonym(s)
Herpes gestationis[a]	Pemphigoid gestationis[a]
Pruritic Urticarial Papules and Plaques of Pregnancy (PUPPP)[a]	Polymorphic eruption of pregnancy[a] Toxemic rash of pregnancy Toxic erythema of pregnancy Late onset prurigo of pregnancy
Prurigo of pregnancy[a]	Prurigo gestationis (Besnier) Early onset prurigo of pregnancy Papular dermatitis of pregnancy Pruritic folliculitis of pregnancy
Cholestasis of pregnancy[a] 1. Prurigo gravidarum 2. Jaundice of pregnancy	Obstetric cholestasis[a]
Inadequately documented	
Linear IgM disease of pregnancy	

[a] Preferred terminology

Modern classifications omit diseases of doubtful existence or relegate them to a second list of dubious importance. Only herpes gestationis (HG), pruritic urticarial papules and plaques of pregnancy (PUPPP), and cholestasis of pregnancy (CP) have withstood the tests of time and are universally accepted as uniquely relevant to pregnancy. But such a strenuous scheme omits those patients with early onset prurigo.

Table 19-2 takes all of these factors into consideration and lists a rationalized classification for the pruritic entities of pregnancy, together with their synonyms. CP would normally be omitted from reviews on the *dermatoses* of pregnancy because there is no primary dermatologic lesion associated with it. But failure to appreciate CP in a woman with widespread excoriations or scratch papules surely, in retrospect, accounts for some of the confusion that has generated such a rich proliferation of terms in the dermatology literature. Prurigo of pregnancy, as defined by Holmes and Black[12] incorporates Besnier's prurigo of pregnancy, Nurse's early onset form of prurigo, and Spangler's papular dermatitis of pregnancy. Holmes and Black thought pruritic folliculitis distinctive, and listed it separately.[12] But because all of the original patients with this entity were thought to have papular dermatitis clinically, and none had complete biochemical investigations, I consider pruritic folliculitis to be in the early onset group. Prurigo of pregnancy is probably not a homogeneous collection of patients and will, no doubt, continue to be debated. Terms in current use by different authors are noted in Table 19-2 by asterisks. "Pruritus gravidarum" and "jaundice of pregnancy" are in quotes because they are not universally agreed on. Linear

Immunoglobulin M (IgM) dermatosis of pregnancy[13] is listed separately because it has not yet withstood the tests of time.

HERPES GESTATIONIS

Definition

In its classical presentation, herpes gestationis is an extremely rare, autoimmune, Immunoglobulin G (IgG)-mediated, complement dependent, vesiculobullous disease of pregnancy, characterized clinically by the rapid progression of intensely pruritic, urticarial lesions on the trunk to a generalized pemphigoid-like eruption, sparing the face, mucous membranes, and usually the palms and soles. It tends to present during the second or third trimester, or occasionally during the immediate postpartum period, exacerbate at the time of delivery, then spontaneously regress over weeks to months, only to recur earlier and more severely during subsequent gestations.

The term herpes gestationis, first proposed by Milton in 1872, is synonymous with pemphigoid gestationis, which is used preferentially in the United Kingdom.

Epidemiology

An incidence estimate of 1 in 3,000 pregnancies made by Russell and Thorne in 1957[14] is still widely quoted, but clearly errant. This estimate was no doubt exaggerated by the selective referral built into the data base of the investigators. More recent estimates from different groups are in close agreement: Kolodny estimated an incidence of 1 in 10,000 deliveries, but his data actually showed only 2 occurrences in 113,000 deliveries.[15] Holmes and colleagues[16] counted 2 cases in 84,000 consecutive deliveries in England and Shornick and colleagues[17] estimated an incidence of 1 in 50,000 deliveries in the greater Dallas area. These incidences are probably all overestimates, but are considerably closer to the experience of the dermatologic community than previous estimates.

The disease respects no particular racial boundaries, although there is some evidence that its incidence may vary according to the incidence of the various HLA types in different populations.[18]

Etiology

The disease is presumed to be autoimmune, caused by a well-characterized anti-basement membrane zone (BMZ) antibody, the so-called "HG factor." In fact, HG is currently defined by the immunofluorescent finding of complement (C) in a smooth, linear band along the cutaneous basement membrane zone in a clinically compatible situation. The use of split skin specimens, chemically separated through the lamina lucida, reveals the immunoreactants to be on the epidermal side. Immunoelectron microscopy reveals a location similar to bullous pemphigoid (BP) antigen. There is a "serum factor" which causes the deposition of C in this location. Because this factor was initially erroneously thought to be heat labile,[19] it was thought *not* to be an immunoglobulin, but this has been clearly and repeatedly shown to be incorrect. The HG factor is an IgG.[20] There is no evidence that it differs in structure from other IgGs. It is found by direct immunofluorescence (IF) approximately 25 percent of the time, although it may be demonstrable more often if more refined techniques are used.[20,21] Using indirect, complement added IF, HG factor is demonstrable in the majority of cases. The IgG (HG factor) appears to be an IgG1[20,22] and is specific for an antigen similar to (but not necessarily identical with) the BP antigen, now known to be the hemidesmosome of the basal keratinocyte.[23] There are differences in preferential binding of HG antibody to the 180 kD protein over the 240 kD protein typically found in BP;[24,25] it is not yet clear that the antigens of BP and HG are identical. It may be that the HG and BP antibodies simply recognize different epitopes of the same protein. Pathophysiologically, the antibody fixes to the basement-membrane zone, triggering complement activation via the classical complement pathway. Chemoattraction of eosinophils and their subsequent degranulation follows. It is presumably proteolytic enzymes released from eosinophilic granules that serve to dissolve the bond between epidermis and dermis. There is no evidence that the *antigen* in HG is aberrant. The antigen appears to be a normal component of normal skin, as evidenced by the ability of HG antibody to fix complement to the skin of those without disease. It would thus appear that it is the production of antibody that is the deviant step in the cascade of events leading to disease. The production of antibody is at least a second step, however, as a breakdown of the regulatory process must precede it. Bonagura and colleagues[26] have noted in a single case a marked decrease in anti-idiotype antibody (the natural down regulator of antibody production) to anti-HLA antibodies during the later stages of pregnancy, followed by an increase as the disease remits. This is exactly the opposite of what happens during normal pregnancy, where there is an increase in anti-idiotype antibodies as the pregnancy progresses. This may explain the increased incidence of anti-HLA antibodies in those with a history of HG.[27] What initiates the production of auto-antibody remains enigmatic, but as HG is exclusively a disease of pregnancy (or trophoblastic tumors), recent attention has focused on immunogenetics and the potential for cross reactivity between placental tissues and skin.

Immunogenetic studies have revealed a marked increase in the HLA antigens DR3 and DR4: 61[28] to 80 percent[16] have DR3, 52 to 53 percent have DR4, and 43 to 50 percent have the simultaneous presence of both. It is not known how the presence of these antigens contributes to the development of HG. It is noteworthy that patients with neither antigen can have clinically indistinguishable disease, so the presence of the characteristic HLA antigens alone is not sufficient to produce disease.[28]

There appears to be a mild increase in the HLA antigen DR2 in the husbands of women with HG and it may be that immunologically primed women simply react more strongly to those with disparate antigens.[27] This might be implied by the additional finding that anti-HLA antibodies occur at a higher frequency in those with a history of HG than in normal multiparous controls, but other explanations have been suggested. Perhaps studies of the rare families in which skip pregnancies occur will provide some additional insight into the role the husband's antigens play in the initiation of disease.

It has recently been shown that the HG antibody binds to amnionic basement membrane.[29,30] This finding is not unexpected, as amnion is derived from fetal ectoderm and is antigenically similar to skin, with both pemphigoid and pemphigus antigens represented.[31] But there is an additional finding in the placental tissue of those with HG that appears to be unique. Within the villous stroma of chorionic villi, adjacent to the maternal decidua, these women show an increase in MHC class II antigens (DR, DP, DQ) together with an increased number of lymphocytes near the site of immune attack.[32,33] The MHC antigens expressed are incomplete: DR and DP are well represented, but there is little or no DQ and no evidence of cells comparable to monocytes or macrophages.[33–35] This situation implies ongoing immune response, but not that of classical antigen–antibody reactivity (where all three antigens are represented). Gonwa and colleagues[36] have shown that mononuclear cells that incompletely express class II molecules function poorly as antigen presenting cells, but are potent mediators of autoimmune, allogeneic reactions. It has therefore been proposed that HG is a disease initiated by the aberrant expression of MHC class II antigens (of paternal haplotype) that serve to initiate an allogeneic response to placental BMZ, which then cross reacts with skin.[37] Whether this is actually the case will require considerably more work to ascertain, but as a hypothesis fitting all of the available data, such a theory holds particular interest.

Clinical and Laboratory Manifestations

HG may present during any pregnancy, not just the first. Once it has developed, however, it tends to occur earlier and be more severe during any subsequent gestation. There have recently been reported well documented cases of disease-free pregnancies in those with a previous history of HG, however, and the true risk of recurrence, although certainly occurring in the majority of cases, is not universal.[17,38]

The disease typically presents with exasperating pruritus alone or with intensely pruritic, urticarial lesions during the second or third trimester. First trimester onset has been reported. Fifty percent of cases begin on the abdomen, often within or immediately adjacent to the umbilicus. The other 50 percent begin with typical lesions, but in an atypical distribution (onset on the extremities or even the palms or soles). Facial involvement is distinctly uncommon and mucosal disease nearly nonexistent. Misdiagnosis as allergic contact dermatitis or drug rash is common. The exaggerated degree of pruritus progressing in short order to vesiculobullous disease is the gold standard of clinical HG. The clinical presentation and course, however, are extremely variable. Many patients experience spontaneous resolution during the later part of gestation, only to flare dramatically at the time of delivery. Others may initially present within hours of parturition. Still others may have trivial, nonvesicular disease during one pregnancy, only to suffer exaggerated and characteristic disease during a subsequent gestation. Exacerbation at the time of delivery is characteristic, occurring in the majority of patients. As the disease fades, mild recurrences with menstruation are common. Recurrence with the use of oral contraceptives occurs in at least 25 percent of patients. There are occasional reports of prolonged disease following delivery, even years following parturition, but the majority of patients experience spontaneous regression over weeks to months.

The newborn may be affected with mild cutaneous involvement 10 percent of the time, but typically the disease is self-limited, resolving spontaneously over days to weeks. IF on fetal skin may be positive despite a lack of clinically apparent disease. There is controversy as to whether there is any increase in fetal morbidity or mortality associated with HG, but such might be expected if our concept of HG as a disease initiated by allogeneic attack within the placenta is correct. Holmes and Black[39] have reported an increase in small for gestational age births in women with HG, suggesting at least some placental insufficiency. A more recent study confirmed a slight tendency for small-for-gestational-aged children and revealed a slight tendency for prematurity in those pregnancies affected by HG: 16 percent of deliveries associated with HG occurred before 36 weeks and 32 percent before 38 weeks, compared to 2 percent and 11 percent, respectively in the same women during unaffected pregnancies.[40] These findings were not related to the use of systemic steroids, as there was no difference between those treated and those not treated. No increase in spontaneous abortions or fetal mortality were noted.

Routine laboratory investigations tend to be unhelpful. Occasional patients develop peripheral eosinophilia and it has been suggested that the severity of disease tends to be reflected by the degree of peripheral eosinophilia.[41] Anti-BMZ antibody titers do not correlate with the extent or severity of disease, nor is there any apparent correlation between HLA type and clinical activity.[28] There is a higher incidence of anti-HLA antibodies in patients with HG than normal, multiparous women, but there is no evidence that these are clinically relevant.[27] One additional study found an increased incidence of antithyroid antibodies,[16] but clinically apparent thyroid dysfunction has rarely been reported. One might actually expect a high incidence of other autoimmune disease in women with a history of HG, given their increase in HLA DR3, but such is not historically obvious. Antinuclear antigens and complement levels are normal. Acute phase reactants may be increased.

The histopathology in HG classically shows a subepidermal vesicle with lymphocytes and eosinophils in a perivascular distribution within the dermis. Eosinophils may be seen lined up along the dermal–epidermal junction, and typically fill the vesicular space. Classical histopathology is seen in the minority of cases; nonspecific changes with a mixed infiltrate containing eosinophils is more often encountered.

The sine qua non for the diagnosis of HG is the finding during active disease of C3 with or without IgG in a linear band along the BMZ of perilesional skin. In salt split specimens, antibody deposition is found along the base of the epidermal fragment, similar to the staining seen in BP. Indirect IF only occasionally shows IgG deposition in a similar pattern, however, this antibody typically shows the capacity to fix C to the BMZ, even when the antibody itself is not discernable.

Physical Examination

Early features include intensely pruritic, hive-like lesions on the trunk or extremities. Fifty percent of patients experience the initial onset of lesions on the abdomen or within the umbilicus itself. The other 50 percent have more atypical onsets, but the development of blisters should alert the physician to the possibility of HG. Progression to vesiculobullous disease is nearly invariant and usually occurs within days to weeks of the initial onset of pruritus. Cases without blisters during the initial involved pregnancy have been reported, followed by more typical disease during subsequent gestations. The degree of pruritus typically defies description and is far beyond objective findings. The palms and soles are generally spared and the disease almost never involves the face or mucosal surfaces.

Differential Diagnosis

Early in onset HG may be confused with PUPPP. This is particularly troublesome given the possibility of urticarial HG, rare though it may be. More typically, the rapid and relentless progression to vesiculobullous lesions excludes alternative considerations. The most frequent error in initially suspect situations is to confuse HG with allergic contact dermatitis or drug rashes. IF then becomes the key to differentiation, although the clinical course is usually distinctive enough to differentiate these entities.

Management

Topical steroids and antihistamines are usually ineffective, but are occasionally helpful, and may temporize until delivery. Systemic steroids remain the cornerstone of therapy. Most patients respond to 0.5 mg/kg of prednisone daily. Maintenance therapy, generally at a lower dose, may or may not be required throughout gestation; many patients actually experience spontaneous regressions during the third trimester, only to flare again with parturition.

Alternatives to steroids (dapsone, pyridoxine, Ritodrine) or adjuvants (gold, methotrexate, cytoxan, cyclophosphamide, plasmapheresis) have been reviewed.[42] None are particularly useful prior to term, and the experience with each has been variable at best.

PRURITIC URTICARIAL PAPULES AND PLAQUES OF PREGNANCY

Definition

PUPPP is an idiopathic, intensely pruritic, urticarial or papular dermatosis that tends to occur during the later part of the third trimester or immediate postpartum period, most commonly in primiparous women. Although vesiculation may be seen in PUPPP, PUPPP contrasts with HG because it does not progress to bullous disease nor display immunoreactants at the dermal–epidermal junction on IF. It tends to remit spontaneously within days of parturition, and only occasionally recurs during subsequent gestations. PUPPP is synonymous with "toxic erythema of pregnancy"[16] and also incorporates the poorly characterized terminology of Bourne's toxaemic rash of pregnancy[6] and Nurse's late onset prurigo of pregnancy.[7] Holmes and Black[43] and Holmes[44] have made a compelling argument that the terminology be changed to "polymorphic eruption of pregnancy," but unfortunately, this terminology has not yet gained universal support.

Epidemiology

The seminal paper on PUPPP by Lawley and colleagues in 1979[8] provided a significant clarification of previously conflicting and overlapping schemes for classifying the dermatoses unique to pregnancy. Prior descriptions by Bourne, then Nurse, although widely quoted, were without benefit of histopathologic or laboratory investigations and intrinsically confusing. Lawley's clarification unified Bourne's "toxaemic rash of pregnancy" and Nurse's late onset form of "prurigo gravidarum."

PUPPP is the most common of the specific dermatoses of pregnancy. Its incidence is unknown, but has been estimated to be as common as 1 in

160 deliveries.[44] It has been reported to occur predominantly in primiparous women (75–85%), but first onset after multiple normal gestations has been noted. Based on the available reports, it is unclear whether those who first develop PUPPP after multiple normal gestations do so after a change in paternal influence as seen in HG. Once disease occurs, it tends *not* to recur during subsequent pregnancies, although one group has noted recurrence in up to 50 percent of cases.[16] There is no known association between PUPPP and any other cutaneous or systemic disease. There are no maternal or fetal morbidities, and only a single report of involvement of the newborn.[45]

Etiology

The cause of PUPPP remains unknown. Investigations to date have been exclusionary. Liver function, hormone levels, cortisol metabolism, direct, and indirect IF are normal. Recent reference has been made to an increase in maternal weight gain or the frequency of twinning associated with PUPPP and it has therefore been suggested that rapid, late stretching of the abdominal skin may somehow be etiologic.[46,47] It is interesting to note that Bourne made similar observations in his original series of patients with toxaemic rash of pregnancy in 1962.[6]

Clinical and Laboratory Manifestations

Onset is abrupt, generally in the last 2 or 3 weeks of pregnancy, and often within striae distensae. Pruritus is generally intense and occurs coincident with the rash. Rapid spreading to the trunk or extremities is the rule, but like HG, involvement of the face is exceptional. Lesions may be papular or urticarial, although fine vesicles may be seen in up to 40 percent of cases.[44] Bullae are not a feature of PUPPP. The incidence of vesiculation in PUPPP together with the broad range of clinical presentations in these patients has lead Holmes and Black[43,44] to propose the terminology "polymorphic eruption of pregnancy."

The histopathology of urticarial or papular lesions shows nonspecific perivascular lymphocytic infiltrates with variable degrees of dermal edema. There may be neutrophils or a variable number of eosinophils within the infiltrate. The epidermis is often normal, although there may be spongiosis, parakeratosis, or even eosinophilic spongiosis.

Laboratory investigations help only to exclude concurrent problems. Liver function tests are normal. Urine or serum human chorionic gonadotropins and cortisol metabolism are normal. Direct IF of lesional skin may show C within vascular walls, but the finding of a linear band of C3 or IgG along the BMZ indicates the alternative diagnosis of HG. HLA typing shows no difference between those with PUPPP and normal controls.[16]

Differential Diagnosis

Drug rashes must remain highly suspect. Fortunately, pregnancy is generally a time of limited drug use. Toxic erythemas of viral origin are usually apparent within the context of associated symptoms. The most important differential is the rare urticarial form of HG. The only way to exclude this is by IF.

Management

The majority of reported patients have benefited from the use of potent topical corticosteroids and oral antihistamines, but occasional women may require systemic steroids. As resolution is typically spontaneous, rapid, and complete, often within 7 to 10 days of delivery, a conservative approach to management seems justified.

PRURIGO OF PREGNANCY

Definition

Prurigo of pregnancy affects about 1 in 300 pregnancies[48] and is characterized by the onset of discrete, pruritic, excoriated papules in a localized or generalized distribution during the second or third trimester. Lesions may or may not be follicular. Disease may last for weeks to months postpartum, and recurrence during subsequent gestations is variable. By definition, liver function tests are normal and IF fails to reveal immunoreactants at the dermal–epidermal junction, but accurate classification of published patients is not always possible, as most cases have been incompletely evaluated.

Prurigo of pregnancy is a clarification of Besnier's prurigo gestationis, Nurse's early onset form of prurigo and Spangler's papular dermatosis of pregnancy. Pruritic folliculitis of pregnancy belongs in this group clinically, being separated only by its histopathology. As noted earlier, as those with pruritic folliculitis were thought clinically to have papular dermatitis but did not have the appropriate laboratory investigations to exclude it, it is unclear what the precise relationship between these entities is. It seems likely that "prurigo of pregnancy" is a heterogeneous group, classified together because of extensive clinical overlap, incomplete evaluation and failure to identify alternative etiologies.

Etiology

The etiology is unknown. As it is likely that this group is heterogeneous, multiple pathways may be relevant. Black has suggested that the findings in many of these patients may be the result of prurigo gravidarum in women with the atopic diathesis.[48]

Clinical and Laboratory Manifestations

Prurigo of pregnancy typically presents during the second or third trimester with discrete scratch papules, predominantly on extensor surfaces. Typical lesions are .5 to 1.0 cm in size, with or without a central crust. Pustules or follicular pustules may be seen, but blisters are not.

Neither Nurse nor Spangler reported histopathologic findings. Rahbari[49] summarized the results of 16 biopsies referred to his histology laboratory, but the diagnosis was confirmed only by clinical suspicion. Because both papules and vesicles were reported from the referring clinicians, and the results of laboratory investigations were not available, it is likely that his cases were drawn from a heterogeneous group. Pathology typically revealed mild acanthosis, parakeratosis, focal exocytosis, and crust formation. There was extensive dermal edema with scattered eosinophils and neutrophils within the mixed lymphohistiocytic infiltrate. There was capillary endothelial damage, but without vasculitis. Holmes and Black[12] reported similar histology without neutrophils or eosinophils, together with negative direct and indirect IF. Zoberman and Farmer[11] reported similar findings in their retrospective study describing pruritic folliculitis of pregnancy, except that their six patients had clinically follicular lesions showing intraluminal pustule formation containing neutrophils, lymphocytes, mononuclear cells, and variable numbers of eosinophils. Four patients who had IF had negative results.

Laboratory findings are inconsistently described.

Physical Examination

Except for widespread excoriations and excoriated papules, generally on extensor surfaces, the physical examination is normal.

Differential Diagnosis

The first differential is between a specific dermatosis of pregnancy and the wide variety of pruritic entities unrelated to gestation. Bites, especially scabies, should be excluded. All patients should have normal liver function studies and serum bile acids. Drug-induced disease should be excluded.

Management

Prurigo of pregnancy is maddening but benign, and requires only symptomatic treatment. As there is no evidence of maternal or fetal risk, there is no indication for intervention.

CHOLESTASIS OF PREGNANCY

Definition

CP is a genetically linked, estrogen-dependant alteration in liver function resulting in cholestasis, with or without jaundice. The mechanism by which this happens is unknown. The tendency is generally manifested by presentation in the third trimester with intense pruritus. The diagnosis is confirmed by the finding of increased serum bile acids in the absence of alternative explanations. Thus, the features of the disease are (1) symptoms of cholestasis relating to pregnancy with no history of exposure to hepatitis or hepatotoxic drugs, (2) the presence of generalized pruritus with or without jaundice, (3) demonstration of biochemical abnormalities consistent with cholestasis, (4) disappearance of signs and symptoms following pregnancy, and (5) recurrence during a subsequent gestation.

There appears to be no *maternal* morbidity or mortality associated with CP, other than the potential for malabsorption. *Fetal* risks do, however, appear increased. It is generally accepted that there is an increased tendency for premature labor, fetal stress, and fetal deaths.[50,51]

Cholestasis of pregnancy is reasonably divided by some into those with jaundice (cholestatic jaundice of pregnancy) and those with pruritus and other biochemical abnormalities without hyperbilirubinemia (pruritus gravidarum).[52]

Epidemiology

Jaundice occurs in approximately 1 in every 1,500 pregnancies.[53] Cholestasis of pregnancy is the second most common cause of gestational jaundice, viral hepatitis being more common. It is estimated that CP accounts for approximately 20 percent of cases of obstetric jaundice, although the frequency depends on the demographics of the area. Obstetric cholestasis is particularly common in Scandinavia, Northern Europe, and Chile, but distinctly uncommon in Asians or blacks. A positive family history is seen in up to 50 percent of those affected, and normal relatives (male or female) of those affected frequently show impaired BSP clearance under the influence of estrogens. A Mendelian dominant inheritance associated with the HLA A31, B8 haplotype has been proposed.[54]

Etiology

A single biochemical anomaly explaining CP has yet to be elucidated.

Plasma volume increases dramatically during pregnancy, while blood volume increases only modestly. Hepatic blood flow tends to stay constant, but as a percentage of cardiac output, it decreases. By term, blood flow to the liver decreases from 35 percent of cardiac output to 29 percent.[54] Some argue that this relative fall in flow decreases clearance of toxins, including estrogens.[53]

Estrogens increase biliary cholesterol concentration and secretion and impair hepatic capacity to transport anions like bilirubin, bile salts, and BSP. Some authors have argued that bile secretion is blocked in CP through inhibition of membrane (Na, K)-ATPase or directly at the level of the tight junction. More recently it has been proposed that estrogens mediate their effect via the regulation of actin molecules, which function intracellularly to mediate bile secretion.[55]

Clinical and Laboratory Manifestations

Patients typically present in the last trimester of otherwise uneventful pregnancies, although initial presentation as early as 8 weeks has been reported. Intense, generalized pruritus is invariably the presenting symptom. Symptoms tend to be worse at night and worst on the trunk, palms, and soles, and tend to persist for the duration of the pregnancy. No further symptoms may arise. Up to 50 percent of patients, however, develop dark urine, light colored stools or jaundice within 2 to 4 weeks. Unlike pruritus, which may wax and wane, jaundice tends to stabilize shortly after presentation. Symptoms disappear within 24 to 48 hours of delivery; jaundice resolves in 1 to 2 weeks. Recurrence during subsequent pregnancies is nearly invariant, and follows a similar course. Recurrences with the use of oral contraceptives are also routine.

Increased serum bile acids are the sine qua non, and are typically 3 to 100 times normal. In those without jaundice, elevated serum bile acids may be the only identifiable laboratory abnormality (prurigo gravidarum). Conjugated (direct) bilirubin is increased, but rarely above 2 to 5 mg per dl. Alkaline phosphatase, GGT, and cholesterol are unreliable during pregnancy, but AST remains within four times normal, even in those with CP. Higher elevations reflect hepatic injury of alternative cause. Serum abnormalities do not parallel fetal risk, and are only useful to confirm the presence or absence of disease. Hepatic ultrasonography is normal. Liver biopsy is not indicated for uncomplicated CP, but if done, shows centrilobular cholestasis, which may be patchy or mild, but can be severe with bile thrombi found within dilated canaliculi. Hepatocellular necrosis and portal inflammation are not seen.

Physical Examination

The physical exam is normal, although mild hepatomegaly may be seen when jaundice is present.

Differential Diagnosis

Viral hepatitis is more common, and should be excluded by appropriate serology.

There is, by definition, no primary dermatitis associated with CP. The finding of cutaneous inflammation or concurrent (particularly organ specific) symptoms should also provoke a search for alternative causes.

Failure of pruritus to stop within days of delivery, or the persistence of elevated liver function tests suggest underlying primary biliary cirrhosis.

Management

Treatment of the patient is symptomatic. Cholestyramine or phenobarbitol may be useful for relatively modest elevations of serum bile acids, but their use is disputed. Phototherapy using UVB may be useful. There is a tendency for these women to subsequently develop cholelithiasis or gallbladder disease.

If intrahepatic cholestasis lasts for several weeks, vitamin K absorption may be impaired, leading to a prolonged prothrombin time. Without exogenous vitamin K, fetal prothrombin activity can be negligible or absent, leading to a high incidence of intracranial hemorrhage. The prothrombin time should therefore be routinely monitored, and intramuscular vitamin K administered as necessary.

The incidence of fetal risks is controversial, and appropriate management is therefore debated. Meconium staining and premature labor occur with frequencies as high as 45 percent.[56] Fetal distress and increased stillbirths are also reported, with mortality in some series as high as 13 percent. Some authors argue for weekly amniocentesis after 30 weeks, with delivery on signs of meconium staining or when the lecithin–sphingomyelin ratio shows maturity.[51] Others argue for delivery at 38 weeks to avoid later risks.

INADEQUATELY DOCUMENTED ENTITIES

Linear IgM Dermatosis of Pregnancy

Alcalay and colleagues[13] described a single case characterized by intensely pruritic, follicular papules and pustules showing nonspecific histopathology (without evidence of folliculitis), but bright, linear IgM along the BMZ by IF. The lesions began during the 37th week of gestation and resolved within 6 weeks of delivery of a normal male. Repeat IF following resolution of the rash was negative. Liver function studies and the biochemical investigations reported in papular dermatitis were not done.

REFERENCES

1. Winton GB: Skin diseases aggravated by pregnancy. *J Am Acad Dermatol* 20:1–13, 1989.
2. Winton GB, Lewis CW: Dermatoses of pregnancy. *J Am Acad Dermatol* 6:977–998, 1982.
2a. Davies JHT: Prurigo annularis. *Br J Dematol* 53:143, 1941.
2b. Bierman SM: Autoimmune progesterone dermatitis. *Arch Dermatol* 107:896–901, 1973.
3. Spangler AS, Reddy W, Bardawil WA, et al: Papular dermatitis of pregnancy. A new clinical entity? *JAMA* 181:577–581, 1962.
4. Besnier E, Brocq L, Jacquet L: La pratique dermatologique 1:75. Masson et Cie, Paris, 1904.
5. Costello MJ: Eruptions of pregnancy. *NY State J Med* 41:849, 1941.
6. Bourne G. Toxemic rash of pregnancy. *Proc R Soc Med* 55:462–464, 1962.
7. Nurse DS: Prurigo of pregnancy. *Aust J Dermatol* 9:258–267, 1968.
8. Lawley TJ, Hertz KC, Wade TR, et al: Pruritic urticarial papules and plaques of pregnancy. *JAMA* 241:1696–1699, 1979.
9. Michaud RM, Jacobson D, Dahl MV: Papular dermatitis of pregnancy. *Arch Dermatol* 118:1003–1005, 1982.
10. Nguyen LQ, Sarmini OR: Papular dermatitis of pregnancy: A case report. *J Am Acad Dermatol* 22:690–691, 1990.
11. Zoberman E, Farmer ER: Pruritic folliculitis of pregnancy. *Arch Dermatol* 117:20–22, 1981.
12. Holmes RC, Black MM: The specific dermatoses of pregnancy. *J Am Acad Dermatol* 8:405–412, 1983.
13. Alcalay J, Ingber A, Hazaz B, et al: Linear IgM dermatosis of pregnancy. *J Am Acad Dermatol* 18:412–415, 1988.
14. Russell B, Thorne NA: Herpes gestationis. *Br J Dermatol* 69:339–357, 1957.
15. Kolodny RC: Herpes gestationis: A new assessment of incidence, diagnosis, and fetal prognosis. *Am J Obstet Gynecol* 104:39–45, 1969.
16. Holmes RC, Black MM, Dann J, et al: A comparative study of toxic erythema of pregnancy and herpes gestationis. *Br J Dermatol* 106:499–510, 1982.
17. Shornick JK, Bangert JL, Freeman RG, et al: Herpes gestationis: Clinical and histologic features of twenty-eight cases. *J Am Acad Dermatol* 8:214–224, 1983.
18. Shornick JK, Meek TJ, Nesbitt LT, et al: Herpes gestationis in blacks. *Arch Dermatol* 120:511–513, 1984.
19. Provost TT, Tomasi TB: Evidence for complement activation via the alternate pathway in skin diseases. I. Herpes gestationis, systemic lupus erythematosus and bullous pemphigoid. *J Clin Invest* 52:1779–1787, 1973.
20. Kelly SE, Cerio R, Bhogal BS, et al: The distribution of IgG subclasses in pemphigoid gestationis: PG factor is and IgG1 autoantibody. *J Invest Dermatol* 92:695–698, 1989.
21. Holubar K, Konrad K, Stingl G: Detection by immunoelectron microscopy of immunoglobulin G deposits in skin of immunofluorescence negative herpes gestationis. *Br J Dermatol* 96:569–571, 1977.
22. Carruthers JA, Ewins AR: Herpes gestationis: Studies on the binding characteristics, activity and pathogenetic significance of the complement-fixing factor. *Clin Exp Immunol* 31:38–44, 1978.
23. Mutasim DF, Takahashi Y, Labib RS, et al: A pool of bullous pemphigoid antigen(s) is intracellular and associated with the basal cell cytoskeleton-hemidesmosome complex. *J Invest Dermatol* 84:47–53, 1985.
24. Morrison LH, Labib RS, Zone JJ, et al: Herpes gestationis autoantibodies recognize a 180-kD human epidermal antigen. *J Clin Invest* 81:2023–2026, 1988.
25. Kelly SE, Bhogal BS, Wojnarowska F, et al: Western blot analysis of the antigen in pemphigoid gestationis. *Br J Dermatol* 122:445–449, 1990.

26. Bonagura VR, Rohawsky-Kochan C, Reed E, et al: Perturbation of the immune network in herpes gestationis. *Hum Immunol* 15:211–219, 1986.

27. Shornick JK, Stasny P, Gilliam JN: Paternal histocompatibility (HLA) antigens and maternal anti-HLA antibodies in herpes gestationis. *J Invest Dermatol* 81:407–409, 1983.

28. Shornick JK, Stasny P, Gilliam JN: High frequency of histocompatibility antigens HLA-DR3 and DR4 in herpes gestationis. *J Clin Invest* 68:553–555, 1981.

29. Ortonne JP, Hsi BL, Verrando P, et al: Herpes gestationis factor reacts with the amniotic epithelial basement membrane. *Br J Dermatol* 117:147–154, 1987.

30. Kelly SE, Bhogal BS, Wojnarowska F, et al: Expression of pemphigoid gestationis-related antigen by human placenta. *Br J Dermatol* 118:605–611, 1988.

31. Robinson HN, Anhalt GJ, Patel HP, et al: Pemphigus and pemphigoid antigens are expressed in human amnion epithelium. *J Invest Dermatol* 83:234–237, 1984.

32. Borthwick GM, Sunderland CH, Holmes RC, et al: Abnormal expression of HLA-DR antigen in the placenta of a patient with pemphigoid gestationis. *J Repro Immunol* 6:393–396, 1984.

33. Borthwick GM, Holmes RC, Stirrat GM: Abnormal expression of Class II MHC antigens in placentae from patients with pemphigoid gestationis: Analysis of Class II MHC subregion product expression. *Placenta* 9:81–94, 1988.

34. Kelly SE, Fleming S, Bhogal BS, et al: Immunopathology of the placenta in pemphigoid gestationis and linear IgA disease. *Br J Dermatol* 120:735–743, 1989.

35. Kelly SE, Black MM, Fleming S: Antigen-presenting cells in the skin and placenta in pemphigoid gestationis. *Br J Dermatol* 122:593–599, 1990.

36. Gonwa TA, Pickers LJ, Raff HN, et al: Antigen presenting capabilities of human monocytes correlates with their expression of HLA-DS, an Ia determinant distinct from HLA-DR. *J Immunol* 130:706–714, 1983.

37. Kelly SE, Black MM, Fleming S: Hypothesis. Pemphigoid gestationis: A unique mechanism of initiation of an autoimmune response by MHC class II molecules? *J Pathol* 158:81–82, 1989.

38. Holmes RC, Black MM, Jurecka W, et al: Clues to the aetiology and pathogenesis of herpes gestationis. *Br J Dermatol* 109:131–139, 1983.

39. Holmes RC, Black MM: The fetal prognosis in pemphigoid gestationis (herpes gestationis). *Br J Dermatol* 110:67–72, 1984.

40. Shornick JK, Black MM: Fetal risks in herpes gestationis. *J Am Acad Dermatol* 26:63–68, 1992.

41. Lawley TJ, Stingl G, Katz SI: Fetal and maternal risk factors in herpes gestationis. *Arch Dermatol* 114:552–555, 1978.

42. Shornick JK: Herpes gestationis. *J Am Acad Dermatol* 17:539–556, 1987.

43. Holmes RC, Black MM: The specific dermatoses of pregnancy: A reappraisal with special emphasis on a proposed simplified clinical classification. *Clin Exp Dermatol* 7:65–73, 1982.

44. Holmes RC: Polymorphic eruption in pregnancy. *Sem Dermatol* 8:18–22, 1989.

45. Uhlin SR: Pruritic urticarial papules and plaques of pregnancy. Involvement of mother and infant. *Arch Dermatol* 117:238–239, 1981.

46. Yancey KB, Hall RP, Lawley TJ: Pruritic urticarial papules and plaques of pregnancy. Clinical experience in twenty-five patients. *J Am Acad Dermatol* 10:473–480, 1984.

47. Cohen LM, Capeless EL, Krusinski PA, et al: Pruritic urticarial papules and plaques of pregnancy and its relationship to maternal-fetal weight gain and twin pregnancy. *Arch Dermatol* 125:1534–1536, 1989.

48. Black MM: Prurigo of pregnancy, papular dermatitis of pregnancy, and pruritic folliculitis of pregnancy. *Sem Dermatol* 8:23–25, 1989.

49. Rahbari H: Pruritic papules of pregnancy. *J Cut Pathol* 5:347–352, 1978.

50. Reyes H: The enigma of intrahepatic cholestasis of pregnancy: Lessons from Chile. *Hepatol* 2:87–96, 1982.

51. Fisk NM, Storey GNB: Fetal outcome in obstetric cholestasis. *Br J Obstet Gynaecol* 95:1137–1143, 1988.
52. Desmet VJ: Cholestasis: Extrahepatic obstruction and secondary biliary cirrhosis. In MacSween RNM, Anthony PP, Scheuer PJ (eds): Pathology of the Liver. New York, Churchill Livingstone, 1987, p 408.
53. Rustgi VK: Liver disease in pregnancy. *Med Clin NA* 73:1041–1047, 1989.
54. Lunzer MR: Jaundice in pregnancy. *Baillieres Clin Gastroenterol* 3:467–483, 1989.
55. Reyes-Romero MA: Are changes in expression of actin genes involved in estrogen-induced cholestasis? *Med Hypoth* 32:39–43, 1990.
56. Fisk NM, Bye WB, Storey GNB: Maternal features of obstetric cholestasis: 20 years experience at King George V Hospital. *Aust NZ J Obstet Gynaecol* 28:172–176, 1988.

THE ITCHES OF HIV INFECTION AND AIDS

Clay J. Cockerell

INTRODUCTION

Patients who suffer infection with the human immunodeficiency virus (HIV) are prone to develop a number of cutaneous abnormalities. Pruritus, unfortunately, complicates many of these conditions, and while it may seem to be of relatively minor significance in the context of the more severe life threatening illnesses these patients face, it nevertheless poses a serious problem. Itching may be persistent and result in substantial morbidity. In fact, the quality of life of an individual suffering from relentless pruritus may be so greatly deteriorated as to lead to suicidal ideation. Furthermore, pruritus may be the presenting sign of HIV infection, whether there are skin lesions or not.[1,2] It is therefore important to be aware of itching as a complication of HIV infection, be it either the full-blown acquired immune deficiency syndrome (AIDS) or the AIDS-related complex (ARC). Without knowledge of the numerous conditions that may lead to this symptom, therapeutic endeavors most likely will be fruitless.

Although the pathophysiology of itching has been described elsewhere in this book, there are certain mechanisms that may be more applicable to the patient with HIV disease. Although these individuals may develop any cutaneous disorder that afflicts immunocompetent individuals, such as type I immediate hypersensitivity reactions, it has recently been demonstrated that patients with AIDS and HIV disease have elevated serum levels of immunoglobulin E (IgE) directed to HIV-1.[3] Furthermore, this antibody increases in titer as CD4 (T helper) cell numbers fall. Elevated serum levels of IgE are found in a number of pruritic conditions, such as atopic dermatitis, and the same mechanisms that lead to itching with atopy may be operational in these patients.[4] Basophils from HIV-infected patients also demonstrate enhanced degranulation in vitro[5] and a similar phenomenon in vivo would be expected to result in excessive release of pruritogenic compounds such as histamine. Basophil hyperreleasability suggests that mast cells in tissue might be hyperreleasable as well, leading to cutaneous manifestations of histamine release. Indeed, eosinophils are commonly observed in histologic sections taken from inflammatory skin conditions of patients with HIV infection, possibly an indication of mast cell granule release.[6]

Abnormality of peripheral nerves also may be important in pruritus in HIV-infected individuals. HIV can infect cells other than those of the lymphoreticular system, particularly fibroblasts and neurons.[7] It is conceivable that infection of peripheral nerves by HIV could lead to stimulation of pathways associated with pruritus either directly or indirectly. Furthermore, neural viral infection could lead to direct release of Substance P, a compound known to be associated with itching.[8] Stress has been linked to release of Substance P and degranulation of mast cells[9,10] and in the setting of hyperreleasable mast cells in an HIV-infected host this could be a significant factor in inducing pruritus.

Finally, the epidermis is commonly abnormal in these individuals. This in turn leads to abnormal barrier function, enhancing the effects of irritants and cutaneous allergens. This might again potentiate mast cell degranulation as well as lead to synthesis of prostaglandins and other substances that could cause or potentiate pruritus.[11,12]

Patients with HIV disease may develop any of the numerous well described conditions associated with pruritus ranging from infections and infestations to systemic diseases. Such conditions are often caricatures of those found in immunocompetent individuals both in morphology and symptomatology. In addition, certain inflammatory skin diseases have been noted with greater frequency in the HIV-infected host and seem to be peculiarly associated with HIV disease. These conditions may be grouped broadly into infections and infestations, noninfectious inflammatory dermatoses, and systemic diseases associated with pruritus. These will be discussed in sequence and, finally, principles of therapy will be specifically addressed.

INFECTIONS AND INFESTATIONS

Probably the most common infectious condition that leads to pruritus in patients with HIV disease is scabies. Scabies may assume a number of unusual clinical manifestations, many of which are distinct from those in fully immunocompetent hosts. The classic "itchy red bump disease" may be observed, characterized by dome-shaped papules with small burrows in the usual distribution such as the groin and the finger webs. In debilitated individuals, thickened keratotic plaques of Norwegian scabies may be encountered. When scraped for microscopic examination innumerable mites are found. However, another manifestation is a widespread eruption of fine erythematous macules and papules that involves the extremities, trunk, and the head and neck with a clinical appearance similar to an inflammatory dermatosis.[13] Such cases may be misdiagnosed as atopic dermatitis or as drug eruptions.[13] When scrapings are eventually performed, innumerable mites similar to the number seen in Norwegian scabies are usually identified. Biopsies characteristically demonstrate an inflammatory infiltrate of lymphocytes and numerous eosinophils in the dermis with slight epidermal hyperplasia, spongiosis, and a slightly thickened cornified layer containing myriad mites.[14] The reason for the development of this widespread scabetic eruption is not clear but may be related to the diminution in Langerhans' cell number known to be present in these individuals.[15] One last form of scabies that may be seen rarely is a widespread eruption of follicular pustules.[16]

Treatment of all the different forms of scabies is similar to that in immunocompetent individuals; however, in our experience, post scabetic "id" reactions and papular urticaria are quite common following such treatment and may persist for many months after all mites have been eradicated.[17] Treatments with systemic antihistamines such as doxipen in high doses accompanied by topical corticosteroid preparations and antipruritic emollients may have to be continued for months. We recently encountered an individual who had an eruption of pruritic, urticarial papules that persisted for over 1 year following treatment for scabies. No mites could be identified with repeated scrapings. Finally, nodular scabies leading to either pruritic pseudolymphomata and/or prurigo nodularis may supervene.

In addition to scabies, *Demodex folliculorum* has also been postulated to cause a pruritic folliculitis in patients with HIV disease.[18] Such eruptions have been reported to consist of pruritic papules and pustules with an appearance similar to folliculitis. The condition was thought to be due to Demodex because pustules when examined microscopically were shown to contain numerous Demodex mites. The condition resolved following treatment with 1 percent lindane lotion. Metronidazole gel (Metrogel®) as well as oral metronidazole 250 mg by mouth twice daily is also effective.

Superficial fungal infections may also lead to pruritus in HIV-infected individuals. Widespread dermatophytosis with extensive involvement of trunk, extremities, and groin may occur and may be associated with either pronounced or minimal inflammation. The morphology of this condition may be unusual and examples of thick, verrucous crusted plaques with erythema and eruptions of widespread pustules have been encountered.[19] Extensive *tinea capitis* and Majocchi's granuloma may both arise in the setting of HIV disease and may be extremely pruritic. Causative organisms are generally the same as those that cause disease in immunocompetent hosts but on occasion an unusual pathogen such as *Scopulariopsis brevicaulis* will be encountered.[20] Although the pruritus generally resolves following eradication of the causative fungus, id reactions and papular urticaria may occasionally develop. Candidiasis, especially in intertriginous areas, may be extremely pruritic as a consequence not only of maceration and irritation, but perhaps also as a consequence of the fungal infection itself. Candidal infection, especially when present in the oropharynx, is associated with CD4 cell numbers of less than 100 per mm^3,[21] a sign of profound immunodepression. In addition to intertrigo, *C. Albicans* may also infect other areas such as the nail leading to nail dystrophy and paronychia, the oral commisures leading to verrucous papules and nonhealing fissures, and other areas occasionally leading to thickened verrucous lesions with features of candidal granuloma.[17] Although topical antifungal agents may have some efficacy in treating these conditions, systemic antifungal agents such as ketoconazole, fluconazole, or itraconazole are often required for eradication.

Folliculitis may cause pruritus whether it is due to infection with truly pathogenic bacteria such as staphylococci or organisms not considered pathogens such as "diphtheroids."[22] Folliculitis may be very widespread and commonly fails to respond to treatment with systemic antibiotics and topical antiseptic washes.[23] Patients often excoriate and rub affected follicles extensively, leading to prurigo nodularis. Prurigo nodularis is notoriously difficult to treat in immunocompetent individuals; in patients with HIV disease it may be even more so. An additional complication that may supervene is cutaneous ulceration with secondary bacterial infection, which can become systematized.

Prurigo nodularis may also occur as a complication of insect bite reactions. Penneys and others have postulated that such eruptions arise at the sites of previously injected mosquito salivary gland antigens as a consequence of an immunologic "recall" reaction due to the B-cell activation commonly present with HIV infection.[24] The resultant intense pruritus leads to secondary rubbing and excoriation with the eventual clinical lesions of prurigo nodularis. We have observed other insect bite reactions, such as those due to fire ants, become persistent and pruritic, eventuating in prurigo nodularis.[25] (For further discussion of prurigo nodularis, see Chap. 7.)

Although cutaneous viral infections are not commonly associated with itching, occasionally herpetic infections, either herpes simplex or herpes zoster, may lead to tingling and pruritic sensations at the onset of an eruption. This is most likely secondary to irritation of affected nerves. Varicella, which is frequently unusual in presentation and quite severe in these patients, often leads to severe pruritus.[26,27] It is important to treat those with herpes-virus infections with systemic acyclovir, often in high doses, to avoid potential serious complications such as disseminated disease, scarring, and postherpetic neuralgia.[28]

In addition to herpes-virus infections, other systemic viral infections such as measles and the acute exanthem of HIV infection may on occasion be associated with mild pruritus. We have evaluated four individuals at our institution with measles all of whom had mild pruritus associated with generalized dryness of the skin.[29] In no case did our patients develop serious sequelae. The acute exanthem of HIV infection has been recently described in patients with HIV disease.[30–33] Clinically, this eruption may have an appearance similar to other morbilliform eruptions such as those associated with infectious mononucleosis,[32] a roseola-like eruption with erythematous macules and papules involving the face, trunk, and extremities associated with pharangytis and myelopathy,[34] and, finally, a vesico-pustular eruption with involvement of the mucous membranes.[33] These eruptions are thought to develop anywhere from 1 to 3 weeks following exposure to HIV and may be the earliest marker of the infection.[32] Patients usually do not experience striking pruritus but may have mild itching as with other viral exanthems. It is unclear if the eruption itself is specific, but in patients at risk for HIV disease, the development of any viral exanthem should serve as a warning that HIV infection may be imminent. Histologically, two patterns have been described. One is that characteristic of most viral exanthemata, namely a superficial perivascular infiltrate of lymphoctyes and histiocytes with slight spongiosis of the epidermis.[35] The second shows a folliculitis and perifolliculitis with focal epidermal spongiosis and epidermal necrosis.[36] The infiltrate in the second pattern consists primarily of lymphocytes with occasional neutrophils.

NONINFECTIOUS INFLAMMATORY DERMATOSES

A number of noninfectious conditions occur with increased frequency in the setting of HIV infection, many of which are associated with severe pruritus. Such conditions may be divided into three groups: those in which the epidermis is abnormal, those in which the epidermis is unaffected, and those associated with abnormality of follicles.

Pruritic Dermatoses with Epidermal Abnormality

One of the most common cutaneous manifestations of HIV infection is a seborrheic dermatitis-like eruption which may be found in up to 83 percent of HIV-infected individuals.[19] This condition is distinct from seborrheic dermatitis found in individuals who are not immune suppressed. The eruption is usually extensive, commonly involving the entire face, and on occasion, the trunk and extremities (Fig. 20-1).[37,38] The eruption initially consists of fine erythematous papules that tend to coalesce to form plaques. These are often indurated with prominent scale and crust on the surface. In some cases, the plaques may become quite thick and almost verrucous. Pruritus, while usually not severe, is not uncommon, especially when the eruption is florid. The pathogenesis of this condition is somewhat controversial. Some maintain

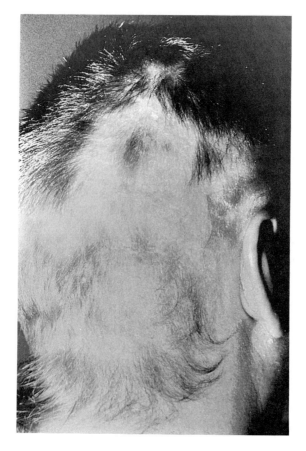

Figure 20-1 Seborrheic dermatitis may be quite pruritic and result in scratching with secondary alopecia as depicted here.

that the process is analogous to psoriasis. Stress, either metabolic or emotional in origin, may lead to the de novo development of or exacerbation of a preexisting condition, similar to flares of seborrheic dermatitis in patients with neurologic disorders.[39] Indeed, central nervous system (CNS) infection with HIV may be important in the development of seborrheic dermatitis in these patients. Others have posited that the eruption is caused by fungal infection with *Pityrosporum ovale*.[19,40] While in some cases numerous fungal spores may be demonstrated in infundibula of follicles and within the cornified layer histologically, in others, little if any fungi are seen. Treatment with topical corticosteroid preparations and antiseborrheic shampoos may be efficacious. In some cases, however, the process may be refractory to therapy. Treatment with topical and/or systemic antifungal preparations may yield benefit in selected instances.[40]

We have observed several patients with seborrheic dermatitis and HIV infection who flared following discontinuation of zidovudine (AZT) therapy. Although the reasons behind this remain unknown, it is tempting to speculate that direct HIV infection of the skin may be playing a role in the development of this condition.

Psoriasiform dermatitides other than seborrheic dermatitis have been observed in these patients, many of which may be quite pruritic. Although the name "psoriasiform dermatitis of AIDS" has been suggested,[41] a number of different inflammatory processes may assume psoriasiform appearances clinically and histologically. True psoriasis vulgaris may worsen in patients with HIV infection and improve following the administration of AZT.[42,43] Just as with other psoriasiform processes, psoriasis may on occasion be pruritic. Because psoriasiform dermatoses in these individuals may be caused by a number of different processes, it is important to perform biopsies, cultures, and serologic studies where appropriate to establish the correct diagnosis. Treatment of true psoriasis in these patients may be quite problematic, the usual topical treatments with tar and corticosteroids being ineffective. Because of the immunocompromise already present, methotrexate must be used with extreme caution, if at all. In addition, etretinate may afford some benefit.[41]

Patients with HIV infection are commonly xerotic and may have acquired ichthyosis. Just as in any patient with severe xerosis, cracking of the skin with marked pruritus can result. It is important that patients avoid excessive exposure to soap and water and apply emollients liberally to alleviate this problem.

Atopic dermatitis may arise de novo in a few patients with HIV infection, and individuals with longstanding atopic dermatitis may experience severe flares of their disease.[44] Such flares seem to occur with greater frequency when the total CD4 cell count falls below 100 to 150mm^3.[19] The precise reason for this is unclear but may in part be related to abnormal release of cytokines such as gamma interferon with a consequent failure to keep the diathesis in check.[45] In some cases, the "atopic dermatitis" is not truly atopic dermatitis at all but represents an atopic dermatitis-like condition.[46] Clinically, these eruptions may have features similar to atopic dermatitis without either a family or personal history of atopy. In addition, histopathologic findings are often not typical of those seen in classic atopic dermatitis. Treatment of atopic dermatitis and atopic dermatitis-like conditions in these patients consists of administration of antihistamines, application of emollients, and avoidance of precipitating factors such as excessive bathing. Until underlying immune deficits are improved, however, the condition often persists regardless of therapy.

A number of other conditions have also been associated with HIV infection and pruritus. Both florid persistent pityriasis rosea[19] and transient acantholytic dermatosis (Grover's disease)[47] have been seen with increased frequency in these patients. HIV-infected patients with Grover's disease are usually younger than immunocompetent counterparts. In addition, the eruption may be persistent rather than transient and may last for many months.[47] Histopathologic findings are similar to those of classic Grover's disease, although the number of eosinophils and plasma cells within the inflammatory cell infiltrate may be exaggerated.[48]

Lichen planus and lichenoid dermatitis induced both by drugs and ultraviolet radiation have also been described.[49,50] We have encountered several cases of chronic photodermatitis with lichenoid morphologies thought to have been induced by drugs. These eruptions were extremely resistant to treatment and flared following minimal exposures to ultraviolet irradiation. One case of true hypertrophic lichen planus has been described in an HIV-infected individual,[49] but we have yet to see a significant increase in the number of cases of lichen planus in our patient population. In addition to lichenoid photodermatitis, chronic psoriasiform photodermatitides analogous to persistent light reactions have been reported.[51] Such eruptions are thought to be "recall" reactions to photoallergens to which the patient had been sensitized previously. Extreme photoprotection is often required in such individuals to ameliorate the problem.

Although delayed-type hypersensitivity is diminished in patients with HIV disease, occasionally allergic contact dermatitis may be encountered.[52] The clinical findings may be bizarre with unusual distributions and morphologies. Even when an excellent history of allergen exposure is present, patch testing may fail to reveal positive results. Such eruptions are usually strikingly pruritic and require application of potent topical corticosteroid ointments.

A number of drug reactions may result in pruritic dermatoses. The most common ones encountered in patients with HIV infection are morbilliform in nature and the most common agents to which these individuals are sensitive include trimethoprim-sulfamethoxazole (Bactrim®), clindamycin, cephalexin, diphenylhydantoin, and ansamycin (Rifabutin®).[53,54] Drug hypersensitivity may lead to more serious complications including erythema multiforme and toxic epidermal necrolysis both of which may be heralded by a pruritic erythematous eruption.[19,55] It is important in such cases to discontinue the offending agent as soon as possible and to administer systemic antihistamines and sometimes systemic corticosteroids.

Chronic irritation may also be associated with pruritus. Patients suffering from longstanding diarrhea such as that which occurs in the Gay Bowel Syndrome may develop chronic perianal irritation with lichen simplex chronicus. Once again, in spite of application of topical antipruritic and topical anti-inflammatory agents, the problem may continue until the underlying process is reversed. Patients with extensive condyloma acuminata may have low grade inflammation and drainage in perianal locations leading to a similar phenomenon.[56]

A condition known as papular dermatitis of AIDS, which is characterized by the presence of small skin-colored to pinkish papules distributed on the upper trunk, neck, and face, may be pruritic.[57] When tissue from this eruption is examined microscopically, different histologic patterns have been observed, some suggestive of papular urticaria and others suggestive of spongiotic dermatitis.[57] This condition may not in truth represent a single disease but may be comprised of several different entities. Pruritus is variable in extent and may range from minimal to severe.

Dermatitis herpetiformis[58] and bullous pemphigoid[59] have been linked to HIV disease, although the strength of the association is questionable. We have had the opportunity to evaluate two individuals with AIDS and dermatitis herpetiformis both of whom responded to treatment with diaminodiphenyl-sulfone (Dapsone). One of them had an eruption that was so extensive it required hospitalization, however. Histologic findings were similar to those seen in immunocompetent individuals.

Pruritic Dermatoses with Normal Epidermis

Patients with HIV disease may develop a number of pruritic urticarial eruptions in which the epidermis is unaffected. One of the most common is acute and chronic urticaria.[60] Clinical courses may be similar to those of immunocompetent patients, but the problems of diagnosis and treatment may be compounded in the setting of compromised immunity. Certain etiologic agents, such as hepatitis B, infectious mononucleosis, amebiasis, and strongyloidiasis, are more frequent in the HIV-infected patient[61] and must not be overlooked. Urticarial allergic eruptions due to drug hypersensitivity are also common and may occur with any of the medications these patients may receive.[54,60] Finally, leukocytoclastic vasculitis, which occurs with increased frequency in HIV-infected patients, may exhibit an urticarial morphology.[60,62] Noninfectious conditions such as periodontal disease[63] and connective tissue disorders[64,65] occur with greater frequency in these patients and may both be associated with urticaria. Because of the elevated serum IgE levels and hyperreleasability of histamine-containing cells[3,5] urticarial eruptions may be extremely refractory to therapy. Treatment consists of identification of and elimination of underlying causes as well as the administration of systemic antihistamines. Treatment with systemic corticosteroids should be avoided because of their serious side effects.

Another disorder that has been observed in HIV-infected patients is the hypereosinophilic syndrome.[66] Skin manifestations may consist of pruritic urticarial plaques, which may be very widespread. One case progressed to an erythroderma. Patients characteristically manifest a marked eosinophilia of greater than 1500 eosinophils/mm^3. Therapy with psoralen plus ultraviolet A may be beneficial.

Macular amyloidosis may also be encountered in these patients. We have seen three cases involving both caucasians and hispanics in our patient population, all of which were associated with striking pruritus which led to rubbing and excoriation with eventual clinical appearances of lichen amyloidosus and prurigo nodularis. The reason some patients with HIV disease develop macular amyloidosis is not clear, but it may be related to resolution of a preexisting lichenoid dermatitis or photodermatitis. Individually necrotic keratinocytes, possibly as a consequence of the diminished number of Langerhans cells, are seen commonly in skin biopsies from inflammatory conditions in HIV-infected individuals[6] and superficial deposits of amyloid may be arising from breakdown products of dyskeratotic cells. Patients usually present with brown to slate-gray reticulated patches that may be localized or quite extensive.[67] Treatment is ineffective but some relief of pruritus may be achieved with administration of antihistamines and application of topical lotions containing pramoxine, menthol, and/or phenol.

Patients also may develop pruritus as a primary idiopathic process.[1,68] Just as in patients with other systemic diseases, pruritus without a cutaneous eruption may be a presenting sign of HIV infection.[1] It is important in the general evaluation of a patient with idiopathic pruritus to consider this diagnosis and perform HIV testing where appropriate. Furthermore, patients with HIV infection may be under severe stress, a factor that may induce or exacerbate pruritus.[69] Until underlying emotional or metabolic stresses are alleviated, it is unlikely that the pruritus will resolve.

Certain systemic diseases associated with pruritus may occur with increased frequency in patients with HIV disease. Hepatic disease may occur due to infectious agents such as hepatitis B virus or *Mycobacterium avium intracellulare.*[70] Other infectious agents such as cytomegalovirus (CMV), herpes simplex virus, and Epstein-Barr virus may cause hepatitis with associated pruritus.[70] Acalculous cholecystitis may also occur as a consequence of CMV or cryptosporidium infection leading to biliary obstruction with consequent cutaneous deposition of bile salts and pruritus.[71,72] The liver may also be damaged by drugs such as trimethoprim-sulfamethoxazole (Bactrim®), isoniazid, rifampin, and ketoconazole.[73-75]

In addition, renal disease is not uncommon in these individuals. The kidney may be affected coincidentally, as through unrelated diabetes mellitus, or through direct infection with HIV.[76,77] Furthermore, renal disease may develop concomitantly with HIV infection, as, for example, in heroin-related nephropathy.[78] Regardless of the etiology, renal disease may lead to uremia with attendant pruritus. Lymphomas of several different varieties are increased in incidence in this setting[79-81] and may be associated with itching either secondary to a pruritic paraneoplasic phenomenon or to a circulating pruritogenic factor as in Hodgkin's disease[82,83] (see also Chap. 21). It is obviously important to exclude the coexistence of any underlying systemic abnormality with appropriate diagnostic tests.

Pruritic Dermatoses with Abnormalities of the Follicle

Abnormality of the hair follicle may be the source of pruritus in some instances. Bacterial folliculitis occurs with increased frequency in these indi-

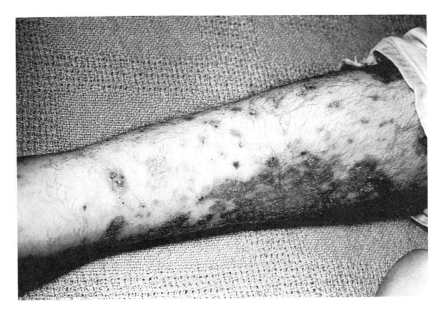

Figure 20-2 Widespread excoriations may be due to underlying eosinophilic pustular folliculitis as depicted here. Note the coexistent plaque of Kaposi's sarcoma adjacent to which these lesions had arisen.

viduals (vide supra). Eosinophilic pustular folliculitis is characterized by a widespread eruption of follicular papules and pustules with marked pruritus.[84,85] Patients often experience such severe pruritus at the time of presentation that few if any intact pustules may be present and only excoriations and lichen simplex chronicus may be noted.[86] The pathophysiology of this condition is unknown, but when lesions are biopsied, the histopathologic findings are distinct from those of bacterial and other types of pustular folliculitis in that the follicle is filled with myriad eosinophils predominantly in the infundibulum.[87] On occasion, there may be follicular rupture with eosinophils in a perifollicular location, sometimes associated with a mixed inflammatory cell infiltrate with granulomatous features. Treatment of this condition with antihistamines and topical antipruritic agents is usually futile. Fortunately, however, ultraviolet B (UVB) phototherapy is highly efficacious in alleviating the symptoms.[86] Patients are treated at gradually increasing exposures to UVB until the pruritus and the eruption abate. Such treatment should be undertaken with some caution, however, as UVB exposure may lead to a decrease in the number and function of Langerhans' cells and CD4 cells.[88] In addition, one study has demonstrated that exposure of HIV-infected lymphocytes in vitro to UVB irradiation led to increased virus expression.[89] A prudent measure to take in treating patients with this condition is to shield all nonaffected areas.

Perforating folliculitis may also be encountered. The pathogenesis of this condition is controversial, and many hold that this represents little more than prurigo papules occurring in the background of pruritus of another cause. Others postulate that *Pityrosporum ovale* infection of follicles plays a role in eliciting this phenomenon.[50] Treatment with ketoconazole, fluconazole, or itraconazole may result in improvement in some cases.

DIAGNOSIS AND TREATMENT

In order to precisely diagnose the cause of pruritus in an HIV-infected individual, it is important to recognize that there may be myriad causes. Ancillary tests such as scrapings and cultures will readily identify infectious processes such as mites of scabies and fungal organisms. Patch testing to identify allergic contact dermatitis may be valuable but should be undertaken with the caveat that these individuals have diminished cell mediated immunity, which may lead to falsely negative test results. Biopsies are important as certain inflammatory diseases, such as urticarial vasculitis and eosinophilic folliculitis, can only be diagnosed with certainty via histopathology. In all cases it is important to alert the histopathologist that a given individual is at risk for HIV disease or is so infected. With such information in mind, the pathologist is more likely to perform special tests in search of infectious agents.[6] Furthermore, immunofluorescence studies may be required.

It is important not to underestimate the importance of careful histories, cutaneous examinations, and systemic evaluations in these patients as severe life threatening diseases may be present and not fully manifest. Clinical–pathologic correlation in which clinical findings are wedded to those of the laboratory ultimately may be the only way to arrive at accurate diagnoses. In some cases, a precise diagnosis may be elusive.[6]

Treatment is best directed at underlying diseases if those can be identified. For example, individuals with pruritus secondary to fungal infections will often respond well to eradication of the ongoing process. The same is true with individuals suffering from underlying lymphomas and hepatic and renal abnormalities. When offending agents can be identified, such as drugs and allergens, it is important to eliminate those as well. In addition, administration of antiviral agents such as AZT and dideoxyinosine (DDI) may lead to immune enhancement and a consequent diminution of symptoms secondary to virucidal effects.[90,91]

It is important to understand that some treatments should be avoided in these patients or if they are to be used, only with very careful and close monitoring. Methotrexate for psoriasis and Reiter's syndrome[92] may lead to worsening of the immune compromise these patients already face with acceleration of death.[76] Although ultraviolet therapy is often quite beneficial,[86,93,94] its indiscriminate use should be avoided as it may lead to worsened immunodepression, elicitation of photoallergic processes, and development of cutaneous malignancies.[88] Topical corticosteroids, while quite beneficial in some cases, should also be used with caution as these may also worsen immunodepression.

The topical agents most commonly used in these patients are corticosteroid creams and ointments, emollients such as lactic acid lotions and petrolatum products, soothing topical antipruritic agents such as pramoxine, and lotions and ointments containing menthol and phenol. Finally, scabicidal agents such as gamma benzene hexachloride and 5 percent precipitated sulfur and antifungal creams containing clotrimazole, cyclopirox, and econazole are commonly dispensed. Such topical therapy may have some benefit in those who are relatively immunocompetent, but in those more profoundly immunocompromised, that is, with CD4 positive cell counts less than 100 cells/mm^3, they may be completely ineffective.[19] Systemic treatments that may yield some benefit include antihistamines of various classes. As a general rule, we tend to begin with agents such as chlorpheniramine and increase the dosage to as much as is tolerated by the patient before adding additional agents or changing. Astemizole, while sometimes effective in urticarial eruptions, is usually not effective in eradicating pruritic symptoms. In general, the greater the antipruritic effect of an antihistamine, the greater the tendency to produce sleep, a side effect that may be poorly tolerated by many individuals. Cholestyramine may be beneficial in patients with cholestasis.[95] Activated charcoal tablets and naloxone may also be efficacious in some cases.[96,97]

It is important to support patients through the virtually inevitable discouragement that develops in the face of persistent pruritus requiring longstanding treatment. Psychotherapy and group support sessions may be necessary to fend off depression and suicidal ideation.[98]

CONCLUSION

Pruritus in patients with HIV disease is a serious problem for a number of reasons. It is important to recognize that it may be a symptom of a number of different conditions many of which may be serious. It also may be a presenting sign of HIV disease and for that reason, clinicians should be attuned to this possibility and not hesitate to take careful histories about risk factors for HIV infection. It is important that dermatologists recognize the importance of their role in early diagnosis of HIV disease, especially in light of recent studies that show the efficacy of treating asymptomatic HIV-infected individuals with AZT.[99] The dermatologist is an important caretaker of the patient with HIV disease and given his or her unique abilities in diagnosis and treatment of skin disease, he or she may be able to significantly lessen the severe morbidity posed by this maddening symptom.

REFERENCES

1. Shaprio RS, Samorodin C, Hood A: Pruritus as a presenting sign of acquired immunodeficiency syndrome. *J Am Acad Dermatol* 16:1115–1117, 1990.
2. Liautaud B, Pape JW, DeHovitz JA, et al: Pruritic skin lesions: A common initial presentation of acquired immunodeficiency syndrome. *Arch Dermatol* 125:629–632, 1989.
3. Levy JA: Changing concepts in HIV infection: Challenges for the 1990's. Opening Ceremony Address at the 6th Annual International Conference on AIDS, San Francisco, CA, June 20, 1990.
4. Dahl MV: The Immune System in Health and Disease in Moschella SL, Hurley HJ (eds): *Dermatology*. Philadelphia, Saunders. 1985, pp 201–208.
5. Miadonna A, Zeggieri E, Tedeschi A, et al: Enhanced basophil releasability in subjects infected with human immunodeficiency virus. *Clin Immunol Immunopathol* 54:237–246, 1990.
6. Cockerell CJ, Rao BK: Histologic patterns of unusual inflammatory dermatoses in patients with human immunodeficiency virus infection. Poster presentation. VII International Conference on AIDS, San Francisco, CA, June 17, 1991.
7. Tateno M, Gonzalez-Scarano F, Levy JA: Human immunodeficiency virus type 1 can infect CD4 negative human fibroblastoid cells. *Proc Natl Acad Sci* 11:4287–4290, 1989.
8. Marx JL: Brain peptides. Is Substance P a transmitter of pain signals? *Science* 205:1886, 1979.
9. Matis WL, Lauker RM, Murphy GF: Substance P induces the expression of an endothelial-leukocyte adhesion molecule by microvascular endothelium. *J Invest Dermatol* 94:492–495, 1990.
10. Klein LM, Lauker RM, Matis WL, et al: Degranulation of human mast cells induces an endothelial antigen central to leukocyte adhesion. *Proc Natl Acad Sci* 86:8972–8976, 1989.
11. Martin J: Pruritus. *Int J Dermatol* 24:634–639, 1985.
12. Hagermark O, et al: Potentiation of itch and flare responses in human skin by prostaglandins E_2 and F_2 and a prostaglandin endoperoxide analog. *J Invest Dermatol* 69:527–530, 1977.
13. Sadick N, Kaplan MH, Pahwa SG, et al: Unusual features of scabies complicating human T-lymphotropic virus type III infection. *J Amer Acad Dermatol* 15:482–486, 1986.
14. Glover R, Young L, Goltz RW: Norwegian scabies in acquired immunodeficiency syndrome: Report of a case resulting in death from associated sepsis. *J Amer Acad Dermatol* 16:396–399, 1987.
15. Belisto DV, Sanchez MR, Baer RL, et al: Reduced Langerhan's cell Ia antigen and ATPase activity in patients with the acquired immunodeficiency syndrome. *N Engl J Med* 310:1279–1282, 1984.
16. Cockerell CJ: Personal observation.
17. Fisher BK, Warner LC: Cutaneous manifestations of the immunodeficiency syndrome. *Int J Dermatol* 26:615–630, 1987.
18. Ashack RJ, Frost NL, Norins AL: Papular pruritic eruption of Demodex folliculitis in patients with acquired immunodeficiency syndrome. *J Am Acad Dermatol* 21(2 Pt. 1):306–307, 1989.
19. Kaplan MH, Sadick N, McNutt S, et al: Dermatologic findings and manifestations of acquired immunodeficiency syndrome (AIDS). *J Am Acad Dermatol* 16:485–506, 1987.
20. Moore MK: Skin and nail infections caused by non-dermatophyte filamentous fungi. *Mykosen suppl.* 1,28, 1978.
21. Klein RS, Harris CA, Smal CB, et al: Oral candidiasis in high-risk patients as the initial manifestation of the acquired immunodeficiency syndrome. *N Engl J Med* 311:354–358, 1984.
22. Sindrup JH, Lisby G, Weismann K: Skin manifestations in AIDS, HIV infection, and AIDS-related complex. *Int J Dermatol* 26:267–272, 1987.

23. Farthing CF, Staughton RCD, Rowland Payne CME: Skin disease in homosexual patients with acquired immune deficiency syndrome (AIDS) and lesser forms of human T cell leukaemia virus (HTLV III) disease. *Clin Exp Dermatol* 10:3–12, 1985.
24. Penneys NS, Nayar JK, Bernstein H, et al: A chronic pruritic eruption in patients with AIDS associated with increased antibody titers to mosquito salivary gland antigens. *J Am Acad Dermatol* 21:421–425, 1989.
25. Cockerell CJ: Non-infectious inflammatory skin diseases in HIV-infected individuals. *Dermatol Clin,* 9:531–541, 1991.
26. Alessi E, Cusini M, Zerboni R, et al: Unusual varicella zoster virus infection in patients with the acquired immunodeficiency syndrome. *Arch Dermatol* 124:1011–1012, 1988.
27. Perronne C, Lazanas M, Leport C, et al: Varicella in patients infected with the human immunodeficiency virus. *Arch Dermatol* 126:1033–1036, 1990.
28. Janier M, Hillion B, Baccard M, et al: Chronic varicella zoster infection in acquired immunodeficiency syndrome. *J Am Acad Dermatol* 18:584–585, 1988.
29. Cockerell CJ: Personal Observation, 1990.
30. Cooper DA, Gold J, Maclean P, et al: Acute AIDS retovirus infection. Definition of a clinical illness associated with seroconversion. *Lancet* 1(8428):537–540, 1985.
31. Rustin MHA, Ridley CM, Smith MD, et al: The acute exanthem associated with seroconversion to human T-cell lymphotropic virus III in a homosexual man. *J Infect* 12:161–163, 1986.
32. Kessler HA, Blaauw B, Spear J, et al: Diagnosis of human immunodeficiency virus infection in seronegative homosexuals presenting with an acute viral syndrome. *JAMA* 258:1196–1199, 1987.
33. Calabrese LH, Proffitt MR, Levin KH, et al: Acute infection with the human immunodeficiency virus (HIV) associated with acute brachial neuritis and exanthematous rash. *Ann Intern Med* 107:849–851, 1987.
34. Lindskov R, Lindhardt BO, Weismann K, et al: Acute HTLV-III infection with roseola-like rash. *Lancet* 1(8478):447, 1986.
35. McMillan A, Bishop PE, Dennis A, et al: Immunohistology of the skin rash associated with acute HIV infection. *AIDS* 3:309–312, 1989.
36. Brehmer-Anderson E, Torssander J: The exanthema of acute (primary) HIV infection. Identification of a characteristic histopathological picture? *Acta Derm Venereol* (Stockh) 70:85–87, 1990.
37. Mathes BM, Douglass MC: Seborrheic dermatitis in patients with acquired immunodeficiency syndrome. *J Am Acad Dermatol* 13:947–951, 1985.
38. Soeprono FF, Schinella RA, Cockerell CJ, et al: Seborrheic-like dermatitis of acquired immunodeficiency syndrome. *J Am Acad Dermatol* 14:242, 1986.
39. Burton JL, Cartlidge M, Shuster S: Effects of L-dopa on the seborrhea of parkinsonism. *Br J Dermatol* 88:475–479, 1973.
40. Ford GP, Farr PM, Ive FA, et al: The response of seborrheic dermatitis to ketoconazole. *Br J Dermatol* (suppl. 3)26:25, 1984.
41. Sadick NS, McNutt NS, Kaplan MH: Papulosquamous dermatoses of AIDS. *J Am Acad Dermatol* 22:1270–1277, 1990.
42. Duvic M, Johnson TM, Rapini RP, et al: Acquired immunodeficiency syndrome-associated psoriasis and Reiter's syndrome. *Arch Dermatol* 123:1622–1632, 1987.
43. Johnson TM, Duvic M, Rapini RP: AIDS exacerbates psoriasis. *N Engl J Med* 313:1415, 1985.
44. Ball LM, Harper JI: Atopic eczema in HIV-seropositive hemophiliacs. *Lancet* ii:627–628, 1987.
45. Parkin JM, Eales I-J, Galazka AR, et al: Atopic manifestations in the acquired immunodeficiency syndrome: Response to recombinant interferon gamma. *Br Med J* 294:1185–1186, 1987.
46. Cockerell CJ: Atopic dermatitis-like and seborrheic dermatitis-like eruptions in HIV infected patients. *Clin Dermatol* 9:49–51, 1991.

47. Muhlemann MF, Anderson MG, Paradinas FJ, et al: Early warning skin signs in AIDS and persistent generalized lymphadenopathy. *Br J Dermatol* 114:419–424, 1986.
48. Cockerell CJ: Personal observation.
49. Pardo RJ, Kerdel FA: Hypertrophic lichen planus and light sensitivity in an HIV-seropositive patient. *Int J Dermatol* 27:642–644, 1988.
50. Viraben R, Dupre A: Lichenoid granulomatous papular dermatosis associated with human immunodeficiency virus infection: An immunohistochemical study. *J Amer Acad Dermatol* 18:1140–1141, 1988.
51. Toback AC, Longley J, Cardullo AC, et al: Severe chronic photosensitivity in association with acquired immunodeficiency syndrome. *J Amer Acad Dermatol* 15:1056–1057, 1986.
52. Knobler RM: Human immunodeficiency virus infection. *Dermatol Clin* vol 7, no. 2, 1989.
53. Gordin FN, Simon GL, Wofsy CD, et al: Adverse reactions to trimethoprim-sulfamethoxazole in patients with the acquired immunodeficiency syndrome. *Ann Intern Med* 100:495, 1984.
54. Farthing CF, Brown SE, Staughton RCD: *A Colour Atlas of AIDS.* London, Wolfe Medical Publications Ltd., 1986, pp 24–37.
55. Kalter DC, Tschen JA, Klimar M: Maculopapular rash in a patient with acquired immunodeficiency syndrome. *Arch Dermatol* 121:1455–1460, 1985.
56. Cockerell CJ: Personal observation.
57. James WD, Redfield RR, Lupton GP, et al: A papular eruption associated with human T-cell lymphotropic virus type III disease. *J Am Acad Dermatol* 13:563–566, 1985.
58. Mitsuhashi Y, Hohl D: Dermatitis herpetiformis in a patient with acquired immunodeficiency syndrome-related complex. *J Amer Acad Dermatol* 18:583, 1988.
59. Levy PM, Balavoine JF, Salomon D, et al: Ritodrine responsive bullous pemphigoid in patients with AIDS-related complex. *Br J Dermatol* 114:635–636, 1986.
60. Friedman-Kien AE: *Color Atlas of AIDS.* Philadelphia, Saunders. 1989, pp 93–124.
61. Glatt AE, Chirgwin K, Landesman SH: Treatment of infections associated with human immunodeficiency virus. *N Engl J Med* 318:1439–1448, 1985.
62. Velji AM: Leukocytoclastic vasculitis associated with positive HTLV-III serologic findings. *JAMA* 256:2196–2197, 1986.
63. Silverman S Jr, Migliorati CA, Lozada-Nur F, et al: Oral findings in people with or at high risk for AIDS: A study of 375 homosexual males. *J Am Dent Assoc* 112:187–192, 1986.
64. Ulirsch RC, Jaffe ES: Siogren's syndrome-like illness associated with the acquired immunodeficiency syndrome-related complex. *Human Pathol* 1063–1068, 1987.
65. de Clerck LS, Couttenye MM, de Broc ME, et al: Acquired immunodeficiency syndrome mimicking Siogren's syndrome and systemic lupus erythematosis. *Arthr Rheum* 31:272–275, 1988.
66. May LP, Kelly J, Sanchez M: Hypereosinophilic syndrome with unusual cutaneous manifestations in two men with HIV infection. *J Am Acad Dermatol* 23:202–204, 1990.
67. Bernhard JD: Macular amyloidosis, notalgia paresthetica, and pruritus: Three sides of the same coin? *Dermatologica* 183:53–54, 1991.
68. Penneys NS: *Skin Manifestations of Aids.* New York, Lippincott. 1989, pp 138–140.
69. Bernhard JD: Cutaneous sensation and the pathophysiology of pruritus. In Soter NA and Baden HP (eds.) Pathophysiology of Dermatologic Diseases, 2d ed. New York, McGraw-Hill. 1991, pp 73–82.
70. Lebovics E, Thung SN, Schaffner F, et al: The liver in the acquired immunodeficiency syndrome. A clinical and histologic study. *Hepatology* 5:293–298, 1985.
71. Kavin N, Jonas RB, Chowdhury L, et al: Acalculous cholecystitis and cytomegalovirus infection in the acquired immunodeficiency syndrome. *Ann Intern Med* 104:53–54, 1986.
72. Blumberg R, Kelsey P, Perrone T, et al: Cytomegalovirus and cryptosporidium-associated acalculous gangrenous cholecystitis. *Am J Med* 76:1118–1123, 1984.
73. Wharton JM, Coleman DL, Wofsy CB, et al: Trimethoprim-sulfamethoxazole or pentamidine for *Pneumocystis carnii* pneumonia in the acquired immunodeficiency syndrome: A prospective randomized trial. *Ann Intern Med* 105:37–44, 1986.

74. Zimmerman HJ: *Hepatotoxicity, the Adverse Effects of Drugs and Other Chemicals on the Liver.* New York, Appleton-Century-Crofts, 1978.
75. Lewis JH, Zimmerman HJ, Benson GD, et al: Hepatic injury associated with ketoconazole therapy: Analysis of 33 cases. *Gastroenterology* 86:503–513, 1984.
76. Rao TKS, Friedman EA, Nicastri AD: The types of renal disease in the acquired immunodeficiency syndrome. *N Engl J Med* 316:1062–1068, 1987.
77. Bourgoignie JJ, Meneses R, Pardo V, et al: The nephropathy related to acquired immunodeficiency syndrome. *Adv Nephrol* 17:113–126, 1988.
78. Rao TKS, Nicastri AD, Friedman EA: Natural history of heroin associated nephropathy. *N Engl J Med* 290:19–23, 1974.
79. Haskal ZJ, Lindan CE, Goodman PC: Lymphoma in the immunocompromised patient. *Radiol Clin North AM* 28(4):885–899, 1990.
80. Serrano M, Bellas C, Campo E, et al: Hodgkin's disease in patients with antibodies to human immunodeficiency virus. *Cancer* 65(10):2248–2254, 1990.
81. Myskowski P, Straus DJ, Safai B: Lymphoma and other HIV-associated malignancies. *J Am Acad Dermatol* 22(6 Pt 2)1253–1260, 1990.
82. Olsson H, Brandt L: Relief of pruritus as an early sign of spinal cord compression of Hodgkin's disease. *Acta Med Scand* 206:319, 1979.
83. Gilbert HS, Warner RR, Wasserman LR: A study of histamine in myeloproliferative disease. *Blood* 18:795, 1966.
84. Soeprono FF, Schinella RA: Eosinophilic pustular folliculitis in patients with acquired immunodeficiency syndrome. *J Am Acad Dermatol* 14:1020, 1986.
85. Colton AS, Schachner L, Kowalczyk AP: Eosinophilic pustular folliculitis. *J Am Acad Dermatol* 14:469–474, 1986.
86. Buchness MR, Lim HW, Hatcher VA, et al: Ultraviolet B phototherapy of eosinophilic pustular folliculitis in patients with the acquired immunodeficiency syndrome. *N Engl J Med* 318:1183–1185, 1988.
87. Cockerell CJ: Cutaneous manifestations of HIV infection other than Kaposi's sarcoma: Clinical and histologic aspects. *J Am Acad Dermatol* 22:1260–1269, 1990.
88. Harber LC, Bickers DR: *Photosensitivity Diseases.* 2d ed, Toronto, Dekcer. 1989, pp 46–53.
89. Valerie K, Delers A, Bruck C, et al: Activation of human immunodeficiency virus type 1 by DNA damage in human cells. *Nature* 333 (6168):78–81, 1988.
90. Fischl MA, Richman DD, Greico MH, et al: The efficacy of azidothymidine (AZT) in the treatment of patients with AIDS and AIDS-related complex: A double-blind, placebo-controlled trial. *N Engl J Med* 317:185–191, 1987.
91. Rozencweig M, McLaren C, Beltangady M, et al: Overview of phase 1 trials of 2',3'-dideoxyinosine (ddI) conducted on adult patients. *Rev Infect Dis* (suppl 5)12:s570–s576, 1990.
92. Winchester R, Bernstein DH, Fischer HD, et al: The co-occurrence of Reiter's syndrome and acquired immunodeficiency. *Ann Intern Med* 106:19–26, 1987.
93. Pardo J, Bogaert MA, Penneys NS, et al: UVB phototherapy of the pruritic papular eruption of the acquired immunodeficiency syndrome. *J Am Acad Dermatol* 26:423–428, 1992.
94. Gorin I, Lessana-Leibowitch M, Fortier P, et al: Successful treatment of the pruritus of human immunodeficiency virus infection and acquired immunodeficiency syndrome with psoralens plus ultraviolet A therapy. *J Am Acad Dermatol* 20:511–513, 1989.
95. Lottsfeldt Fl, Krivit N, Aust JB, et al: Cholestyramine therapy in intrahepatic biliary atresia. *N Engl J Med* 269:186–189, 1963.
96. Pederson JA, Matter BJ, Czerwinski AW, et al: Relief of idiopathic generalized pruritus in dialysis patients treated with activated oral charcoal. *Ann Intern Med* 93:446, 1980.
97. Bernstein JE, Swift R: Relief of intractable pruritus with naloxone. *Arch Dermatol* 15:1366, 1979.

98. Kendall J, Gloersen B, Gary P, et al: Doing well with AIDS: Three case illustrations. *Arch Psychiatr Nurs* 3:159–165, 1989.

99. Volberding PA, Lagakos SW, Koch MA, et al: Zidovudine in asymptomatic human immunodeficiency virus infections: A controlled trial in persons with fewer than 500 CD4 positive cells per cubic millimeter. *N Engl J Med* 322:941–949, 1990.

TWENTY-ONE
PRURITUS AND MALIGNANCY

Barry D. Goldman and Howard K. Koh

Cancer is the most feared cause of pruritus. Case reports have linked almost every type of malignancy to pruritus, but the true relationship between cancer and itching is unclear. Whether patients presenting with generalized pruritus should be fully evaluated for malignancy is the subject of considerable controversy. The fact that both malignancy and pruritus are more common in the elderly complicates the debate. In this chapter, we describe the clinical features of pruritus in the presence of malignancy, review proposed mechanisms for its pathophysiology, and discuss epidemiologic studies of the prevalence of malignancy in patients with generalized pruritus. Then, in separate sections, we review studies on pruritus related to specific malignancies, present considerations for evaluating patients with pruritus for malignancy, and discuss the treatment of pruritus in cancer patients.

CLINICAL FEATURES

Pruritus was first linked to lymphoma and carcinoma about the turn of the 20th century.[1] The association between pruritus and malignancy (lymphoma and carcinoma) has since been described by many researchers, and most clinicians believe in the existence of a link. Pruritus may be seen in advanced malignancy or it may be an early sign. The intensity and extent of pruritus do not correlate with the extent of tumor involvement.

The pruritus of carcinoma may differ from the pruritus of lymphoma. Cormia, in his classic description of pruritus associated with carcinoma, noted that the itching is moderate to severe, changes in intensity over time, occasionally changes locations on the body, and fails to respond to topical therapy.[2] In his patients, the pruritus predominantly involved the upper trunk and extensor aspects of the upper extremities, as well as the anterior surfaces of the lower legs. The skin was free of visible primary lesions, although some patients had secondary "scratch papules" on the lower legs. Cormia described four typical cases in which pruritus preceded the diagnosis or recurrence of cancer and noted that a range of malignancies was responsible. The pruritus usually preceded the diagnosis of carcinoma by less than a year, often just weeks.

In contrast, pruritus may precede the diagnosis of lymphoma, especially Hodgkin's disease, by as much as 5 years.[3] It can be intolerably severe and continuous, and it is often accompanied by a burning sensation.[4] It is often most intense at night.[3] The itching commonly starts on the lower extremities, at times associated with ichythyosiform changes, before becoming generalized. Newbold found that most patients with Hodgkin's disease and generalized pruritus have a mediastinal mass.[4] In localized Hodgkin's disease, the pruritus tends to occur in the area drained by the lymphatics invaded by the disease.[4]

In lymphoma, scratching may lead to the appearance of papules, prurigo nodules, and lichenification, sometimes misdiagnosed as papular urticaria, neurotic excoriation, or infestation.[5] Excoriations often appear on the upper and lower extremities but rarely on the face or neck.[6] Scratching may cause erosions, excavations and denuded areas, which may heal with hyperpigmented scars. In contrast to other neoplasms, the uncommon cutaneous nodular lesions in Hodgkin's disease are usually pruritic.[7] An ill-defined hyperpigmentation of the skin can also occur.[8] Andrade and colleagues suggested that the presence of intense pruritus, prurigo-like papules, and hyperpigmentation, even in the absence of adenopathy, should alert clinicians to search for Hodgkin's disease.[9]

In early lesions of cutaneous T-cell lymphoma (CTCL; mycosis fungoides), the pruritus may be intense but the cutaneous lesions slight, making the clinical diagnosis difficult. It is often the exasperating itch that first awakens the suspicion that the eruption, which may simulate psoriasis, eczema, or some other common dermatosis, may in fact be CTCL.[7] Localized or generalized pruritus can precede the lesions of CTCL by as many as 10 years.[10]

Parapsoriasis, a benign, asymptomatic eruption of erythematous or tawny, slightly scaly plaques, can evolve into CTCL. One long-term study of parapsoriasis associated the intensification of the accompanying pruritus in 6 of 13 patients (46%) with clinical progression to CTCL.[11] McDonald suggested that physicians suspect CTCL in any patient with dermatitis and extreme pruritus.[12] Itching is usually seen with early stage (patch and plaque) CTCL, while the tumor stage of CTCL tends to have heavily infiltrated, but nonpruritic, lesions. Shapiro suggested that plaques with dermal infiltration that itch intensely are a manifestation of "lymphoblastoma," differentiating this from nonpruritic cutaneous infiltrates, such as syphilis, tuberculosis, leprosy, and deep mycotic infection.[7] Lyell concurred, maintaining that intense pruritus associated with lesions characterized by an unexpected degree of infiltration is a chief indicator of CTCL.[8] Sezary syndrome, the leukemic variant of CTCL, is a generalized exfoliative dermatitis characterized by intense pruritus, lymphadenopathy, and an atypical mononuclear cell population in the skin and peripheral blood.[13]

Pruritus accompanying leukemia tends to be widespread at onset but is usually less severe than that seen in lymphoma.[2] As in lymphoma, however, pruritus can precede the diagnosis by several years.[14] Nodules and plaques of leukemia cutis are generally nonpruritic, although exceptions have been noted.[15]

A common theme for all these malignancies is that pruritus frequently clears rapidly when the malignancy is treated. The return of pruritus may herald recurrence of the tumor. The persistence or recurrence of itching months, or even years, following an apparent cure of a malignancy suggests that the destruction or removal of the primary tumor was incomplete or that metastasis has supervened.[2] As pruritus may constitute the only evidence of recurrence or progression of the malignancy, it is an important warning symptom.

PATHOGENESIS

The pathophysiology of pruritus in the presence of malignancy is not known. We also do not know whether carcinoma and lymphoma cause pruritus through the same mechanisms. Several hypotheses have been raised, as described in the following paragraphs.

In pruritus linked to malignancy, direct tumor invasion of the skin has not been demonstrated. Suggested mechanisms of pruritus include the propositions that it results from an immune response prompted by microscopic cutaneous implants of the tumor,[16] from toxic products of necrotic tumor cells entering the systemic circulation,[7] from an allergic reaction to tumor-specific antigens,[17] and from production of chemical mediators of pruritus by the tumor.[18] Cormia and colleagues suggested that pruritus might be due to increased proteolytic activity, although he found normal levels of proteases in patients with carcinomatosis or malignant lymphomas.[19]

Histamine has also been postulated by some to play a role in the pathogenesis of cancer-related pruritus.[3] However, Burtin and colleagues demonstrated decreased skin response (itching, wheals, and flares) to intradermal histamine in patients with solid tumors and concluded that the presence of a tumor decreased skin sensitivity to histamine.[20] Sabolovic and colleagues found decreased histamine levels in the blood in patients with malignant tumors.[21] This suggests that histamine is not involved in itching due to carcinoma. In addition, antihistamines are often of little benefit to pruritic cancer patients, except for their sedative effects.

In carcinoid syndrome, serotonin has been implicated in pruritus.[22] Serotonin could induce pruritus by direct action, by vasodilation decreasing the threshold for itching, or via histamine and bradykinin release.[23] Megel further postulated that proteinase release secondary to local changes in histamine content are responsible.[22]

In Hodgkin's disease, it has been suggested that an autoimmune response to lymphoid cells may cause the release of pruritogens like leukopeptidases and bradykinins.[7] Others speculate that the eosinophilia seen in the pleomorphic infiltrate of Hodgkin's disease is linked to histamine release.[24] Amhot and Green suggested a role for high serum levels of IgE, which, like the pruritus, responded to treatment of the lymphoma in their patients.[25] Pruritus is absent in areas supplied by transected nerves secondary to compression of the lumbar cord, suggesting a peripheral, not central nervous system, origin.[26] Clinically, the xerosis and ichthyosiform changes regularly seen in Hodgkin's disease probably contribute to pruritus.

The pruritus in CTCL appears to be associated with the degree of histologic epidermotropism by the neoplastic and inflammatory cell infiltrates, a feature more often seen in early stage disease. Rosychuk speculated that pruritus may stem from the release of pruritogenic mediators close to the naked dermoepidermal nerve endings.[27] Others postulate that the pruritus may be due to the release of leukopeptidases and cellular products created by host resistance to the malignant cells.[28] Again, this concept is in accord with the higher frequency of pruritus in the patch and plaque stages of CTCL, where host resistance is still effective, and the relative lack of pruritus in the tumor stage, where resistance begins to wane and malignant cells are more numerous.[28] In patients with Sezary syndrome, Totterman and colleagues found that episodes of pruritus were correlated with the appearance of circulating clonal T-cells expressing certain T-cell activation markers.[29] Totterman postulated that the pruritus in his patient may have been due to the production or release of soluble T-cell lymphokines such as interleukin 2.[29,30]

Pruritus does not occur in most cases of chronic granulocytic leukemia even though it is often characterized by the presence of large numbers of circulating, histamine-containing basophils, perhaps because of functional abnormalities of those cells.[3]

While these specific theories are intriguing, none have been proven. Indeed, in some cases, the pruritus may be due simply to the nonspecific debilitating effects of the carcinoma on the patient, making the skin more susceptible to external irritants.

THE PREVALENCE OF MALIGNANCY IN GENERALIZED PRURITUS

While almost every type of malignancy has been associated with pruritus, few long-term studies have substantiated a statistically significant relationship, a fact that was recognized 30 years ago.[10]

We identified eight studies that attempted to define the prevalence of malignancy in patients presenting to dermatologists with generalized pruritus, excluding patients with identifiable primary skin lesions.[8,31–37] A summary of these studies is presented in Table 21-1. In the first six studies, encompassing 384 patients, 30 patients (8%) had or were eventually diagnosed with cancer. Of the cancer patients, 13 (43%) had lymphoproliferative disease, with an

Table 21-1 Generalized pruritus and prevalence of malignancy

Study (author, year, country)	Number of patients	Patients with malignancy number (%)	Patients with lympho-proliferative malignancy number (%)	Cancers diagnosed before evaluation for pruritus	Comparison group?
Forman, 1954[31] Britain	64	3 (4.2)	2 (3.1)	?	no
Rajka, 1966[32] Sweden	34	9 (26.5)	6 (17.6)	?	no
Lyell, 1972[8] Scotland	74	7 (2.7)	1 (1.4)	?	no
Beare, 1976[33] Ireland	43	3 (6.9)	1 (2.3)	2	no
Kantor and Lookingbill, 1983[34] USA	44	5 (11.3)	1 (2.3)	3	yes[a]
Paul, Paul and Jansen, 1987[35] Finland	125	8 (6.4)	2 (1.6)	4	yes[b]
Olumide and Oresanya, 1987[36] Nigeria	268	4 (1.5)	2 (0.7)	?	no
Rantuccio, 1989[37] Italy	447	3 (0.7)	2 (0.5)	?	no

[a] 44 age- and sex-matched psoriatic patients
[b] age- and sex-matched prevalence of malignancy as determined by Finnish Cancer Registry

especially high prevalence of Hodgkin's disease (8 patients). Only 17 of the 384 patients (4%) seen for generalized pruritus had or developed an underlying carcinoma. In the three studies that indicated when the malignancy was diagnosed, 9 of the 16 cancers had been diagnosed before referral to a dermatology clinic.

Kantor and Lookingbill's retrospective study used a comparison group.[34] They compared the prevalence of malignancy among 44 patients with generalized pruritus with that among 44 age- and sex-matched controls with psoriasis. Five of the patients with pruritus (11%) had cancer, three of them diagnosed before the dermatology referral. Hence, two patients in the study group were found to have a malignancy on followup, compared to 1 of the 44 controls. Of note, these authors originally identified 50 patients seen for generalized pruritus, but they were able to follow up on only 44; it is possible that some of or all of the other six patients also had cancer.

Only Paul and colleagues supply the average age of the study population, an important consideration in light of the relationship of age to cancer.[35] In this Finnish study, the authors followed 125 patients (mean age of 52) for over 6 years. Eight patients (6%) had a malignancy, with four diagnosed before referral to the dermatologist. However, the number of expected malignancies in a population of that age and size was also eight, so the results were not significantly different. On the other hand, lymphoma was observed in 2 of the 125 patients, compared with an expected prevalence of less than 1 in 1000.

The two other studies summarized in Table 21-1, which were larger than the first six, show an even lower prevalence of malignancy among patients with pruritus. Olumide and Oresanya studied 268 patients in Nigeria with generalized pruritus and no obvious skin disease.[36] Filiariasis was responsible for more than half the cases. They found cancer in four patients (1%), two of whom had Hodgkin's disease. The results of this study, however, may not apply to non-African people. Rantuccio observed three cancers among 447 patients (less than 1%) with pruritus followed over 18 years; two of these malignancies were lymphoproliferative.[37] This study was reported in a brief letter and lacked details concerning screening, investigation, and followup.

On the whole, all these studies suggest that while patients presenting to dermatologists with complaints of generalized pruritus have a relatively low prevalence of malignancy, rates of lymphoma appear relatively high. We note, however, that these studies all suffer shortcomings. First, the method and length of follow up were not always described or differed from study to study, making comparisons difficult. Second, the patient populations varied; some investigators evaluated hospitalized patients, others included outpatients and still others included those with visible skin lesions.[8] Finally, some of these studies were retrospective.

The ideal study should be prospective. It should enroll a large number of patients with clearly defined, standardized eligibility criteria, such as persistent, unexplained, generalized pruritus for at least 2 months, unresponsive to topical and oral therapy. Patients with cancer diagnosed before referral to the study should be noted. An appropriate sex- and age-matched control group should be selected, with both groups followed and evaluated in the same manner. Power calculations are necessary for proper statistical evaluation. Followup should be long term (at least 5 years) and dropouts should be minimized, with vital status of all subjects identified at the end of the study. Until these criteria are met, there will be continued debate about the validity of the present published studies.

We should also stress that patients with pruritus from malignancy may not present to dermatology clinics. Also, the number of cases of pruritus would probably increase if more attention were paid to the symptom by nondermatologist physicians. Cancer patients visit other specialists, prompted by obvious nondermatologic symptoms.[36] In particular, many patients with pruritus and an underlying carcinoma are likely to have complaints such as weight loss, jaundice, fever, or malaise, which would require general medical evaluation. Hence, the prevalence of malignancy-related pruritus in the general patient population might differ significantly from that found in selected patients referred to regional medical centers or dermatologists,[8,38] making an association of pruritus with malignancy based solely on studies of patients seen in dermatology clinics even harder to demonstrate.

PRURITUS AND LYMPHOPROLIFERATIVE DISEASE

If we now examine those malignancies complicated or associated with pruritus, by far the strongest link is with lymphoproliferative disorders, especially Hodgkin's disease. Because the older literature often refers to lymphoproliferative disease with outdated terminology such as undefined "reticuloses," "lymphoblastomas," and "lymphosarcomas," assessing the relevance of such studies to current medical practice can be difficult. The prognostic value of pruritus in Hodgkin's disease is the subject of debate, although its recurrence after the malignancy has been treated is an important warning sign. We shall now examine the role of pruritus in Hodgkin's disease, non-Hodgkin's lymphoma, cutaneous T-cell lymphoma, and leukemia (lymphocytic and non-lymphocytic).

Hodgkin's Disease

The association of pruritus with Hodgkin's disease is so strong that pruritus was considered as a "B" symptom in the staging scheme of this lymphoma until 1971. Over 30 years ago, Bluefarb reviewed the prevalence of pruritus during the clinical course of Hodgkin's disease.[39] Bluefarb summarized 12 studies, reprinted in Table 21-2, finding an average prevalence of about

Table 21-2 The prevalence of pruritus during clinical course among patients with Hodgkin's disease[a]

Study	Number of cases	Prevalence of pruritus (%)
Adlercreutz[40]	30	30.0
Bersack[41]	224	13.4
Burger and Lehman[42]	54	18.5
Burnan[43]	173	31.8
Cole[44]	34	23.5
Colrat[45]	13	84.6
Desjardins and Ford[46]	135	6.7
Goldman and Victor[47]	212	11.6
Jackson and Parker[48]	220	29.0
Longcope[49]	86	3.5
Weinberg[50]	12	58.3
Ziegler[51]	70	11.4

[a]From Bluefarb[39]

26 percent, with a range from 4 to 85 percent.[40–51] We have reviewed 10 studies published since Bluefarb's, noting both the prevalence of pruritus and whether the symptom was a presenting one.[6,52–60] The results are listed in Table 21-3. About 35 percent of Hodgkin's disease patients had pruritus during their clinical course. Roughly 15 percent presented with pruritis, either alone or with other symptoms. Most important, 7 percent presented with pruritus as the sole symptom before the diagnosis of lymphoma.

A few investigators have tried to define a subset of patients with Hodgkin's disease most likely to have pruritus. Kaplan suggested that pruritus tends to occur more frequently in women than men, although the occurrence of B symptoms in general is distinctly more prevalent among males.[6] Chawla and colleagues found pruritus to be more associated with nodular sclerosis than other forms of Hodgkin's disease.[55] Other clinicians have suggested that pruritus may be more common in older patients and in those in the terminal stages of Hodgkin's disease.[3] Both the frequency and the intensity of the pruritus seem to heighten as the underlying disease progresses.[3] Gobbi and colleagues noted that pruritus often parallels the course of Hodgkin's disease and may disappear in remission and reappear in exacerbation.[61]

Investigators have debated the prognostic value of pruritus in Hodgkin's disease, with some finding no effect, others indicating an adverse effect, and still others determining that only severe pruritus had an adverse effect. As mentioned, pruritus was considered to be a B symptom of Hodgkin's disease (along with fevers and night sweats) from 1965 to 1971. Following several studies showing that pruritus had a negligible impact on survival (in both regionally localized and more advanced stages of Hodgkin's disease),[55,56] pruritus was replaced by weight loss as a B symptom.

Table 21-3 The prevalence of pruritus as a presenting symptom and during the clinical course among patients with Hodgkin's disease

Study	Number of patients	Present on diagnosis (total) (%)	(sole symptom) (%)	(severe) (%)	Present during clinical course (%)	Effect on prognosis
Cohen et al., 1964[52]	388	9	—	—	—	—
Ultmann, 1966[53]	135	15	—	—	—	—
Lobell et al., 1966[54]	78	18	—	—	—	none
Chawla et al., 1970[55]	523	15	—	—	30	none
Tubiania et al., 1971[56]	224	33	—	—	—	none
Kaplan, 1972[6]	445	15	—	—	—	none
Amblard et al., 1973[57]	94	8	7	—	40	—
Lee and Spratt, 1974[58]	163	11	—	—	—	worse
Feiner et al., 1978[59]	99	N.A.	—	6	—	worse[a]
Gobbi et al., 1985[60]	635	15	7	5	—	worse[a]

[a] Adverse effect found for severe pruritus only.

Subsequently, Gobbi and colleagues[61] and Feiner and colleagues[59] found that severe pruritus, as opposed to mild pruritus, had a major impact on survival in Hodgkin's disease and was superior to night sweats for identifying patients who require more aggressive therapy. They distinguished severe from mild pruritus, with the former characterized by multiple excoriations, generalized and symmetric presentation, and ineffectiveness of local and systemic antipruritic agents[59,61]; originally, Feiner also included response of the pruritus to radiotherapy or chemotherapy as a criterion for severe pruritus but this was later dropped. Feiner found that out of 99 patients with Hodgkin's disease, all 6 who presented with severe pruritus had a much lower 5-year survival than stage-matched patients without pruritus. Three patients placed in the A category who presented with severe pruritus alone had an atypical aggressive clinical course more characteristic of patients with B symptoms.[59] Gobbi and colleagues found that patients with severe, generalized pruritus had a statistically significant shorter survival time than did those with mild or no itching.[61] These authors also questioned whether Hodgkin's disease can be in stage 1A or 1B with localized involvement if generalized pruritus is present.

On the whole, we believe that these studies indicate that severe, persistent, generalized pruritus is a poor prognostic sign in Hodgkin's disease, and its return after treatment is a useful indicator of the presence of the underlying disease. Gobbi and colleagues suggested that severe pruritus should replace night sweats as a B symptom.[60] However, as severe pruritus is much less common (5%) than other symptoms, we feel it should be reconsidered as an addition to, rather than as a replacement for, night sweats.

Non-Hodgkin's Lymphoma

Pruritus is not as common a manifestation of non-Hodgkin's lymphoma. Roughly 2 percent of patients will complain of pruritus at presentation, and another 10 percent will have pruritus at some time during the course of the disease.[62,63] Pruritus appears more frequently in well differentiated lymphocytic lymphoma.[62] The pruritus may be localized or generalized. Prurigo-like papules, sometimes resembling dermatitis herpetiformis, have been described.[39] The pruritus is less continuous than that of Hodgkin's disease and usually disappears after removal of the nodal disease.[39]

The effect of pruritus on the prognosis of non-Hodgkin's lymphoma is unknown. Generalized pruritus may herald the reappearance of the lymphoma, however, sometimes preceding clinical lymphadenopathy by many months.

Cutaneous T-Cell Lymphoma

Pruritus is a considerable cause of morbidity and even mortality in CTCL, as secondary infections in the excoriations of pruritic skin are potentially lethal.[64] Degos and colleagues found pruritus in 79 percent of patients with CTCL.[65] In another study, 69 percent of 337 patients (233) had pruritus; moreover, in this analysis, deaths due to CTCL were twice as common among those with pruritus, although information on the stage of disease was not available.[66]

Leukemia

Pruritus is not common in leukemia. Two large studies on acute leukemia did not even list pruritus as a symptom,[67,68] making it unlikely that pruritus is a common occurrence in that disease. When it does occur, it is more common in chronic and in lymphocytic leukemia than it is in acute or granulocytic leukemia.[10] Bonvalet and colleagues estimated the prevalence to be 5 percent with chronic lymphocytic leukemia (CLL).[69] Some of the past reported association of pruritus with CLL may, in part, be due to confusion with Sezary syndrome. As a rule, nodules and plaques determined to be leukemia cutis are nonpruritic.[69]

PRURITUS AND CARCINOMA

Pruritus is a symptom of many solid tumors, although its prevalence with individual carcinomas is not well established. A temporal sequence of remission on tumor removal and relapse with recurrence of the tumor is helpful in attributing the pruritus to a particular tumor.[70] However, most clinical series of cancer patients fail to include pruritus as a symptom. Either oncologists do not consider pruritus an important symptom compared to other constitutional complaints, or it is simply not a common occurrence. Also, patients may not mention itching unless specifically asked, as other problems may seem more urgent. Still, even in patients with advanced tumors, unrelenting pruritus can be the principal subjective complaint.[71]

True cutaneous metastases of malignant tumors do not cause itch. Anecodotal evidence suggests that the appearance of generalized pruritus in carcinoma is a bad prognostic sign and tends to occur in older patients in the terminal stages of disease.[3,16] Metastases to the liver or to the area of the porta hepatis may lead to itching due to cholestasis, as discussed in the following section.

Gastrointestinal Cancer

Gastrointestinal malignancies may cause pruritus, in most cases because of extrahepatobiliary obstructive disease. The pruritus ranges from mild and variable to severe and chronic, leading some patients to contemplate suicide.[72] Usually, the pruritus is generalized with particular involvement of the palms and soles, the extensor surfaces of the extremities, and the upper trunk.[72] The butterfly sign, an area of relative hypopigmentation seen on unreachable areas of the back, may serve as a clue to chronic obstructive hepatobiliary disease in patients with generalized pruritus.[73]

In one study, half of 38 patients with carcinoma of the ampulla of Vater presented with pruritus.[74] In another study, Baker and colleagues found pruritus to be present in 20 percent of patients with cancer of the head of the pancreas and 40 percent of patients with cancer of the ampulla of Vater or extrahepatic bile duct.[75] Of note, in both studies, pruritus was not seen in the absence of jaundice. Schoenfield found pruritus with extrahepatic obstruction in 75 percent of patients with malignant lesions and in 50 percent of patients with benign disorders.[76] Pruritus usually precedes jaundice in primary biliary cirrhosis, while the reverse is true in cancer of the bile duct.[77] Pruritus is more common in jaundiced patients who suffer from extrahepatobiliary obstruction than in patients with infectious hepatitis or cirrhosis.[3]

In Hodgkin's disease, involvement of the periportal lymph nodes may also cause pruritus as a result of biliary obstruction.[39]

The cause of pruritus in malignant extrahepatobiliary obstruction is uncertain, although elevated levels of bile acids in the blood and skin have been implicated. The pruritus seems related to jaundice; abdominal malignancies that do not cause jaundice are associated with pruritus only rarely, and surgical or medical treatment of jaundice relieves the itch. Levels of bile acids, however, fail to correlate with the intensity or even the presence of pruritus.[72] The spontaneous disappearance of pruritus in patients with hepatic disease should be considered a poor prognostic sign, indicating severe deterioration in liver function.[70] (See also Chap. 16.)

Tumors of the Central Nervous System

Pruritus has also been associated with tumors of the brain. In a study by Andreev and Petkov,[17] 13 of 77 patients (17%) complained of pruritus. Most characteristic was pruritus of the nostril, observed in six patients (8%) with advanced brain tumors infiltrating the base of the fourth ventricle, which subsided after removal of the tumor in two cases. The pruritus was generalized in the other seven patients. The nasal pruritus was sometimes extremely severe, causing patients to scratch their nose even while asleep or rub their nose on a pillow if in restraints. This particular type of pruritus has not been observed with other malignancies.[17] Much earlier, Wartenberg also reported two cases of brain tumors causing increased intracranial pressure in which intense pruritus of the nostrils was present.[78] However, in a survey of half a dozen neurologists and neurosurgeons, only one was aware of this association.[79]

Lung Cancer

Pruritus rarely occurs as the presenting symptom of carcinoma of the bronchus. Thomas and Harrington noted five cases in the literature, the first in 1927.[80] We found only one series on lung cancer that mentioned pruritus as a symptom; 1 of 280 patients presented with pruritus.[81] In marked contrast to lymphoproliferative diseases, the longest interval between the onset of pruritus and time of lung cancer diagnosis was only 10 weeks. Thomas and Harrington demonstrated ectopic parathyroid hormone (PTH) in the serum of a patient with pruritus and oat cell carcinoma of the lung and suggested that pruritus may have been due to PTH production from the tumor.[80]

Other Carcinomas

Mengel reported that pruritus is an occasional symptom of carcinoid syndrome.[22] The itch, which was extremely distressful, was partly relieved by serotonin blockers. As Federspiel and colleagues noted pruritus in only 1 of 35 patients (3%) with gastrointestinal carcinoid,[82] this symptom cannot be considered common.

Pruritus has also been described in association with multiple endocrine neoplasia II (Sipple's syndrome), in which parathyroid hyperplasia and elevated histamine levels were found.[3] Nunziata and colleagues described a hereditary localized pruritus of the scapular region that affected certain members of one family who later went on to develop Sipple's syndrome.[83] (See also, discussion of notalgia paresthetica in Chap. 12.)

Pruritus with hyperpigmentation occurs more frequently with carcinomas of the gastrointestinal tract than with tumors in other locations.[7] The cause of this paraneoplastic pigmentation is unknown. Pruritus has been present in 40 percent of patients with the sign of Leser–Trelat, the sudden appearance or increase in size of itchy seborrheic keratoses heralding the occurrence of malignancy.[84] Pruritus has also been reported as a precursor symptom of breast cancer and carcinoma of the stomach, uterus, prostate, and thyroid.[85]

OTHER MALIGNANCIES

Pruritus has been noted as an occasional presenting symptom of myelomatosis.[86] It has also been reported as a feature of renal disease secondary to myelomatosis, but is not considered to be a common symptom. Polycythemia rubra vera has a well-known association with pruritus, present in 20 to 50 percent of the cases.[3] Known as "bath pruritus," owing to its occurrence immediately after bathing, the pruritus may be generalized or occur around the head and neck. Episodes last from a few minutes to an hour. The pathogenesis may be related to increased serum histamine levels from the increased number of circulating basophils. Polycythemia is covered in greater detail in Chap. 17.

EVALUATION AND TREATMENT

The following subsections describe the evaluation for cancer in patients with pruritus, considerations in evaluating pruritus in a patient in whom cancer has been diagnosed, and treatment for pruritus in the presence of a malignancy.

Evaluation for Malignancy in Patients with Pruritus

Because pruritus is a nonspecific symptom much more commonly related to skin and other systemic disorders than it is to carcinoma, a diagnosis of cancer must obviously be established by means other than recognition of the itching state.[10] As already noted, studies of generalized pruritus have failed to note a higher than expected overall number of cancers but have shown a disproportionate number of lymphoproliferative neoplasms, with an especially high prevalence of Hodgkin's disease. Hence, we reason that, in the absence of other systemic complaints or physical exam findings, and after other benign and systemic causes have been ruled out, the workup should be directed first toward uncovering a lymphoproliferative malignancy.

Patients should be questioned for the date of onset as well as the location of the pruritus. The character of the itch may be important as a burning sensation may suggest Hodgkin's disease. Constitutional complaints such as fevers, weight loss, night sweats, anorexia, and fatigue should be sought. A comprehensive physical exam should include a thorough search for lymph-node enlargement, hepatomegaly, and splenomegaly. The presence of ich-thyosis with pruritus may be suggestive of Hodgkin's disease. Eczematous or psoriasiform pruritic plaques with a degree of induration may be CTCL.

An initial laboratory evaluation for malignancy should consist of a chest x-ray, a complete blood cell count with differential and peripheral blood smear, and liver function tests. A chest x-ray could help detect mediastinal adenopathy in patients with Hodgkin's disease. A complete blood cell count with a differential and a peripheral blood smear may uncover an occult hematologic malignancy or perhaps confirm a suspicion of polycythemia vera.[38] Liver function tests might detect evidence for malignant extrahepa-tobiliary obstruction or primary or metastatic liver tumors.

Once this basic search is done, other signs may be of value. Changes in skin color are important. Erythroderma could raise consideration of lym-phoproliferative malignancies such as Sezary syndrome. Jaundice could in-dicate a gastrointestinal malignancy. Hyperpigmentation can occur in both lymphoma and carcinoma. Purpuric scratch marks may indicate a hema-tologic malignancy. The stool, because of its easy accessibility, can be screened for occult blood, and a pelvic exam should be considered. Vickers reported generalized pruritus and low serum iron without anemia as a harbinger of "reticulosis."[87] Hence, he recommended obtaining serum iron as part of an evaluation, and if low, pursuing intensive investigation for lymphoma includ-ing lymphangiography and laparotomy, although a chest X-ray and CT scan of abdomen might reveal the same information today. This topic is covered further in Chapter 17.

Beyond this, any further workup should be directed by positive findings. Certainly, a patient with pruritus who has been treated for a tumor in the past should have a thorough reevaluation for the recurrence of that malig-nancy, even if pruritus was not part of the earlier history. Only after all possible etiologies for persistent generalized pruritus have been excluded should an evaluation for an occult carcinoma be considered. Some suggest closely following adult patients with atopic dermatitis and high serum IgE, as they can develop Hodgkin's disease within a few years.[88]

If no etiology is found and the pruritus persists, the physical exam should be repeated, at an interval depending on the severity of symptoms, response to therapy and suspected pathology. Selected laboratory tests should be obtained at 6-month intervals when symptoms persist, even if no diagnosis is made after an extensive evaluation. As pruritus may precede a diagnosis of malignancy by many years, patients should be followed serially over time. However as efforts for cancer detection will generally not be cost effective, an uncritically chosen battery of tests should be avoided.[34] Unfortunately, the present medicolegal environment makes it difficult to determine when a workup is sufficient.[89] Because physicians have been sued for not identifying Hodgkin's disease in patients presenting with generalized pruritus, it may be wise in cases of persistent intractable pruritus for physicians to re-evaluate and consult with other medical colleagues.[38]

Workup for Pruritus in Cancer Patients

Dermatologists may be asked to see hospitalized cancer patients because of intractable pruritus. The presence of pruritus in a patient with cancer does not necessarily imply a link between the two, and other causes must be investigated. Hospitalized patients may develop miliaria, contact dermatitis, scabies, and itching due to excessively dry skin, to name but a few. Bedridden patients may also develop irritation, and, rarely, allergy to bed sheets,[90] but both are less common than supposed. Some investigators have reported that dermatitis herpetiformis,[91] transient acantholytic disease (Grover's disease),[92] and bullous pemphigoid[93] may occur in association with malignancy. Anhalt and colleagues have recently reported a variety of pemphigus in cancer patients, which they have named paraneoplastic pemphigus.[94] In these disorders, itching may be accompanied by vesicles, bullae, erosions, or small itchy red papulo-vesicles and excoriated papules.

In general, if the itching is well localized, it is unlikely to be related to the underlying malignancy and another etiology should be sought.[95] However, there are several exceptions. Pruritus of the nostrils can be associated with brain tumors, patients with Hodgkin's disease can complain of mild localized pruritus, pruritus vulvae has been reported in patients with carcinoma of the cervix, and pruritus ani may accompany rectal or sigmoid colon cancer.[95] Racz noted that in cancer of the prostate, persistent itching at the scrotal and perineal region may focus attention on the disease.[71]

Medications or treatments for cancer patients may also cause pruritus. Morphine, doxorubicin (adriamycin), and radiation therapy can all cause pruritus.[96]

Treatment of Pruritus

While reviews on the treatment of pruritus in cancer patients are available,[95,96] there are few clinical studies on the efficacy of antipruritic agents in this population. Pruritus associated with cancer is improved only slightly or not at all by various types of local antipruritic agents or by systemic steroids, antihistamines, or tranquilizers. As we have already noted, the most valuable treatment is the removal or arrest of the underlying carcinoma although, even then, pruritus may not disappear.

The present day standard treatment is to start with customary topical therapy, which is considered nonspecific for cancer patients: rehydration, ensuring adequate fluid intake, maintaining high humidity, and avoiding temperature extremes.[95] Wet dressings may be helpful, as it cools by evaporation. Topical steroids may be helpful. Other agents include camphor and menthol, which may provide a cooling sensation. Topical local anesthetics are not recommended, as they are not very effective and have a high frequency of allergic sensitization.

Antihistamines of the H1 blocking type are widely used. However, their indiscriminate use should be discouraged in this setting as studies have found cancer patients less sensitive than normal to histamine-induced itching.[20] Racz found phenothiazines, especially chlorpromazine, to be helpful in patients unresponsive to other therapies.[71] Cimetidine may have a role in histamine-related itching and has been effective in some patients with lymphoproliferative disease.[97] If the pruritus is intractable, alternative nonspecific methods of treatment such as ultraviolet light B, cholestyramine, naloxone, charcoal, and transcutaneous nerve stimulation should be considered.[95] (See also Chap. 26.)

Treatment of pruritus in the presence of Hodgkin's disease is best accomplished by treating the lymphoma. After this, there is no standard therapy. One study noted substantial improvement in the pruritus in four patients when cimetidine, an H2 antagonist, was used.[97] Although cimetidine has not been shown to be effective in other types of itching and H2 agonists do not produce itching, Bernhard offers several hypotheses as to why cimetidine may be effective for pruritus in this case: The pruritogen in Hodgkin's disease may be different from that of other types of pruritus, cimetidine may block the synthesis of the pruritogen, or H2 activity may simply cause itching in Hodgkin's disease but not in other conditions.[5]

In patients with CTCL, symptomatic relief of itching has been achieved by radiation therapy, nitrogen mustard, PUVA, photopheresis, and other measures that act against the underlying tumor. Antihistamines are sometimes helpful. Treatment of the disease with total-skin electron beam can first cause a transient exacerbation of pruritus (in patients with more than 50% of affected skin), followed later by its diminution.[98] This occurrence may be due to an extreme sensitivity of the CTCL cells to radiation, leading to cell necrosis. While cyclosporin A has been noted to relieve the pruritus of CTCL rapidly,[29] its long-term effects on the disease process are unclear and its nephrotoxic effects preclude its routine use. Compounds containing menthol have been found to have excellent local antipruritic effects in CTCL. Cimetidine has improved pruritus in some patients.

A variety of other treatments for pruritus in malignancy have been reported. Treatment with cyproheptadine, a potent H1 antihistamine and antiserotonin agent, proved effective in one patient with gastric carcinoid tumors.[3] Hypnosis has been used successfully in one patient with leukemia and pruritus.[99] Bonnekoh and colleagues reported success with PUVA when treating a patient with bronchial carcinoma who developed generalized pruritus 2 years after diagnosis.[100] For pruritus secondary to malignant extrahepatic obstruction, a variety of treatments are listed in Chap. 16. More detailed recommendations for symptomatic treatment of pruritus are given in Chaps. 26 and 27.

SUMMARY

Our review finds that the malignancies associated with generalized pruritus are disproportionately represented by lymphoproliferative disorders, especially Hodgkin's disease. Also, clinical series of patients with Hodgkin's disease, non-Hodgkin's lymphoma, and CTCL consistently note a certain percentage of patients with pruritus. Prognostically, several studies show that severe pruritus appears to be an adverse symptom in Hodgkin's disease.

The link between pruritus and carcinoma is less strong. It is based on their temporal relationship and on the occasional clearance of pruritus after the malignancy is treated. Most clinical series of patients with carcinoma fail to mention pruritus as a symptom, and when they do, pruritus is distinctly uncommon. Many clinicians maintain that the association is simply coincidental. The clinical appearance of the itch, with few exceptions, is relatively nonspecific for any particular type of malignancy. The intensity of pruritus in carcinoma fails to correlate with the tumor burden, as pruritus can occur prior to diagnosis or in the terminal stages.

In the absence of other systemic complaints or physical exam findings, we recommend that the workup of a patient with generalized persistent pruritus should first be directed toward uncovering a lymphoproliferative malignancy. A search for carcinoma should ensue only on an individualized basis and should be directed by the patient's specific signs and symptoms.

The treatment of cancer-related pruritus should be directed toward treatment of the tumor. Symptomatic measures should be employed whenever necessary and possible. Other causes of itching in cancer patients, such as drugs and dermatological diseases, should be considered.

Future research must generate more data on the true prevalence of malignancy in patients who present with generalized pruritus. Finding a specific marker for neoplastic disease in the presence of pruritus would be useful. Finally, discovering the mechanisms and mediators of pruritus in malignancy offers the best hope for guiding treatment and prevention of this condition in the future.

ACKNOWLEDGMENTS

We thank Mary Beth Mercer, MPH, for her assistance on this project, Cynthia Barber, MPH, for her review of the manuscript, and Claudia Arrigg, MD, and John Kraiden, MD for their unending encouragement and support.

REFERENCES

1. Becker SM, Kahn D, Rothmam S: Cutaneous manifestations of internal malignant tumors. *Arch Dermatol Syph* 45:1069–1080, 1942.
2. Cormia FE: Pruritus, an uncommon but important symptom of systemic carcinoma. *Arch Dermatol* 92:36–39, 1965.
3. Botero F: Pruritus in systemic disease. *Cutis* 21:873–880, 1978.
4. Newbold C: Skin markers of malignancy. *Arch Dermatol* 102:680, 1970.
5. Bernhard JD: Itching as a manifestation of noncutaneous diseases. *Hosp Pract* (Off Ed) 22:81–95, 1987.
6. Kaplan HS: *Hodgkin's Disease.* Cambridge, Mass., Harvard University Press. 1972, pp 262–263.
7. Shapiro AL: Itching(pruritus), in Green A. (ed): *Signs and Symptoms.* New York, McGraw-Hill. 1970, pp 960–982.
8. Lyell A: The itching patient, a review of the causes of pruritus. *Scott Med J* 17:334–348, 1972.
9. Andrade R, Gumport SL, Poplkin GL, et al: *Cancer of the Skin,* vol. 1. Philadelphia, Saunders. 1976, pp 1230, 1240–1241.
10. Winkelmann RK: Dermatologic clinics. 1. Comments on pruritus related to systemic disease. *Proc Staff Meet Mayo Clin* 36:187–196, 1961.
11. Fleischmajer R, Pascher F, Sims CF: Parapsoriasis en plaques and mycosis fungoides. *Dermatologica* 131:149, 1965.
12. McDonald C: Mycosis fungoides: A malignant cutaneous lymphoma. *Conn Med* 33(1): 37–41, 1969.
13. Wieselthier JS, Koh HK: Sezary syndrome: Diagnosis, prognosis, and critical review of treatment options. *J Am Acad Dermatol* 22:381–401, 1990.
14. Peterson AO, Jarratt M: Pruritus and nonspecific nodules preceding myelomonocytic leukemia. *J Am Acad Dermatol* 2:496–498, 1980.
15. Czarnecki D, Downes N, O'Brien T: Pruritic specific cutaneous infiltrates in leukemia and lymphoma. *Arch Dermatol* 118:119–121, 1982.
16. Schoenfeld Y, Weiberg A: Generalized pruritus in metastatic adenocarcinoma of the stomach. *Dermatologica* 155:122–124, 1977.
17. Andreev VC, Petkov I: Skin manifestations associated with tumors of the brain. *Br J Dermatol* 92:675, 1975.
18. Beaff D: Pruritus as a sign of systemic disease; report of metastatic small cell carcinoma. *Arizona Med* 37:831–833, 1980.
19. Cormia F, Dougherty J, Unrau S: Proteolytic activity in dermatoses: Studies of blood of patients with pruritus. *J Invest Dermatol* 30:21, 1958.
20. Burtin C, Noirot C, Giroux C, et al: Decreased skin response to intradermal histamine in cancer patients. *J All Clin Immunol* 78(1 pt 1):83–89, 1986.
21. Sabolovic D, Dubrav D, Culo F, et al: Histamine levels in the blood in patients with malignant tumors. *Lijec Vjesn* 111:185-7, 1989.
22. Mengel CE: Cutaneous manifestations of the malignant carcinoid syndrome. *Ann Intern Med* 58:989–993, 1963.

23. Gilchrest BA: Pruritus, pathogenesis, therapy, and significance in systemic disease states. *Arch Intern Med* 142:101–104, 1982.
24. Cormia FE, Domonkos AN: Cutaneous reactions to internal malignancy. *Med Clin North Am* 49:655–680, 1965.
25. Amhot P, Green L: Atrophy and immunoglobulin E concentrations in Hodgkin's disease and other lymphomas. *Br Med J* 6109:327, 1978.
26. Boudin G, Castaigne P, Lemenager F: Les manifestations neurologiques de la maladie de Hodgkin: Deductions sur les voies nerveuses sensitives par ou chemine le prurit. *Sem Hop Paris* 26:3455–3459, 1950.
27. Rosychuk RA: Endocrine, metabolic, internal, and neoplastic causes of pruritus in the dog and cat. *Vet Clin North Am—Small Animal Prac* 18(5):1101–1110, 1988.
28. Rosenberg FW: Cutaneous manifestation of internal malignancy. *Cutis* 20:227–234, 1977.
29. Totterman TH, Scheynius A, Killander A, et al: Treatment of therapy-resistant Sezary syndrome with cyclosporin-A; suppression of pruritus, leukaemic T cell activation markers and tumor mass. *Scand J Haematol* 34:196–203, 1985.
30. Gaspari AA, Lotze MT, Rosenberg SA, et al: Dermatologic changes associated with inter-leukin 2 administration. *JAMA* 258:1624, 1987.
31. Forman L: Pruritus and its management. *BMJ* 2:365–367, 1954.
32. Rajka G: Investigation of patients suffering from generalized pruritus with special reference to systemic diseases. *Acta Derm Venerol* (Stockh) 46:190–194, 1966.
33. Beare J: Generalized pruritus; a study of 43 cases. *Clin Exp Dermatol* 1:343–352, 1976.
34. Kantor G, Lookingbill DP: Generalized pruritus and systemic disease. *J Am Acad Dermatol* 9:375–382, 1983.
35. Paul R, Paul R, Jansen CT: Itch and malignancy prognosis in generalized pruritus: A 6-year follow-up of 125 patients. *J Am Acad Dermatol* 16(6):1179–1182, 1987.
36. Olumide Y, Oresanya F: Generalized pruritus as a presenting symptom in Nigeria. *Int J Dermatol* 26(3):171–174, 1987.
37. Rantuccio F: Incidence of malignancy in patients with generalized pruritus. *J Am Acad Dermatol* 21(6):1317, 1989.
38. Lober C: Should the patient with generalized pruritus be evaluated for malignancy? *J Am Acad Dermatol* 19:350–352, 1988.
39. Bluefarb SM: *Cutaneous Manifestations of the Malignant Lymphomas.* Springfield, Ill, Charles C. Thomas. 1959, pp 242–255.
40. Adlercreutz E: Till kannedomen om lymfogranulomatosens klinik. *Finska Laksallsk Handl* 76:587, 1934.
41. Bersack SR: Hodgkin's disease-incidence and prognosis; a statistical correlation with the clinico-pathologic picture. *Arch Intern Med* 73:232, 1944.
42. Burger RE, Lehman EP: Hodgkin's disease: Review of 54 cases. *Arch Surg* 43:839, 1941.
43. Burnam CF: Hodgkin's disease with special reference to its treatment by irradiation. *J Am Med Assoc* 87:1445, 1926.
44. Cole HNL: The cutaneous manifestations of Hodgkin's disease: Lymphogranulomatosis. *J Am Med Assoc* 69:341, 1917.
45. Colrat AL: L'adenie eosinophilique prurigene-lymphogranulomatose. *These de Lyon* 282, 1920–21.
46. Desjardins A, Ford F: Hodgkin's disease and lymphosarcoma; clinical and statistical study. *JAMA* 81:925–927, 1923.
47. Goldman LB, Victor AW: Hodgkin's disease: An analysis of 212 cases. *JAMA* 114:1611, 1940.
48. Jackson Jr H, Parker Jr F: Hodgkin's disease. Involvement of certain organs. *N Y State J Med* 232:547, 1945.
49. Longcope WT: Hodgkin's disease, in Osler Sir William (ed): *Modern Medicine,* 3d ed. Philadelphia, Lea and Febiger. 1972, vol 5, p. 226.

50. Weinberg F: Lymphogranuloma tuberculosum. *Ztschr Klin Med* 85:99, 1917.
51. Zeigler K: *Die Hogkinische Krankheit.* Jena, Germany, G. Fischer, 1911.
52. Cohen BM, Smetana HF, Miller RW: Hodgkin's disease: Long survival in a study of 388 World War II Army cases. *Cancer* 17:856–866, 1964.
53. Ultmann J: Clinical features and diagnosis of Hodgkin's disease. *Cancer Res* 19(3): 297–307, 1966.
54. Lobell M, Bogg DR, Wintrobe MM: The clinical significance of fever in Hodgkin's disease. *Arch Intern Med* 117:335–342, 1966.
55. Chawla PL, Stutzman L, Dubois RE, et al: Long survival in Hodgkin's disease. *Am J Med* 48:85–91, 1970.
56. Tubiana M, Attie E, Flamant R, et al: Prognostic factors in 454 cases of Hodgkin's disease. *Cancer Res* 31:1801–1809, 1971.
57. Amblard P, Schaerer R, Scotto J, et al: Les manifestations cutanees de la maladie de Hodgkin. A propos de l'etude systematique de 94 sujets proteurs de cette affection. *Sem Hop Paris* 49:3073–3078, 1973.
58. Lee Y, Spratt JS: *Malignant Lymphoma: Nodal and Extranodal Diseases.* New York, Grune & Stratton 1974, pp 18–20.
59. Feiner AS, Mahmood T, Wallner SF: Prognostic importance of pruritus in Hodgkin's disease. *J Am Med Assoc* 240:2738–2740, 1978.
60. Gobbi PG, Cavalli C, Gendarini A, et al: Reevaluation of prognostic significance of symptoms in Hodgkin's disease. *Cancer* 56:2874–2880, 1985.
61. Gobbi PG, Attardo-Pinarinello G, Laltiazio G, et al: Severe pruritus should be a B symptom in Hodgkin's disease. *Cancer* 51:1934–1936, 1983.
62. Rosenberg S, Diamond H, Jaslowitz B, et al: Lymphosarcoma: A review of 1269 cases. *Cancer Res* 31–47, 1961.
63. Molander DW: *Lymphoproliferative Diseases.* Springfield, Ill, Charles C Thomas. 1975, pp 116, 235.
64. Holowach S, McFadden ME, Supik K: Mycosis fungoides; a nursing perspective. *Oncol Nurs Forum* 11(1):20–28, 1984.
65. Degos R, Civatte J, Touraine R, et al: Anatomicoclinical comparison of 129 malignant cutaneous reticulopathies. *Ann Dermatol Syph* (Paris) 92:121, 1965.
66. Lamberg SI, Green S: Status report of 376 mycosis fungoides patients at 4 years: Mycosis fungoides cooperative group. *Cancer Treat Rep* 63:701–707, 1979.
67. Boggs DR, Wintrobe MM, Cartwright GE: The acute leukemias: Analysis of 322 cases and review of the literature. *Cancer Res* 163–170, 1973.
68. Rivers SL, Whittington RM, Gendel BR, et al: Acute leukemia in the adult male. II. Natural History. *Cancer* 16:249–258, 1963.
69. Bonvalet D, Foldes C, Civate J: Cutaneous manifestations in chronic lymphocytic leukemia. *J Dermatol Surg Oncol* 10:4; 1984.
70. Jorizzo JL: The itchy patient, a practical approach. *Prim Care* 10:339–353, 1983.
71. Racz S: Itching in malignant tumorous diseases and its treatment with phenothiazine derivatives. *Acta Unio Intern Contral Cancrum* 16:910–912, 1960.
72. Garden J, Ostrow J, Roenigk H: Pruritus in hepatic cholestasis. *Arch Dermatol* 121: 1415–1420, 1985.
73. Goldman R, Rea T, Cinque J: The "butterfly" sign: A clue to generalized pruritus in a patient with chronic obstructive hepatobiliary disease. *Arch Dermatol* 119:183–184, 1983.
74. Makipour H, Cooperman A, Danzi, JT, et al: Carcinoma of the ampulla of vater; review of 38 cases with emphasis on treatment and prognostic factors. *Ann Surg* 183(4):342–344, 1976.
75. Baker RR, Roda CL, Lee JM: Carcinoma of the head of the pancreas and periampullary region. *Hopkins Med J* 132:214, 1973.
76. Schoenfield LJ: The relationship of bile acids to pruritus in hepatobiliary disease. Presented

at a conference on bile salt metabolism. University Cincinnati Med Center, September, 1967.

77. Arov S: *Cancer Manual,* 8th ed. Am Cancer Society. 1990, p 226.
78. Wartenberg RL: Pruritus nasi bei hirntumoren. *Kiln Wchnschr* 11:461–462, 1932.
79. Helm F, Helm J: Cutaneous markers of internal malignancies, in F Helm (ed): *Cancer Dermatology,* Philadelphia, Lea & Febiger. 1979, pp 247–261.
80. Thomas S, Harrington C: Intractable pruritus as presenting symptom of carcinoma of the bronchus; case report and review. *Clin Exp Dermatol* 8:459–462, 1983.
81. Rassam JW, Anderson G: Incidence of paramalignant disorders in bronchogenic carcinoma. *Thorax* 30:86–90, 1975.
82. Federspiel B, Burke AP, Sobin LH, et al: Rectal and colonic carcinoids: A clinicopathologic study of 84 cases. *Cancer* 65:135–140, 1990.
83. Nunziata V, Gianattasio R, DiGiovanni G, et al: Hereditary localized pruritus in affected members of a kindred with multiple endocrine neoplasia type 2A (Sipple's syndrome). *Clin Endocrinol* 30:57–63, 1989.
84. Holdiness MR: The sign of Leser-Trelat; a review. *Int J Dermatol* 25:564–572, 1986.
85. Winkelmann RK, Muller SA: Pruritus. *Ann Rev Med* 15:53–64, 1964.
86. Erskine JG, Rowna RM, Alexandeer J, et al: Pruritus as a presentation of myelomatosis. *BMJ* 12:687–688, 1977.
87. Vickers C: Nutrition and the skin: Iron deficiency in dermatology. In *Proceedings of the Tenth Symposium on Advanced Medicine,* London, Royal College of Physicians, pp 311–314, 1974.
88. Hanifin J, Rajka G: Diagnostic features of atopic dermatitis. *Acta Derm Venerol Suppl* 92:44–47, 1980.
89. Sher TL: Generalized pruritus in a 62-year-old male. *Ann Allergy* 64:422, 1990.
90. Tegner E: Sheet dermatitis. *Acta Derm Venereol* (Stockh) 65:254, 1985.
91. Leonard J, Tucker W, Fry J, et al: Increased incidence of malignancy in dermatitits herpetiformis. *BMJ* 286:16–18, 1983.
92. Manteaux E, Rapini R: Transient acantholytic disease in cancer patients. *Cutis* 46: 488–490, 1990.
93. Stone S, Schroeter A: Bullous pemphigoid and associated malignant neoplasms. *Arch Dermatol* 1113:991–994, 1975.
94. Anhalt G, Kim S, Stanley J, et al: Paraneoplastic pemphigus: An autoimmune mucocutaneous disease associated with neoplasia. *N Engl J Med* 323(25):1729, 1990.
95. Weltman F, Shupack J: Pruritus in cancer patients. Your Patient and Cancer. *Oncology Nurses* fall:10–24, 1984.
96. Dangel RB: Pruritus and cancer. *Oncol Nurs Forum* 13:17–21, 1986.
97. Aymard JP, Lederlin P, Witz F, et al: Cimetidine for pruritus in Hodgkin's disease. *BMJ* 151–152, 1980.
98. Fuller LM, Hagemeister FB, Sullivan MP, et al: *Hodgkin's Disease and Non-Hodgkin's Lymphoma in Adults and Children.* New York, Raven Press. 1988, p 418.
99. Arment P, Milgrom H: Effects of suggestion on pruritus with cutaneous lesions in chronic myelogenous leukemia. *NY State J Med* 67:833–835, 1967.
100. Bonnekoh B, Thiele B, Merk H, et al: Systemic photochemotherapy (PUVA) in acanthosis nigricans maligna: Regression of keratosis, hyperpigmentation and pruritus. *Zeitschr fur Hautkrankheiten* 64(12):1059–1062, 1989.

TWENTY-TWO

OTHER SYSTEMIC CAUSES OF ITCHING

Jeffrey D. Bernhard

The important systemic causes of generalized pruritus are covered in separate chapters in Section IV of this book, and have also been reviewed by Winkelmann and Muller,[1] by Gilchrest,[2] by Denman,[3] by Bernhard,[4,5] by Greaves,[6,7] and in every major textbook of dermatology. Several rare or anecdotal systemic causes of itching are described in Chap. 13, "Pruritic curiosities." For the sake of completeness, several additional "systemic" causes of generalized and localized itching (usually without diagnostic skin lesions) will be enumerated here. Where it seemed necessary, I have erred on the side of redundancy, so some itches here are also mentioned in other relevant chapters. As some of the associations described in this chapter have been reported in single case reports or small series, the possibility of noncausal associations must be borne in mind. The possibility that an unrelated cause, such as medication, is responsible for the observed association must always be considered as well. Some of the conditions listed may lead to generalized itching without a rash. In some, nonspecific papular eruptions, possibly so-called scratch papules or secondary eczematous changes, may be seen. In some, such as scleroderma and the eosinophilia-myalgia syndrome, other characteristic lesions such as sclerosis of the skin will be seen. Given the wide variety of obvious as well as potentially occult causes of generalized itching, and the fact that many of the occult causes are rare, it is important not to subject every patient with pruritus of undetermined origin to an indiscriminately intensive evaluation. This issue is considered in the chapter on pruritus and malignancy by Koh and Goldman (Chap. 21), and a rational evaluation of the patient with generalized pruritus is presented by Kantor in Chap 24.

OTHER "SYSTEMIC" CAUSES OF LOCALIZED OR GENERALIZED PRURITUS

Parasitic infestation

Giardiasis.[8]
Onchocerciasis.[9]
Gnathostomiasis[10]
Hookworm (ancyclostomiasis)
Ascariasis
Trichinosis
Pinworm[11]

Weil's disease/leptospirosis.[12]

Parvovirus infection/erythema infectiosum.[13]

Chemical intoxication

mercury[14]
diaminodiphenylmethane (the Epping jaundice)[15]

Ciguatera fish poisoning.[16,17] Caused by a toxin, symptoms include diarrhea, abdominal pain, nausea, vomiting, paresthesias, pain, sometimes itching, and the bizarre symptoms of temperature reversal and "aching teeth." Itching occurs in as many as 30 percent of cases. "Barracuda should always be approached with caution, whether dead or alive."[18]

Scombroid fish poisoning.[19] Usually a flushing syndrome, sometimes pruritic, but more often a "burning" sensation. Caused by a toxin (saurine) and high concentrations of histamine.

Arteriohepatic dysplasia syndrome.[20,21] A cause of itching in an infant.

Urticaria and angioedema and their various causes.[22] (for example, vibratory angioedema[23])

Sarcoidosis.[24] Itching is not a common presentation of sarcoidosis. One of the more intriguing, but also uncommon, phenomena in sarcoidosis is alcohol-induced skin pain and itching after a shower.[25]

Familial primary cutaneous amyloidosis.[26] In a British family reported by Newton and colleagues, severe pruritus beginning in childhood was a striking feature of primary cutaneous amyloidosis with an autosomal dominant inheritance pattern. Physical changes of the skin were extremely subtle. When four affected family members were examined some years after the onset of itching, physical findings included mottled hypo- and hyperpigmentation, tiny dome-shaped papules, and lichenification.

Hypereosinophilic syndrome.[27,28] May present with a variety of rashes, generalized pruritus, or aquagenic pruritus.

Eosinophilia-myalgia syndrome[29] A variety of skin lesions have been seen in different patients, including morphea-like sclerosis, urticarial and papular lesions, and generalized sclerosis. Patients tend to present with one type of lesion and do not tend to progress from one variety to another (e.g., urticaria to morphea). Pruritic "rashes" have been reported, and patients may present with intense pruritus. Itching may be localized, as in one man whose presenting complaint was intense itching of the back, neck, and arms, along with dyspnea on exertion.[30] Paresthesias and skin pain occur frequently.[31] One woman presented with scalp pain.[32]

Dermatomyositis and amyopathic dermatomyositis.[33,34] The characteristic skin changes in dermatomyositis include heliotrope discoloration of the eyelids, Gottron's papules, periungual erythema/telangiectasia, and a telangiectatic, violaceous erythema, particularly of the face, neck, and trunk. The latter may have poikilodermatous features, and can occur with, without, or as a harbinger of the muscle disease. Photosensitivity is common, and moderate to severe pruritus is very common as well. Some patients describe "irritation" more than itching, especially when fabrics touch the skin.

Scleroderma.[35] Generalized itching is not common in scleroderma but may be noted early on or in very active phases of the disease. In scleroderma or lupus renal disease, itching may occur as a consequence of renal dysfunction.

Lupus erythematosus. Pruritus is not considered a common feature of this disease. Persistent "urticarial-like weals" in systemic lupus are characteristically not itchy. However, I have encountered several patients with discoid lupus erythematosus whose lesions itch when the disease is active, and two patients with systemic lupus erythematosus who claim that generalized itching without a rash is a consistent feature of flares of their disease. The latter are a mother and daughter who describe the symptom as a "very painful type of itch" that usually affects "the same area, thighs, upper arms, top and sides of head" and across the shoulders. B.T. MacKool and J.S. Dover presented a patient with pruritic discoid lupus involving the scalp, arms, and trunk at a meeting of the New England Dermatological Society at Massachusetts General Hospital on April 13, 1991. Bullous lesions of lupus erythematosus are often very itchy as well.

Sjogren's syndrome.[36] Dry skin with decreased sweating and pruritus may be seen.

Congenital or acquired anhidrosis.[37] Anhidrosis may be congenital or may occur in the settings of quinacrine treatment, metal poisoning, miliaria profunda, central nervous system or spinal cord injuries, Sjogren's syndrome, and metabolic or endocrine diseases such as diabetes. The acquired variety can also be "idiopathic," and can be associated with severe generalized pruritus.

Neurofibromatosis.[38] Individual neurofibromata, the segment in segmental neurofibromatosis, or the entire body may itch.

Hemochromatosis.[39] Generalized pruritus was the presenting symptom of idiopathic hemochromatosis in a 70-year-old woman with a 5-year history of ataxia, but no evidence of cholestasis. One patient presented with typical aquagenic pruritus.[40]

Starvation.[41] Six women with anorexia nervosa or bulimia nervosa developed generalized pruritus. In several, itching resolved when body weight returned to healthier levels. The cutaneous examination was normal except for mild dryness (asteatosis).

Fibromyalgia/Fibrositis.[42–45] Some patients with this disorder complain of itching, tingling, or skin pain.

Chronic fatigue syndrome.[46,47] Rashes and itching have been reported in this syndrome but have not been characterized. Some itching in some cases of this disorder may be variants of psychogenic pruritus, and may be described (as in some other cases of psychogenic pruritus), as "skin on fire."[48]

"Total allergy syndrome" "allergic to everything."[49,50] Some patients with this controversial disorder complain of itching. Other synonyms for this disorder include "twentieth-century disease," multiple chemical sensitivities, and ecologic illness.

Neurogenic pruritus, strange skin sensations, pruritic curiosities. Peripheral neuropathies, strokes, brain tumors, brain abscesses, multiple sclerosis, and psychiatric disorders are occasionally accompanied by localized or generalized itching. See Chap. 12, 13, and 25.

Dumping syndrome.[51] A 62-year-old man who had both a Bilroth II gastrectomy for duodenal ulcer and a transthoracic vagotomy many years previously developed severe post-prandial pruritus associated with the dumping syndrome half an hour after meals. Treatment with oral pectin relieved the itching and other post-prandial symptoms.

Pseudouremic pruritus.[52] An epidemic of scabies in a dialysis unit, including a staff nephrologist and three dialysis nurses, after itching in the index case was erroneously chalked up to uremic pruritus. Included here to demonstrate how easy it is to be misled, and how important it is to examine the patient even when you think you know the cause of his or her itch!

REFERENCES

1. Winkelmann RK, Muller SA: Pruritus. *Ann Rev Med* 15:53–64, 1964.
2. Gilchrest BA: Pruritus. Pathogenesis, therapy, and significance in systemic disease states. *Arch Intern Med* 142:101–105, 1982.
3. Denman ST: A review of pruritus. *J Am Acad Dermatol* 14:375–392, 1986.
4. Bernhard JD: Itching as a manifestation of noncutaneous disease. *Hosp Pract* 22:81–95, 1987.
5. Bernhard JD: Pruritus: Clinical aspects, in Fitzpatrick TB, Eisen AZ, Wolff K, Freedberg IM, Austen KF (eds): *Dermatology in General Medicine*, 3d ed. New York, McGraw-Hill. 1987, pp 78–90.
6. Greaves MW: Itching—research has barely scratched the surface. *N Engl J Med* 326:1016–1017, 1992.
7. Greaves MW: Pruritus, in Champion RH, Burton JL, Ebling FJG (eds): *Textbook of Dermatology*, 5th ed. Oxford, Blackwell Scientific Publications. 1992, pp 527–535.
8. Spaulding HS Jr: Pruritus without urticaria in acute giardiasis. *Ann Allergy* 65:161, 1990.
9. Rozenman D, Kremer M, Zuckerman F: Onchocerciasis in Israel. *Arch Dermatol* 120:505–507, 1984.
10. Kagen CN, Vance JC, Simpson M: Gnathostomiasis: Infestation in an Asian immigrant. *Arch Dermatol* 120:508–510, 1984.
11. Buslau M, Marsch WC: Papular eruption in helminth infection—a hypersensitivity phenomenon? *Acta Derm Venereol* (Stockh) 70:526–529, 1990.
12. White JJ, Prevost JV: Weil's disease: Report of three cases, including the morbid anatomy of one case, and a brief review of the pertinent literature. *Ann Intern Med* 15:207–225, 1941.
13. Jacks TA: Pruritus in parvovirus infection. *J R Coll Gen Pract* 37:210, 1987.
14. Muhlendahl KEv: Intoxication from mercury spilled on carpets. *Lancet* 336:1578–1579, 1990.
15. Kopelman H, Robertson MH, Sanders PG, et al: The Epping jaundice. *Br Med J* 1:514–516, 1966.
16. Morris PD, Campbell DS, Freeman JI. Ciguatera fish poisoning: An outbreak associated with fish caught from North Carolina coastal waters. *South Med J* 83:379–382, 1990.
17. Lawrence DN, Enriquez MB, Lumish RM, et al. Ciguatera fish poisoning in Miami. *JAMA* 244:254–258, 1980.
18. Morris JG Jr: Ciguatra fish poisoning: Barracuda's revenge (editorial). *South Med J* 83:371, 1990.
19. Etkind P, Wilson ME, Gallagher K, et al. Bluefish-associated scombroid poisoning: An example of the expanding spectrum of food poisoning from seafood. *JAMA* 258:3409–3410, 1987.

20. Lister DM, Shuttleworth D, Graham-Brown RAC, et al: Alagille's syndrome (arteriohepatic dysplasia). *Br J Dermatol* 115:52, 1986.
21. Ryatt KS, Cotterill JA, Littlewood JM. Generalized pruritus in a baby as a presenting feature of the arteriohepatic dysplasia syndrome. *Clin Exp Dermatol* 8:657–661, 1983.
22. Czarnetzki MB: *Urticaria.* Berlin, Springer-Verlag, 1986.
23. Lawlor F, Kobza Black A, Breathnach AS, et al: Vibratory angioedema: Lesion induction, clinical features, laboratory and ultrastructural findings and response to therapy. *Br J Dermatol* 120:93–99, 1989.
24. Burke M, Hallak A, Almog C: Sarcoidosis presenting with acute pleurisy, hemoptysis, pruritus, and eosinophilia. *Respiration* 51:248–251, 1987.
25. Sharma OP, Balchum OJ: Alcohol-induced pain and itching on hot shower in sarcoidosis. An unusual association. *Am Rev Resp Dis* 106:763–766, 1972.
26. Newton JA, Jagjivan A, Bhogal B, et al: Familial primary cutaneous amyloidosis. *Br J Dermatol* 112:201–208, 1985.
27. van den Hoogenband HM: Skin lesions as the first manifestation of the hypereosinophilic syndrome. *Clin Exp Dermatol* 7:267–272, 1982.
28. Newton JA, Singh AK, Greaves MW, et al: Aquagenic pruritus associated with the idiopathic hypereosinophilic syndrome. *Br J Dermatol* 122:103–106, 1990.
29. Oursler JR, Farmer ER, Roubenoff R, et al: Cutaneous manifestations of the eosinophilia-myalgia syndrome. *Br J Dermatol* 127:138–146, 1992.
30. Silver RM, Heyes MP, Maize JC, et al: Scleroderma, fasciitis, and eosinophilia associated with the ingestion of tryptophan. *N Engl J Med* 322:874–881, 1990.
31. Medsger TA. Tryptophan-induced eosinophilia-myalgia syndrome. *N Engl J Med* 322:926–928, 1990.
32. Scheff RJ, Rollar AR. The eosinophilia-myalgia syndrome. *Ann Intern Med* 112:964–965, 1990.
33. Euwer RL, Sontheimer RD. Amyopathic dermatomyositis (dermatomyositis sine myositis). *J Am Acad Dermatol* 24:959–966, 1991.
34. Grau JM, Hausmann G, Casademont J, et al: Amyopathic dermatomyositis (correspondence related to previous reference and reply). *J Am Acad Dermatol* 26:505–508, 1992.
35. Claman HN: Mast cell changes in a case of rapidly progressive scleroderma—ultrastructural analysis. *J Invest Dermatol* 92:290–295, 1989.
36. Feuerman EJ: Sjogren's syndrome presenting as recalcitrant generalized pruritus. *Dermatologica* 137:74–86, 1968.
37. Kay DM, Maibach HI: Pruritus and anhidrosis. Two unusual cases. *Arch Dermatol* 100:291–293, 1969.
38. McFadden JP, Logan R, Griffiths WAD: Segmental neurofibromatosis and pruritus. *Clin Exp Dermatol* 13:265–268, 1988.
39. Hamilton DV, Gould DJ: Generalized pruritus as a presentation of idiopathic haemochromatosis. *Br J Dermatol* 112:629, 1985.
40. Nestler JE. Hemochromatosis and pruritus. *Ann Intern Med* 98:1026, 1983.
41. Gupta MA, Gupta AK, Voorhees JJ: Starvation-associated pruritus: A clinical feature of eating disorders. *J Am Acad Dermatol* 27:118–120, 1992.
42. Goldenberg DL: Research in fibromyalgia: Past, present and future. *J Rheumatol* 15:992–996, 1988.
43. Hudson JI, Pope HG: Fibromyalgia and psychopathology: Is fibromyalgia a form of "affective spectrum disorder?" *J Rheumatol* (suppl 19) 16:15–22, 1989. [This article is from an entire supplement dedicated to the subject of fibromyalgia.]
44. Arthritis Foundation: *Fibromyalgia (fibrositis),* 3d ed. (pamphlet). Atlanta, Arthritis Foundation, 1989.
45. Csillag C: Fibromyalgia: The Copenhagen declaration. *Lancet* 340:663–664, 1992.
46. Holmes GP, Kaplan JE, Gantz NM, et al: Chronic fatigue syndrome: A working case definition. *Ann Intern Med* 108:387–389, 1988.

47. Gold D, Bowden R, Sixbey J, et al: Chronic fatigue. A prospective clinical and virologic study. *JAMA* 264:48–53, 1990.
48. Shorter E: *From paralysis to fatigue. A history of psychosomatic illness in the modern era.* New York, The Free Press. 1992, p 303.
49. Brodsky CM: "Allergic to everything": A medical subculture. *Psychosomatics* 24:731–742, 1983.
50. American College of Physicians: Clinical ecology, (position paper) *Ann Intern Med* 111:168–178, 1989.
51. Harries AD, Tredree R, Heatley RV, et al. Pruritus as a manifestation of the dumping syndrome. *Br J Dermatol* 107:707–709, 1982.
52. Lempert KD, Baltz PS, Welton WA, et al: Pseudouremic pruritus: A scabies epidemic in a dialysis unit. *Am J Kidney Dis* 5:117–119, 1985.

TWENTY-THREE

DRUG-INDUCED PRURITUS WITHOUT A RASH

Anna M. Sarno
Jeffrey D. Bernhard

Drugs cause a remarkable variety of cutaneous eruptions.[1-4] Exanthems and urticaria may be the most common; fixed drug eruptions are perhaps the most distinctive.[5] Urticaria or angioedema with anaphylaxis, exfoliative dermatitis–erythroderma syndrome, and toxic epidermal necrolysis[6] are the most dangerous of cutaneous reactions to drugs. Drugs can also cause erythema nodosum, erythema multiforme, purpura, and vasculitis. Eczematous, lichenoid, and pityriasis-rosea-like drug eruptions occur, but are not an everyday occurrence even for dermatologists.[7] Drugs can exacerbate psoriasis,[8] acne,[9] and probably other skin diseases as well. Immunologic, pharmacologic, toxic, and other mechanisms, such as direct mediator release, may be involved. In some cases, sunlight interacts with drugs to cause photosensitivity via photoallergic or phototoxic mechanisms.[10] Many, but not all, of these visible eruptions itch, and the reader is referred to references 1 to 5 for thorough treatments and excellent photographs of the *visible* cutaneous drug reactions.

The focus of this chapter is on drug-induced itching *without* skin lesions or a rash. Generalized pruritus is probably one of the least, if not the least, common of adverse cutaneous reactions to drugs. Amongst 15,438 consecutive medical inpatients monitored by the Boston Collaborative Drug Surveillance Program from 1975 to 1982, 358 cutaneous reactions occurred in 347 patients.[11] Of these, only 5 (1.4 percent) were generalized pruritus, ninety-four percent (337) were generalized morbilliform drug exanthems, and 17 (4.8 percent) were urticaria. Acute generalized itching is a common feature of anaphylactic reactions as well. Although similar mechanisms may

Table 23-1 Drugs that *may* cause pruritus[a]

Antibiotics and other anti-infectious agents

miconazole[a]
ampicillin
cephalosporins
colistin
ketoconazole
polymyxin B
sulfonamides
acyclovir
chloroquine[26,27]
halofantrine[28]
other antimalarials
metronidazole
suramin
lomefloxacin

Anesthetic agents, opiates

morphine
heroin
fentanyl
butorphanol

Analgesics, antipyretics,
antirheumatics, nonsteroidal anti-inflammatory
agents (NSAIAs)

gold[29,30] (common)[b,c]
fenoprofen[b]
aspirin
ibuprofen
other NSAIAs[31]

Antigout drugs (not common)

allopurinol
colchicine
probenecid

Neurologic and psychiatric drugs

pyritinol[b]
benzoctamine
imipramine
isocarboxacid
lofepramine
protriptyline

Cytostatic drugs

bleomycin[b]

Cardiovascular drugs

captopril[b]
enalapril
clonidine[b]
amiodarone
beta-blockers (e.g., atenolol)
diazoxide
diphenoxylate
naftazone
dobutamine (scalp)
quinidine[32]

Diuretics

furosemide
hydrochlorothiazide

Gastrointestinal drugs (not common)

phenolphthalein

Antidiabetic drugs (not common)

insulin
sulfonylureas

Miscellaneous

PUVA (photochemotherapy)[33,34]
hetastarch, hydroxyethylstarch[35,37]

Hormones (usually via cholestasis)

progesterones
estrogens
oral contraceptives
dexamethasone

Thyroid drugs

methimazole
propylthiouracil

Anticoagulants

coumarins
heparin
warfarin

Immunotherapeutic agents

aluminum-precipitated pollen extracts

Table 23-1 Continued

Vitamins and vitamin derivatives	Diagnostics
niacin (nicotinic acid)[d]	iodipamide
vitamin B complex	ioglycamic acid
etretinate[36]	iopanoic acid
isotretinoin	
other retinoids (usually with dry skin)	

[a]Modified, condensed, and expanded from Bork K. *Cutaneous Side Effects of Drugs.* Philadelphia, Saunders, 1988: Table 42, pp 314.
[b]May affect more than 5% of persons exposed.
[c]Noteworthy because itching may be the most common and earliest cutaneous reaction to gold salts, because it may precede a cutaneous eruption by some weeks, and because it may resolve even when treatment is continued. Eosinophilia may, or may not, be present.
[d]Also a notable cause of flushing.

involved in some cases, systemic anaphylaxis is, of course, an emergency situation clinically quite distinct from drug-induced, chronic, generalized pruritus.

Table 23-1 provides a list of the major categories of drugs that may cause pruritus, as well as some examples, comments, and pertinent references. It is important to note that reporting of adverse reactions to medications is not very systematic at best and haphazard at worse. Furthermore, drug-induced itching is more difficult to diagnose and is probably underreported compared to other side effects of drugs, which are not that easy to diagnose in the first place.[12] For these reasons and others, the listing in Table 23-1 is not complete, and cannot convey an accurate sense of the true incidence of itching as a side effect of particular drugs.

PATHOPHYSIOLOGY

In theory, drugs can provoke itching *without* a rash in several ways, many of which are analogous to how they cause itching *with* a rash. These include hepatotoxicity,[13] cholestasis,[14] neuropeptide-related effects,[15] photoallergy and phototoxicity,[16] augmented pharmacologic actions,[17] immunologic hypersensitivity,[18] other toxic effects, and of course, idiopathic or idiosyncratic mechanisms. It has been suggested that anything that can cause urticaria can probably also cause itching without a rash through a process of "urticarial diminution."[19] Some drugs, such as systemic retinoids, commonly cause dryness of the skin, and can cause itching through this relatively trivial side effect.

CLINICAL FEATURES

Drug-induced itching is usually generalized, but localized varieties occur. Sometimes only flexor surfaces of the arms and legs are involved; perhaps these areas have a lower itch threshold. Incipient drug reactions in hospitalized patients often begin with itching of the back, suggesting that pressure, friction, and warmth may contribute to the localization of itching and subsequent exanthems if they develop. Sometimes only the scalp (e.g., dobutamine),[20] perineum (e.g., dexamethasone),[21] face (e.g., spinal anesthetic agents),[22] or genital region (e.g., enalapril)[23] may be affected. When rubbing, scratching, and secondary infection occur, nonspecific changes such as excoriations and eczematization may obscure the fact that the primary problem is underlying pruritus. The permutations of such varieties and combinations of events is at the root of the dermatologic dictum that drugs can do anything and should be considered in the differential diagnosis of any rash with any morphology.

DIAGNOSIS

The principles of diagnosis for drug-induced itching are the same as those which apply to the diagnosis of any suspected drug eruption, including the following.

1. History. The interval between the initiation of drug therapy and the onset of itching can be an important clue. While short intervals are characteristic of many cutaneous reactions, data on drug-induced itching alone is scant to say the least. Given the variety of mechanisms that may be involved, intervals of any length may be expected, and this is borne out by our clinical experience. As drug-induced itching may have such an insidious onset, the patient will most often fail to make the connection between it and a particular medication he or she may have been taking for some time.
2. Physical examination. There is no primary eruption. *Secondary* changes such as excoriation, eczematization, lichenfication, the "burnished nail sign,"[24] and infection may be present. Care must be taken to avoid the trap of assuming that the secondary changes are the primary diagnosis.
3. Discontinuation (dechallenge) of suspected medications. The looming question here is how long a break from suspect medication is enough? This subject has never been adequately addressed. In the last analysis, the nature of the reaction and of its presumed mechanism must be considered. It is fair to conclude that relief could be prompt when certain drugs are discontinued, but that a hepatotoxic effect with cholestasis could take weeks or more to resolve.

4. Special tests such as skin biopsy to exclude other disorders, epicutaneous and intracutaneous tests, radioallergosorbent testing (RAST), and liver function tests may be indicated in certain cases. A complete blood count is helpful in the evaluation of generalized pruritus in any event, but eosinophilia is an inconstant feature of drug-induced itching.

5. Rechallenge with suspected medications is not ordinarily recommended for fear of provoking more serious reactions, but may be considered in special situations when the need to use the drug or to know for certain outweighs the risks.

DIFFERENTIAL DIAGNOSIS

The differential diagnosis of pruritus without a rash in a patient taking one or more medications includes the entire spectrum of systemic diseases that can cause pruritus (as described in Section III of this book), as well as occult infestation and a variety of other dermatologic disorders (as discussed in Section II). The clinical challenge can be enormous, because many patients take multiple medications, because an individual patient may be sensitive to more than one medication, and because no one knows exactly how long a drug must be discontinued before it is safe to conclude that it was or was not the cause of the problem. Another problem is that drug-related itching in elderly patients who may be on multiple medications can be very difficult to distinguish from so-called "senile pruritus."[25] In fact, it may not be possible to diagnose the latter until drugs have been excluded as the cause.

TREATMENT

The obvious treatment for drug-induced itching is to eliminate the offending drug. If that is not possible, or if symptomatic measures are required while the drug or its effects are eliminated from the patient's system, a variety of symptomatic measures, such as cooling or emollient lotions, may be considered (see Section V and Chap. 27, in particular).

REFERENCES

1. Bork K: *Cutaneous Side Effects of Drugs.* Philadelphia, Saunders, 1988.
2. Breathnach SM, Hintner H: *Adverse Drug Reactions and the Skin.* Oxford, Blackwell Scientific Publications, 1992.
3. Felix RH, Smith AG: Skin disorders, in Davies DM (ed.): *Textbook of Adverse Drug Reactions,* 4th ed. Oxford, Oxford Medical Publications, 1991, pp 514–534.
4. Wintroub BU, Stern RS, Arndt KA: Cutaneous reactions to drugs, in Fitzpatrick TB, Eisen AZ, Wolff K, et al. (eds.): *Dermatology in General Medicine,* 3d ed. New York, McGraw-Hill. 1987, pp 1353–1366.

5. Fitzpatrick TB, Johnson RA, Polano MK, et al: Section 21: Drug reactions, in: *Color Atlas and Synopsis of Clinical Dermatology; Common and Serious Diseases,* 2d ed. New York, McGraw-Hill, 1992, pp 596–607.
6. Roujeau J-C, Guillaume J-C, Fabre J-P, et al: Toxic epidermal necrolysis (Lyell Syndrome): Incidence and drug etiology in France, 1981–1985. *Arch Dermatol* 126:37–42, 1990.
7. Fox BJ, Odom RB: Papulosquamous diseases: A review. *J Am Acad Dermatol* 12:597–624, 1985.
8. Abel EA, DiCicco LM, Orenberg EK, et al: Drugs in exacerbation of psoriasis. *J Am Acad Dermatol* 15:1007–1022, 1986.
9. Hitch JM: Acneform eruptions induced by drugs and chemicals. *JAMA* 200:879–880, 1967.
10. Bernhard JD: Photosensitivity, in Lebwohl M (ed.): *Difficult Diagnoses in Dermatology.* New York, Churchill Livingstone. 1988, pp 405–417.
11. Bigby M, Jick S, Jick H, et al: Drug-induced cutaneous reactions. A report from the Boston Collaborative Drug Surveillance Program on 15,438 consecutive inpatients, 1975–1982. *JAMA* 256:3358–3363, 1986.
12. Shear NH: Diagnosing cutaneous adverse reactions to drugs. *Arch Dermatol* 126:94–97, 1990.
13. Davis M, Williams R: Hepatic disorders, in Davies DM (ed.): *Textbook of Adverse Drug Reactions,* 4th ed. Oxford, Oxford University Press. 1991, pp 244–304.
14. Zimmerman HJ, Lewis JH: Drug-induced cholestasis. *Med Toxicol* 2:112–160, 1987.
15. Bernstein JE: Neuropeptides and the skin, in Goldsmith LA (ed.): *Physiology, Biochemistry, and Molecular Biology of the Skin,* 2d ed. New York, Oxford University Press. 1991, pp 816–835.
16. Bernhard JD, Parrish JA, Pathak MA, et al: Abnormal responses to ultraviolet radiation, in Fitzpatrick TB, Eisen AZ, Wolff K, et al. (eds.): *Dermatology in General Medicine,* 3d ed. New York, McGraw-Hill. 1987, pp 1481–1507.
17. Wilkin JK, Hammond JJ, Kirkendall WM: The captopril-induced eruption. A possible mechanism: Cutaneous kinin potentiation. *Arch Dermatol* 116:902–905, 1980.
18. Kalish RS: Drug eruptions: A review of clinical and immunological features. *Adv Dermatol* 6:221–237, 1991.
19. Bernhard JD: A theorem of pruritus and urticarial diminution. *J Am Acad Dermatol:* 28:800, 1993.
20. McCauley CS, Blumenthal MS: Dobutamine and pruritus of the scalp. *Ann Intern Med* 105:966, 1986.
21. Zaglama NE, Rosenblum SI, Sartiano GP, et al: Single, high-dose intravenous dexamethasone as an antiemetic in cancer chemotherapy. *Oncology* 43:27–32, 1986.
22. Scott PV, Fischer HB: Spinal opiate analgesia and facial pruritus: A neural theory. *Postgrad Med J* 58:531–535, 1982.
23. Heckerling PS: Enalapril and vulvovaginal pruritus (letter). *Ann Intern Med* 112:879, 1990.
24. Bernhard JD: Clinical aspects of pruritus, in Fitzpatrick TB, Eisen AZ, Wolff K, et al. (eds.): *Dermatology in General Medicine,* 3d ed. New York, McGraw-Hill. 1987, pp 78–90.
25. Bernhard JD: Phantom itch, pseudophantom itch, and senile pruritus. *Int J Dermatol* 31:856–857, 1992.
26. Osifo NG: Chloroquine-induced pruritus among patients with malaria. *Arch Dermatol* 120:80–82, 1984.
27. Ogunranti JO, Aguiyi JC, Roma S. et al: Chloroquine-induced pruritus and sickle cell gene trait in Africans: Possible pharmacogenetic relationship. *Eur J Clin Pharmacol* 43:323–324, 1992.
28. Ezeamuzie IC, Igbigbi PA, Ambakederemo AW, et al: Halofantrine-induced pruritus amongst subjects who itch to chloroquine. *J Trop Med Hyg* 94:184–188, 1991.
29. Almeyda J, Baker H. Cutaneous reactions to anti-rheumatic drugs. *Br J Dermatol* 83:707–711, 1970.

30. Bailin PL, Matkaluk RM: Cutaneous reactions to rheumatological drugs. *Clin Rhem Dis* 8:493–516, 1982.
31. Bibgy M, Stern RS: Cutaneous reactions to nonsteroidal anti-inflammatory drugs. A review. *J Am Acad Dermatol* 12:866–876, 1985.
32. Holt RJ: Uncharacteristic cutaneous reactions induced by quinidine. *Drug Intell Clin Pharm* 16:615–616, 1982.
33. Rogers S, Marks J, Shuster S: Itch following photochemotherapy for psoriasis. *Acta Derm Venereol* 61:178–180, 1981.
34. Roelandts R, Stevens A: PUVA-induced itching and skin pain. *Photodermatol Photoimmunol Photomed* 7:141–142, 1990.
35. Parker NE, Porter JB, Williams HJM, et al: Pruritus after administration of hetastarch (short report). *B M J* 284:385–386, 1982.
36. Rowland Payne CME: Etretinate and nodular prurigo (letter). *Br J Dermatol* 118:135, 1988.
37. Jurecka W, Szépfalusi Z, Parth E, et al.: Hydroxyethylstarch deposits in human skin—a model for pruritus? *Arch Dermatol Res* 285:13–19, 1993.

DIAGNOSTIC EVALUATION OF THE PATIENT WITH GENERALIZED PRURITUS

Gary R. Kantor

INTRODUCTION

In the evaluation of the patient with generalized pruritus, it is imperative to determine if the patient's itching is related to primary dermatologic disease, systemic disease, or other causes. To make this determination, a thorough history and physical examination are necessary. Certain findings can direct the clinician toward the underlying cause. For example, primary skin lesions such as papules or vesicles point toward a primary dermatologic disease whereas lymphadenopathy or hepatomegaly suggest systemic disease. Laboratory evaluation may disclose an etiology such as cholestasis or hyperthyroidism. If pruritus has been present for at least 3 weeks and a cause cannot be determined, the patient has "pruritus of undetermined origin" (P.U.O.). Further dermatologic and medical consultation, diagnostic studies tailored to the individual patient, and time may be required before a definitive underlying diagnosis can be established.

In previous chapters, the dermatologic and systemic diseases associated with pruritus were reviewed. This chapter will address the clinical and laboratory evaluation of the patient who presents with generalized pruritus.

HISTORY

The history of the presenting symptom is crucial to making a diagnosis. Pertinent features of pruritus that can be elicited by history are shown in Table 24-1 and discussed in following sections.

Table 24-1 Historical features of pruritus

A. Descriptive features of pruritus
    1. Onset—e.g., abrupt, gradual
    2. Nature—e.g., continuous, intermittent, pricking, burning
    3. Duration—e.g., days, weeks, months, years
    4. Severity—e.g., interference with normal activities
    5. Time relation—e.g., nighttime, cyclical
    6. Location—e.g., generalized or localized, unilateral or bilateral
    7. Relationship to activities—e.g., occupation, hobbies
    8. Provoking factors—e.g., water, skin cooling, air, exercise
B. Other pertinent historical factors
    1. Medications—prescribed, over the counter, illicit
    2. Allergies—systemic, topical
    3. Atopic history—asthma, hayfever, eczema
    4. Family history of atopy or skin disease
    5. Occupation
    6. Hobbies
    7. Social history—household and other personal contacts
    8. Bathing habits
    9. Pets and their care
    10. Sexual history
    11. Travel history
    12. Prior diagnoses made by physicians or patient (patient's own theory)

The onset, duration, and nature of pruritus help to determine its cause. In the absence of a primary skin disease, acute onset of pruritus over only several days is less suggestive of underlying systemic disease than chronic, progressive generalized pruritus. Localized pruritus is usually not a consequence of systemic disease. Severity of pruritus varies and is much more troublesome to the patient when it interferes with or awakens the patient from sleep. Nocturnal wakening by pruritus in the absence of a primary skin disease may point to an underlying systemic illness; it is said that "psychogenic" generalized pruritus seldom wakens patients from sleep.[1] In most patients, itching worsens at night, especially in the instance of scabies infestation. Cyclical monthly itching may occur with menses.[2] Hemodialysis patients often experience worsening of pruritus during their dialysis.[3] Pruritus may be described as "burning" in dermatitis herpetiformis or "pricking" in polycythemia vera.

The relationship of itching to activities is also important. For example, itching provoked by cooling of the skin after emergence from a bath ("bath pruritus") may be a symptom of polycythemia vera or of idiopathic aquagenic pruritus.[4] Bathing habits need to be explored in depth because overbathing and harsh soap, especially in the setting of dry, winter air, is a frequent cause of itchy skin, especially among the elderly.[5] Reducing the frequency of bathing, lowering the temperature of the bath water, use of moisturizing or gentle cleansing soaps, towel pat drying, and liberal use of moisturizing lotions or

Table 24-2 Some drugs associated with pruritus[a]

Drugs that cause hepatic cholestasis
    Chlorpropamide
    Tolbutamide
    Phenothiazines
    Erythromycin estolate
    Anabolic steroids
    Oral contraceptives
Chloroquine; other antimalarials
Opiates and their derivatives
Aspirin
Quinidine

[a] See also Chap. 23.

creams should eliminate xerosis and aquagenic pruritus of the elderly, but are helpful for alleviating pruritus regardless of the cause. A list of prior diagnoses, including the patient's own theories, as well as past prescribed and self-administered treatment must also be obtained. Topical antihistamines, anesthetics, antibiotics, and various home remedies may actually worsen itching from sensitization and contact dermatitis.

    Systemic medications may produce pruritus without skin lesions due to allergy, hepatic cholestasis, or other mechanisms (see Chap. 23 and Table 24-2).[6] If the patient is allergic to a systemic medication, chemically similar drugs may precipitate pruritus as well. This frequently occurs with the sulfa-based antibiotics and diuretics. The nonsulfa-based diuretics spironolactone and ethycrynic acid may be helpful in this clinical circumstance. Ethylenediamine contact sensitivity precludes the systemic administration of aminophylline (theophylline and ethylenediamine), pyribenzamine (PBZ), and hydroxyzine (Atarax®, Vistaril®). Occupation and the work environment may be pertinent, especially in fiberglass workers.[7] Hobbies and leisure activities should also be explored. Sexual practices, illicit drug use, and other risk factors for acquired immunodeficiency syndrome (AIDS) may also be obtained in the history. Pruritus may be the presenting symptom of AIDS[8,9] (see Chap. 20).

REVIEW OF SYSTEMS

A brief but thorough review of systems will help direct the physical examination and laboratory evaluation (Table 24-3). Particular attention should be given to the patient's general health, constitutional symptoms, and details of the skin and its appendages.

    For example, pruritus may be an early sign of Hodgkin's disease, so the itchy patient who complains of fevers or night sweats should have a chest

Table 24-3 Review of systems for pruritus

General health—e.g., fevers, sweats, chills, fatigue, anorexia, weight change
Skin—e.g., pigmentation, sweating, xerosis, plethora, jaundice
Hair—e.g., texture, loss, growth
Nails—e.g., grooving, curvature, onycholysis, color changes
Eyes—e.g., exophthalmus, color change of sclera and conjunctiva
Endocrine—e.g., temperature intolerance, tremor, polyuria, polydipsia
Hematopoietic—e.g., anemia, bleeding, lymphadenopathy
Gastrointestinal—e.g., nausea, vomiting, change in bowel habits, blood
Genitourinary—e.g., color of urine, urinary frequency, incontinence, menstrual history,
  pregnancies
Neurologic—e.g., headaches, paresthesias, visual disturbances
Mental status—e.g., mood lability, hallucinations, grandiose ideas, sleep disturbances

radiograph without delay. Positive findings in the review of systems should be used to tailor the initial phase of the evaluation earlier rather than later: some elements of the work-up might be initiated on the first visit, while in other instances it is more appropriate to defer some or all of the laboratory evaluation to follow-up visits.

PHYSICAL EXAMINATION

The physical examination often enables the clinician to discriminate primary dermatologic disease from other causes of pruritus. Most patients with pruritus not related to a primary skin disease demonstrate only excoriations or other secondary changes. Some have no detectable skin changes at all, while others have only the mildest evidence of rubbing. In other instances, lesions may occur as a consequence of rubbing, scratching, or secondary infection.[10,11] Misinterpretation of secondary lesions as the cause for itching may delay the evaluation of the patient. (See Fig. 3-1.)

The presence of primary skin lesions such as papules, vesicles, pustules, and the like suggests a dermatologic disorder. If primary skin lesions are seen in the mid upper back, which is not accessible to the patient's hands, the suspicion for a primary skin disorder is great. Chronicity may be determined by pigmentary changes, lichenification, "burnished nails," and other secondary findings.[6] Because persistent scratching produces postinflammatory hyperpigmentation of the skin, a spared area of skin may appear relatively hypopigmented in comparison. This phenomenon occurs in the so-called "butterfly sign," which describes the relative hypopigmentation of the mid upper back due to its inaccessibility from the patient's hands. The "butterfly sign" was originally described in patients with hepatobiliary disease,[12] but may be seen in other pruritic disorders including atopic dermatitis.[13]

Table 24-4 Causes of "generalized" lymphadenopathy[a]

A. Infection
   1. Bacterial—scarlet fever, brucellosis, tularemia, plague, cat-scratch disease
   2. Viral—rubella, rubeola, mononucleosis, HIV
   3. Fungal—sporotrichosis
   4. Spirochetal—syphilis
   5. Protozoal—toxoplasmosis, Chagas disease, kala-azar
B. Neoplasm
   1. Lymphoma—Hodgkin's disease, non-Hodgkin's lymphoma, mycosis fungoides
   2. Leukemia—lymphocytic, myelocytic
   3. Solid tumor metastases
C. Connective tissue disease
   1. Lupus erythematosus
   2. Dermatomyositis
   3. Rheumatoid arthritis
   4. Still's disease
D. Drugs
   1. Phenytoin
E. Metabolic
   1. Neumann–Pick disease
   2. Gaucher's disease
F. Reactive hyperplasia
G. Dermatopathic
   1. Atopic dermatitis
   2. Exfoliative dermatitis
   3. Mycosis fungoides
H. Miscellaneous
   1. Sarcoidosis
   2. Amyloidosis
   3. Serum sickness
   4. Kawasaki's disease

[a] Defined as three or more anatomic lymph node groups.

Meticulous scrutiny of the skin with the aid of a magnifying lens should be performed to exclude scabies infestation, which produces pruritus out of proportion to the clinical findings. The mite is too small to be seen even with a hand lens, but burrows may be detected more easily upon magnification. (See also Chap. 9.) Surveillance skin scrapings for mites may also be useful. Fine to plate-like noninflammatory scaling, particularly on the legs, flanks, and upper trunk are characteristic of xerosis. Xerosis is common in the elderly due to intrinsic aging changes and is a frequent cause of seasonal pruritus where it has been termed "winter itch."

The general physical examination may disclose an undiagnosed systemic disease. Particular attention should be directed to lymphadenopathy and organomegaly. Table 24-4 lists the most frequent causes of lymphadenopathy.

LABORATORY EVALUATION

According to several studies, systemic disease may be associated with generalized pruritus in 16 to 50 percent of patients.[14–17] However, it is difficult to compare the results of these studies because of the variable patient populations, definitions of generalized pruritus, and laboratory studies performed. Regardless, it is clear that generalized pruritus is associated with systemic disease in a significant number of patients.

If no cause for the patient's itching can be found from the history and physical examination (PUO), it may, in some cases, be reasonable to treat the patient conservatively with systemic antihistamines and topical nonsteroidal soothing emollient lotions or creams for 2 weeks. If there is no response to this conservative management, laboratory evaluation is indicated to exclude an underlying systemic disease.

The systemic causes for PUO are shown in Table 24-5 and discussed throughout Section 3 of this book. Diabetes mellitus[18,19] and iron deficiency anemia[20–22] are the subject of reports that both support and refute their

Table 24-5 Systemic diseases associated with generalized pruritus without primary skin lesions

A. Uremia
B. Obstructive hepatobiliary disease
   1. Primary biliary cirrhosis
   2. Drugs (See Table 24-2)
   3. Extrahepatic biliary obstruction
   4. Intrahepatic cholestasis with pregnancy or menses
C. Hematologic disorders
   1. Polycythemia vera
   2. Iron deficiency anemia (see text)
   3. Paraproteinemia and myeloma
   4. Mastocytosis
D. Endocrine
   1. Hyperthyroidism, hypothyroidism (see text)
   2. Diabetes (see text)
E. Neurologic disorders
   1. Infarcts
   2. Brain abscess
   3. Multiple sclerosis
   4. Tumor
F. Lymphoreticular neoplasms
   1. Hodgkin's disease
   2. Lymphoma
G. Visceral malignancy—solid tumors, carcinoid (see text)
H. Miscellaneous—AIDS, Sjogren's syndrome

Also see Chaps. 15–23.

Table 24-6 Suggested screening laboratory evaluation of pruritus

A. CBC with differential white blood cell count
B. Blood urea nitrogen, creatinine
C. Alkaline phosphatase, bilirubin
D. T4, TSH
E. Glucose
F. Stool for occult blood (if age over 40 years)
G. Chest x-ray

relation to generalized pruritus. However, as laboratory evaluation for their disclosure is routine and relatively inexpensive, screening for diabetes and iron deficiency anemia may be prudent. The argument for obtaining a serum ferritin level to address the question of iron deficiency without anemia is considered by Dr. Adams in Chap. 17.

There are no controlled studies in the literature associating hypothyroidism and generalized pruritus. Itching in these patients is presumably due to associated dry skin as return to a euthyroid state with medical treatment does not abate the itch.

The association of generalized pruritus and systemic malignancy is addressed in Chap. 21. The connection of itching and lymphoma is unquestioned. Although several case reports have documented a positive association with carcinomas as well, Paul and colleagues[23] did not find an increased frequency of malignancy in 125 patients with PUO followed for 6 years. They and others[24] do not recommend expensive cancer screening studies for patients with PUO. We believe that evaluation for occult carcinoma should be considered in individual cases if the history, review of systems, or initial screening laboratory examination or chest x-ray point in that direction, and that patients with PUO should be reassessed periodically. Indiscriminate testing should be discouraged.

Table 24-6 shows a cost-effective laboratory screening for the patient with PUO This group of tests is based on the data of an outpatient evaluation of 44 patients with PUO The complete blood count may occasionally reveal eosinophilia. The most likely dermatologic causes for eosinophilia include atopic dermatitis, pemphigoid, eosinophilic cellulitis, eosinophilic fasciitis, urticaria, some drug reactions, scabies, and exfoliative dermatitis. Other causes of eosinophilia are listed in Table 24-7.[25,26]

Most systemic diseases, including underlying malignancy, will be detected or made suspect by history, physical examination, and the screening laboratory tests. If a systemic cause for PUO is not uncovered at the initial screen, but clinical suspicion is high, further laboratory studies may be indicated in *selected* cases (Table 24-8). Expensive and invasive radiologic studies should be performed judiciously. Biopsy of the skin may be helpful and is discussed in Chap. 5.

Table 24-7 Causes of eosinophilia

Nondermatologic
A. Infection
    1. Parasitic—e.g., trichinosis, filiariasis
    2. Fungal—e.g., aspergillosis, coccidioidomycosis
B. Neoplasm
    1. Leukemia—eosinophilic, chronic myelogenous, lymphoblastic
    2. Lymphoma—mycosis fungoides, Sezary syndrome, Hodgkin's disease
C. Drugs—chlorpromazine, aspirin, iodides, sulfonamides
D. Allergic—asthma, rhinitis, anaphylaxis
E. Renal—renal failure (acute or chronic)
F. Miscellaneous—hypereosinophilic syndrome, sarcoidosis, Wegener's granulomatosis, Churg–Strauss allergic granulomatosis, tryptophan related eosinophilia—myalgia syndrome

Dermatologic
A. Atopic dermatitis
B. Bullous pemphigoid
C. Eosinophilic cellulitis
D. Eosinophilic fasciitis
E. Eosinophilic pustular folliculitis
F. Angiolymphoid hyperplasia with eosinophilia
G. Urticaria
H. Scabies
I. Exfoliative dermatitis

Psychogenic causes for generalized pruritus, as discussed by Dr. Koblenzer in Chap. 25, are often clinically evident at the time of presentation. In these instances, referral to a psychiatrist who has an interest or expertise in psychocutaneous medicine may be helpful. However, the possibility of underlying dermatologic or systemic causes of generalized pruritus must be considered as well: the intense discomfort and sleeplessness experienced by some patients can elicit hostile behavior and strange affect. Some patients thought to have delusional parasitosis may have an underlying systemic

Table 24-8 Further laboratory evaluation of pruritus in selected cases

A. Serum iron, ferritin
B. Serum protein electrophoresis, serum immunoelectrophoresis
C. Skin biopsy for special stains (to exclude mastocytosis)
D. Skin biopsy for direct immunofluorescence (to exclude dermatitis herpetiformis, bullous pemphigoid). See Chap. 5.
E. Stool for ova and parasites
F. Urine for 5HIAA and mast cell metabolites
G. Additional radiologic studies

cause. Inappropriate affect or behavior should not preclude a systemic evaluation.

COURSE AND PROGNOSIS

Negative findings on initial evaluation should not discourage the clinician and do not necessarily exclude associated systemic disease. In one study, 4 (9%) of 44 patients were found to have systemic disease on clinical follow-up.[17] Therefore, reassessment and reevaluation is necessary for these patients. The chest x-ray and laboratory tests may need to be repeated every 3 to 6 months if pertinent to the clinical setting. The patient needs support, empathy, and reassurance. In some instances, a psychiatric or psychologic referral for assistance in coping with pruritus is helpful.

The evaluation of a patient with persistent generalized pruritus can be one of the most challenging problems of clinical medicine. It can also be one of the most gratifying, because the detection of a previously undiagnosed systemic disease is of obvious importance, and because its treatment often eliminates the itch.

REFERENCES

1. Bernhard JD: Nocturnal wakening caused by pruritus: Organic or psychogenic. *J Am Acad Dermatol* 23:767, 1990.
2. Dahl MGC: Premenstrual pruritus due to recurrent cholestasis. *Trans St Johns Hosp Dermatol Soc* 56:11–13, 1970.
3. Gilchrest BA, Stern R, Steinman TI, et al: Clinical features of pruritus among patients undergoing maintenance hemodialysis. *Arch Dermatol* 118:154–156, 1982.
4. Steinman HK, Greaves MD: Aquagenic pruritus. *J Am Acad Dermatol* 13:91–96, 1985.
5. Kligman AM, Greaves MD, Steinman HK. Water induced itching without cutaneous signs. *Arch Dermatol* 122:183–186, 1986.
6. Bernhard JD: Clinical aspects of pruritus, in Fitzpatrick TB, Eisen AZ, Wolff K, et al (eds): *Dermatology in General Medicine,* 3rd ed. New York, McGraw-Hill. 1987, chap 8, pp 78–90.
7. Fisher BK, Warkentin JD: Fiberglass dermatitis. *Arch Dermatol* 99:717, 1969.
8. Shapiro RS, Samorodin C, Hood AF: Pruritus as a presenting sign of acquired immuno-deficiency syndrome. *J Am Acad Dermatol* 16:1115–1117, 1987.
9. Liautaud B, Pape JW, DeHovitz JA, et al: Pruritic skin lesions: A common initial presentation of acquired immunodeficiency syndrome. *Arch Dermatol* 125:629–632, 1989.
10. Pedragosa R, Knobel HJ, Huguet P, et al: Reactive perforating collagenosis in Hodgkin's disease. *Am J Dermatopathol* 9:41–44, 1987.
10a. Fina L, Grimalt R, Berti E, et al: Nodular prurigo associated with Hodgkin's disease. *Dermatologica* 182:243–246, 1991.
11. Shelnitz LS, Paller AS: Hodgkin's disease manifesting as a prurigo nodularis. *Pediatr Dermatol* 7:136, 1990.
12. Goldman RD, Rea TH, Cinque J: The "butterfly" sign: A clue to generalized pruritus in a patient with chronic obstructive hepatobiliary disease. *Arch Dermatol* 119:183–184, 1983.

13. Kimura T, Miyazawa H: The "butterfly" sign in patients with atopic dermatitis: Evidence for the role of scratching in the development of skin manifestations. *J Am Acad Dermatol* 21:579–581, 1989.
14. Rajka G: Investigation of patients suffering from generalized pruritus, with special references to systemic disease. *Acta Derm Venereol* (Stockh) 46:190–194, 1966.
15. Lyell A: The itching patient, a review of the causes of pruritus. *Scott Med J* 17:334–338, 1972.
16. Beare JM: Generalized pruritus, a study of 43 cases. *Clin Exp Dermatol* 1:343–352, 1976.
17. Kantor GR, Lookingbill DP: Generalized pruritus and systemic disease. *J Am Acad Dermatol* 9:375–382, 1983.
18. Jelinek JE: The skin in diabetes mellitus: Cutaneous manifestations, complications, and associations, in Kopf AW, Andrude R (eds): *Yearbook in Dermatology.* Chicago, Year Book Medical Publishers. 1970, pp 5–35.
19. Neilly JB, Martin A, Simpson N, et al: Pruritus in diabetes mellitus: Investigation of prevalence and correlation with diabetes control. *Diabetes Care* 9:273–275, 1986.
20. Lewiecki EM, Rahman F: Pruritus, a manifestation of iron deficiency. *JAMA* 236:2319–2320, 1976.
21. Takkunen H: Iron deficiency pruritus. *JAMA* 239:1394, 1978.
22. Tucker WFG, Briggs C, Challoner T: Absence of pruritus in iron deficiency following venesection. *Clin Exp Dermatol* 19:186–189, 1984.
23. Paul R, Paul R, Jansen CT: Itch and malignancy prognosis in generalized pruritus: A 6-year follow-up of 125 patients. *J Am Acad Dermatol* 16:1179–1182, 1987.
24. Lober CW: Should the patient with generalized pruritus be evaluated for malignancy? *J Am Acad Dermatol* 19:350–352, 1988.
25. Eidson M, Philen RM, Sewell CM, et al: L-tryptophan and eosinophilia—myalgia syndrome in New Mexico. *Lancet* 335:645–648, 1990.
26. Gleich GJ, Adolphson CR: The eosinophilic leukocyte: Structure and function. *Adv Immunol* 39:177–253, 1986.

PSYCHOLOGIC AND PSYCHIATRIC ASPECTS

TWENTY-FIVE

PSYCHOLOGIC AND PSYCHIATRIC
ASPECTS OF ITCHING

Caroline S. Koblenzer

INTRODUCTION

The most ubiquitous of cutaneous symptoms, itching occurs under myriad circumstances and can be attributed to myriad causes: not least of these causes is to be found at the interface of psyche and soma, where itching arises as the result of an interaction between the two. As a background, I will discuss the role of skin as a mirror of psychosomatic interaction, and outline the developmental factors that predispose both an individual toward somatization and the skin as the chosen site of somatic expression. I shall outline a nonspecific concept of psychosocial stress and trace specific pathways through which psychosocial stress may be "transduced" into the physical symptom of itching. Thus the reader will have a broader understanding of the evaluation and management of the patient with idiopathic pruritus in its generalized and localized forms and with its sequelae.

SKIN AS MIRROR OF PSYCHOSOMATIC INTERACTION

It does not take a specialist to divine the physiologic changes in the skin that can mirror our shifting emotional states; numerous examples of these changes have found their way into common parlance; the pallor of shock, the blush of shame, the sweat of anxiety, or the itch of annoyance. But it is not only physiologic change that may occur; the evidence is now incontrovertible that pathologic change also may ensue, with the precipitation or exacerbation of physical symptomatology;[1] pruritus exemplifies this fact, par excellence.

DEVELOPMENTAL FACTORS BEHIND SOMATIZATION

Developmental biologists provide some understanding how and why in certain individuals emotional tension is discharged through physiologic pathways, even beyond infancy, in ways that may lead to pathologic change. Before the capacity for language is developed, all tension in the infant is discharged by physical means.[2;3,p6] The mother or primary care giver provides the infant's emotional milieu.[4] When this dyadic relationship is positive, infantile anxiety is modulated through the mother's responses to the infant's cues. Effective modulation of anxiety ensures that later, when the capacity for language has developed, the discharge of emotional tension will be through dreams, fantasy, and play, rather than the more primitive physiologic pathways.[5] In a less favorable environment physiologic discharge persists, leaving the door open for psychosomatic disease to develop.[2;3,p6] It seems likely that the skin is so frequently a vehicle for psychosomatic processes because of the importance of touch in these early mother–child transactions;[4,6] this early experience of touch confers on the skin a special unconscious symbolic significance; vulnerability to somatization acquired through this pathway has been termed "somatic compliance."[7]

In addition to the modulation of affect, these same mother–child transactions contribute to the development of self-esteem and body image through tactile stimulation;[3,pp.3,44;8] both of these psychological constructs are relevant to the genesis of pruritus as a symptom, as is discussed later in this chapter. While impoverished self-esteem is characteristic of the depressive disorders, impaired integrity of body image is associated with somatic delusions and factitial disorders.

THE TRANSDUCTION OF EMOTIONAL EXPERIENCE TO PHYSICAL SYMPTOM

It becomes increasingly clear that psychological factors may affect the course of virtually any physical disease process.[9;10,p.20] Psychosocial stress, seen as "any non-specific event that, by making demands on the organism, sets in motion a non-specific bodily response that leads to a variety of temporary or permanent physiologic, psychologic, or structural changes,"[11] provides a unifying concept of mind–body interaction. The stress may be generated by elements in the environment or arise intrapsychically, through activation of memory traces and associational links with the past. It depends for its power on genetic predisposition, past experience, and current life circumstances.

Certain of the physiologic pathways so activated participate directly in generating the itch sensation, while others contribute to itching secondarily.

Any one of three separate networks may be involved in the transduction of emotional experience into physical symptom. First are the sympathoadrenomedullary and hypothalamic–pituitary–adrenocortical arms of the stress response; the activation of these two arms is intricately orchestrated by the limbic system.[12] They are influenced by genetic and personality factors, and preferentially activated under differing circumstances; they also participate in the modulation of the form and rate of catecholamine synthesis. Second is the potential for stress to affect every phase of immunologic activity; an extensive literature documents this immunomodulating effect.[1,13] Third is activation of the neuropeptides.[14,15] Figure 25-1 depicts schematically the afferent and efferent pathways the activation of which may allow emotional experience to be expressed in structural or functional organic change.

Interestingly, not all of these paths are unidirectional; it is now fairly well established that a lymphocyte–pituitary–adrenal axis parallels the hypothalamic–pituitary–adrenal axis. Activated lymphocytes can secrete corticotropin-releasing factor (CRF), ACTH, and substances that resemble enkephalins, endorphins, calcitonin, vasoactive intestinal peptide (VIP), substance P, thyroid stimulating hormone (TSH), chorionic gonadotropin, growth hormone (GH), follicle stimulating hormone (FSH), and luteinizing hormone (LH). Clearly, immunologically modulated disease processes may have far-reaching physical and emotional sequelae.[16]

SPECIFIC PSYCHOSOMATIC PATHWAYS INVOLVED IN PRURITUS

Direct Pruritogenesis

Pruritus may be precipitated, prolonged, or enhanced by a number of stress-related mediators.

Histamine

Histamine injected intradermally lowers the itch threshold and prolongs the duration of itching in presence of stress.[17,18] These findings are corroborated by limb perfusion studies showing that stress increases the histamine content of the perfusate.[19]

Neuropeptides

Endogenous opioids. These are released both centrally and peripherally as a part of the stress response. They block the sensation of pain, but enhance

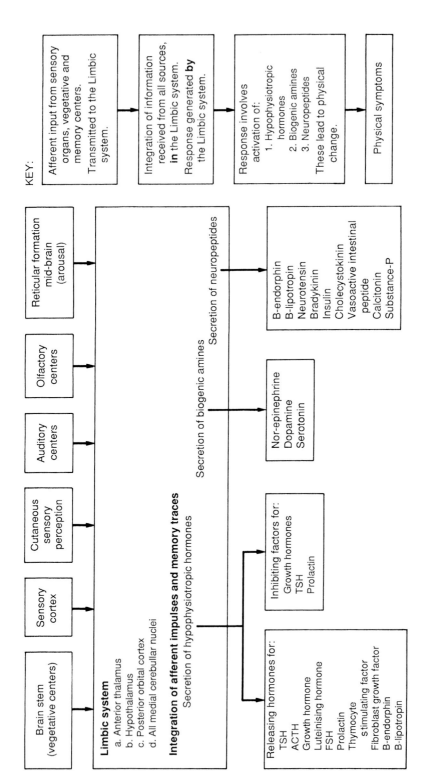

Figure 25-1 Influence of psychological and emotional factors on physiologic function.

itch.[20] This enhancement is supported by the joint findings that patients with liver disease have an elevation of circulating methionine and leucine enkephalin, and that the characteristic pruritus of cholestasis is relieved by opiate antagonists.[21]

A second mechanism may be via the effect of opioids on immunologic function and the generation of immunologically mediated inflammatory reactions. β-endorphin affects both polymorphonuclear leukocyte and natural killer cell activity, increases production of α-interferon and interleukin 2, increases monocyte chemotaxis, and binds to complement.[22]

A third opioid mechanism is the potentiation of histamine-elicited pruritus by methionine enkephalin and β-endorphin, perhaps via the adenylate cyclase system.

Other Neuropeptides

Substance P, VIP, neurotensin, bombesin, cholecystokinin, bradykinin, and calcitonin gene-related peptide (CGRP) all may participate in the stress response, and all may generate pruritus through the medium of histamine release.[15]

Secondary Pruritogenesis

Secondary psychosomatic mechanisms through which itching may be generated or exacerbated include the sweat response, alterations in cutaneous blood flow, and scratching.

The sweat response. Emotional sweating is maximal in the axillae, palms, and soles, but may also be more generalized and is usually associated with chronic anxiety. The irritation and maceration of emotional hyperhidrosis may lead to itching. Sympathetic adrenergic and cholinergic mechanisms are involved, but VIP and Substance P have also been identified at sudomotor nerve endings.[10,p239;23]

Alterations in cutaneous blood flow, and skin temperature. An increase in the cutaneous blood flow by elevating skin temperature may cause itching; this may be secondary to, among other things, the flush of anxiety or embarrassment, the vascular instability of the neurotic adolescent, or the stress of cognitive activity. Opioid mechanisms have been implicated.[24]

Scratching. While scratching may result from itching, it may also be a "derived" activity, representing a displacement of emotional tension into physical activity;[25] for example scratching one's head as an expression of anger or impatience, or the genital scratching of the patient with unresolved sexual conflict; it may also represent "learned behavior."[26] In each case the activity generates further itching; this sensation develops acutely through tissue damage, and the liberation of such chemical mediators of inflammation as prostaglandins and leukotrienes, and chronically through such changes as lichenification, or secondary bacterial infection. Scratching is also discussed in Chap. 6.

THE EFFECT OF PSYCHOLOGICAL FACTORS

That such nonspecific psychological states as anxiety,[27] fatigue,[28] or stress[29] exacerbate itching has long been known; more recently, recognition has been given to the part played by personality configuration and coping style in the expression of stress-related physical symptomatology.[12,22]

In general terms, which particular pathways are activated preferentially depends on the psychologic make-up of the individual and on the light in which that individual views the stressor. The competitive and aggressive individual who feels challenged and copes successfully secretes norepinephrine and is protected from the depression and impaired immunologic responses that may ensue if control of the situation is lost. Those who feel out of control secrete serotonin and dopamine in addition to norepinephrine.[12,30]

More specific to this topic, Fjellner and colleagues have demonstrated experimentally the association, long known to clinical observers, between the stress engendered by uncontrollable situations and the course of pruritic dermatoses.[30–32] These authors found that psychosomatic well-being and the psychosocial factors that shape coping styles could predict whether or not pruritus would be exacerbated by mental stress. Further support comes from two sources: First, depression, dopamine, and serotonin each are associated with pruritic clinical conditions, as is discussed following; second, opioid pathways are activated in situations over which the individual feels no control.[12,32]

THE CLINICAL EXPRESSION OF PSYCHOSOMATIC INTERACTIONS

Generalized Psychogenic Pruritus

Pruritus without associated overt psychopathology. Whitlock[33] summarized the work of early writers on psychogenic pruritus that described putative neurologic abnormalities and postulated specific conflictual issues, usually sexual in nature; it may strike us now as somewhat simplistic. It is difficult to arrive at an accurate estimation of the incidence of psychogenic pruritus because of the possibility of undiagnosed or latent systemic disease, and the paucity of available specific information; it is possible, for example, that those cases in which no cause has been identified are in fact psychogenic. Given these shortcomings, psychogenic factors have been implicated in anywhere from 10 to 40 percent of adults who present with generalized pruritus, and perhaps 100 percent of children.[34–37] Sex incidence is equal and all age groups are represented.[35]

The clinical picture is characteristic; although the prevailing mood may vary, that mood is usually evident at the first meeting; the patient may have a depressive mien with flat affect, overt anxiety, weary resignation, or frustrated impatience. The pruritus of which the patient complains is intolerable, and may be constant or may come in paroxysmal attacks that are at their most severe on retiring; these attacks rather faithfully mirror the emotional state. It is not unusual for the patient to have already exhausted his or her primary care physician and a number of other specialists; often at some level of consciousness, the patient has developed a conviction that no one can be of help. The physician will be told that the patient has tried everything, and the skepticism with which therapeutic suggestions are met will barely be veiled. Objective findings such as excoriations or scarring are often less pronounced than the tenor of the complaint would lead one to expect, while the distress may appear diminished when the patient's attention is diverted. It is often said that psychogenic pruritus seldom disturbs sleep;[38] Gupta and colleagues present evidence, however, to suggest that such psychological factors as depression and alcohol abuse may contribute to nighttime wakening in patients with pruritus.[39]

Psychogenic pruritus has most frequently been associated with the depressive disorders.[10,p214;33,40] In many cases, particularly in older individuals, itching may be present as a so-called "depressive equivalent" in a person who has no awareness of feeling depressed. There is good evidence that depression as encountered in general medicine or primary care does not always conform to the clear cut diagnostic parameters of descriptive psychiatry,[41,42] but a careful enquiry will usually reveal characteristic clinical features, a history of psychosocial stress may be elicited, and resolution can be expected when treatment is so directed. That elevated CSF levels of certain opioids have been demonstrated in depressed patients may help to explain in part this particular expression of depression;[43] further, the feelings of helplessness and hopelessness of the depressed can be viewed in the same light as those feelings that are experienced in circumstances over which the individual feels he or she has no control. These particular feelings, as has been noted, are associated with the secretion of serotonin, dopamine, and opioids and also with pruritus. Pruritus may also accompany anxiety, or it may represent a hysterical conversion reaction, as occurred in a school epidemic reported by Robinson and colleagues.[44]

Cholinergic pruritus, a variant of cholinergic urticaria,[45] and some cases of aquagenic pruritus[46] are other forms in which psychogenic factors play a significant role. Whereas the cholinergic form is usually associated with anxiety, in the author's experience aquagenic pruritus more often represents depression. Adrenergic urticaria and adrenergic pruritus are also associated with stress (see Chap. 18).

Chronic tactile hallucinosis. Chronic tactile hallucinosis[47] refers to an abnormal cutaneous sensation for which no physical cause can be elucidated. The symptom is quite circumscribed and the patient otherwise functions relatively well. The terms used to characterize the perceived sensation vary rather widely, and include burning, sticking, shooting, stabbing, crawling, tingling or freezing; itching also may be described. Whatever, the quality of the sensation, it is invariably said to be "intolerable," intruding on sleep, impairing appetite, curtailing pleasure, and leading to anxiety or depression that may be profound. The patient in most cases will already have consulted numerous specialists in a variety of fields; he or she will have been subjected to a battery of expensive studies, often repeatedly. To the patient's disappointment, and to the physician's frustration, while all findings are normal, no treatment has been effective.

The sensation may be generalized or localized; when it is localized, the face and genitocrural areas are those most commonly affected, and the patient often has devised extreme and idiosyncratic measures for symptom relief. In my experience this condition is significantly more common in women, although no statistics are currently available.

Diagnostically, the underlying psychopathology is either depression or a personality disorder. Chronic tactile hallucinosis is by no means a benign disorder, suicidal ideation is not uncommon, and in Cotterill's report of 28 patients with "Dermatologic Non-Disease," which included some with this syndrome, suicides did occur.[48] Dopamine is the neurotransmitter associated with hallucinatory perception.

Pruritus associated with cutaneous delusions.[10,p108] A delusion is a false belief that is not consistent with the person's educational level or cultural background and that is held unshakably in face of all reason. Delusions are symptomatic of psychosis. Most commonly the delusional patient who presents to the dermatologist has a monosymptomatic hypochondriacal psychosis (delusional disorder somatic type; DSM III R)[49] and functions relatively well otherwise.[50] These patients have a disordered body image (the intrapsychic perception they carry of themselves) indicating some disturbance of the very early mother–child relationship, as described previously; either pruritus or a delusionally motivated need to pick may be a part of the presenting symptom complex. Although a false belief of parasitic infestation is the most commonly encountered, pruritus and attempts to dig out delusional "foreign materials" may also be associated with a false belief that the patient suffers from some form of chemical poisoning, asbestosis, fiberglass contamination, or indeed any life circumstance conveniently available for idiosyncratic, if false, interpretation. The neurotransmitter dopamine has been associated with delusional thinking; dopamine is secreted along with norepinephrine, serotonin, and opioids in situations beyond the individual's control, as noted.

Localized Psychogenic Pruritus

Pruritus associated with cutaneous compulsions.[10,p138] A compulsion is a repetitive action over which the individual has no control, even though he or she fully realizes that it makes no sense. Cutaneous compulsions such as picking, rubbing, scratching, hair-pulling, hand-washing, and the like are symptomatic of an obsessive–compulsive personality configuration, and are frequently associated with an underlying depression; they may occasionally be associated with more severe psychopathology, where the boundaries of the self are blurred and the body image is unstable, as described earlier. Serotonin release has been associated with obsessive–compulsive psychopathology.

Neurotic excoriations. Patients with neurotic excoriations do not form a homogeneous group, and the lesions may result from any one of three common mechanisms. In some, pruritus is not a significant factor. These patients cannot tolerate any interruption in the smooth surface of the skin, which they must pick off; the resultant crusted excoriation presents in turn the same problem, and so the process becomes progressive. Benign keratoses, the keratin plugs of keratosis pilaris, or banal lesions of acne vulgaris may in this way become the focus of a condition that is both progressive and disfiguring.

In others, pruritic lesions such as papular urticaria or folliculitis may attract the attention needed to trigger progressive picking by generating focal pruritus. In each of these two groups, the disorder may start in childhood or adolescence and become habitual. Tension or anxiety may be evident, and depressive features may or may not be prominent. In the third group of patients, the "prurigo" of the European literature,[51] tiny acuminate idiopathic pruritic papules cause intolerable and uncontrollable focal itching. Most commonly distributed on the upper trunk or extremities, these lesions demand paroxysmal scratching, and sometimes ritualized and systematic picking. The attacks occur particularly when the itch threshold is at its lowest, at times of stress, or in the evening. Once started, every lesion must be addressed in turn, and a level of heightened tension experienced by the patient is not relieved until the process of picking is complete; some patients speak freely of the analogy to sexual tension and release. A specific time or location may be designated, and while in some the process is entirely conscious, in others a trance-like state may protect the patient from pain until after the fact. Finger nails, or a shearing force from tangential rubbing may suffice, but in other patients, ancillary help from a knife point or other sharp instrument may be sought.

Onset in this last group of patients is more commonly from middle life on, with depression a prominent feature. This characteristic and pervasive depression may be the legacy of unresolved but profound unconscious anger against figures important in the early life of the patient.[10,p144;52]

The clinical picture is characteristic. Lesions are bilateral, symmetrical, and within easy reach of the hands. All stages of evolution are present concurrently, from tiny papules with superficial excoriations, through clean, saucerized erosions with hypertrophic rim, to atrophic scar, or lesions of prurigo nodularis. Interestingly, Substance P and CGRP, both powerful histamine liberators, have been identified in lesions of prurigo nodularis.[53]

Trichotillomania. Like neurotic excoriations, trichotillomania, an uncontrollable need to pull hairs from scalp, beard, brows, lashes, and pubic or other hairy areas, is considered by many to represent an expression of obsessive–compulsive pathology. The onset is frequently in childhood or adolescence, and in mild cases it may represent a transient response to stress that with empathic handling can readily be outgrown; in others, where a disordered mother–child relationship has been a more prominent feature, the condition may take on the characteristics of a chronic disease, with fluctuations in intensity throughout life.[54] Once started, the patient finds it hard to stop plucking the hairs, and in some, not only ritualization of time and place, but also ritualistic behaviors with the plucked hairs may feature. While some patients note no associated sensation, in others an entirely irresistible itch localized quite accurately to a specific individual hair follicle may set in motion a bout of plucking.

Pruritic secondary effects of compulsive behavior. Examples include the pruritic irritant dermatitis seen commonly in those who frequently and compulsively wash their hands, lip-licking dermatitis, and localized patches of lichen simplex chronicus, from habitual rubbing or scratching.

Other forms of localized psychogenic pruritus. Intractable pruritus in the occipital scalp and anogenital region understandably has deeper and more complex unconscious emotional significance than do the banal patches of lichen simplex chronicus on the extremities that commonly serve as nonspecific outlets for tension release.

Pruritus ani. Pruritus ani has provided a ready source for the elaboration and generalization of theoretical psychoanalytic formulations that one seldom has the opportunity to test in practice. This material has been summarized by Obermayer[55] and Whitlock.[33,p118]

Males predominate in a ratio of 2–4:1, with a peak incidence in the fifth decade. Opinions differ as to the contribution of psychogenic factors in an etiology that by virtue of the ambient conditions is necessarily multifactorial; dermatologists are more likely than gastroenterologists or rectal surgeons to give credence to psychic influences,[10,p221] although most regard these as contributory rather than causal.[56] In my experience, the influence of psychogenic factors is significantly greater than is usually quoted.

Itching, which is often intense, is worst at night, disturbing sleep and engendering feelings of guilt and shame because of the proscription of touching. Patients are frequently anxious, and sweating, maceration, and hemodynamic shifts all play their part in the vicious cycle of itch, scratch, shame, anxiety, sweating, tissue damage, secondary infection, and escalating itch. Extraordinary cleansing rituals, motivated by guilt and shame, may contribute to the tissue damage; although ostensibly in the interests of local hygiene, these rituals both satisfy the demands of unconscious shame and punishment, and also anal erotism.

Although sometimes seen in high achievers with stressful life styles, in my experience pruritus ani is more commonly associated with an obsessive–compulsive character structure and a tendency toward depression. The use of passive–dependency as a defense against unwelcome unconscious feelings of aggression is cited by several authors.[10,p222] Pruritus ani is also discussed in Chap. 11.

Pruritus vulvae et scroti. Genital pruritus, although at least as common, incapacitating, and emotionally disturbing as anal pruritus, has received remarkably little attention in the literature; psychogenic factors similarly are given short shrift. Chronic and intractable vulvar pruritus for example is attributed to psychogenic causes in 1.3 to 7 percent of cases,[57,58] an incidence that to the practicing physician is unrealistically low.

Both vulvar and scrotal pruritus have been associated with sexual frustration; this may arise from either neurotic or realistic sources. Women tend to have hysterical rather than obsessive traits, and although a variety of different unconscious conflictual constellations are described, depression is common. Like anal pruritus, and for similar reasons, itching tends to be worse at night, and scratching expresses both guilt and shame, pleasure and punishment.[55] In the literature, scrotal pruritus has been more directly associated with the more severe forms of sexual dysfunction, and scratching as a form of displaced sexual gratification has been noted.[55] In my experience, depression and guilt are usually the more prominent features, while the sexual overtones tend to remain rather deeply unconscious. By contrast, in younger male patients with sexual insecurity, anxiety may be uppermost. Genital pruritus is also discussed in Chap. 11.

Occipital pruritus. Pruritus of the occipital scalp is most common in older individuals of obsessive–compulsive bent, who have difficulty in handling aggression. Depression is almost universal, often with concomitant anxiety. The itchy scalp is also discussed in Chap. 3, and its differential diagnosis is listed in Table 3-6.

Pruritus in dermatologic disease. The reader is referred to previous sections for a discussion of psychologic influences on physical disease, and the mediation of pruritus. Whereas it is clear that the course of any disease can be influenced by such factors, the two that have received most attention, and in which fluctuations in the degree of pruritus are most clearly discernable, are atopic dermatitis and psoriasis. The stringencies of space require that discussion be confined to these two.

Atopic dermatitis. Itching and erythema are variously quoted as the initiating event in the course of an outbreak of atopic dermatitis, the characteristic eczematous lesions frequently not appearing until scratching has taken place.

The effect of psychological factors on T-cell subsets, on histamine release, and on vascular responses has been discussed; each of these participates in the atopic process. Bradykinin, Substance P, VIP, and met-enkephalin are other affect-sensitive and stress-related pruritogenic neurotransmitters that have been implicated. Once scratching has taken place, the way is open for proteases and other mediators of inflammation to do their work.

From the psychological end, the older literature on atopic dermatitis inculpates specific personality and conflictual constellations. I have summarized this material elsewhere.[10,p281] In recent years more objective information has been sought. Patients with atopic dermatitis demonstrate higher state and trait anxiety than do controls,[59,60] and a greater increase in those sympathetically mediated parameters that lead to a lowering of the itch threshold;[61] conditioning of the scratch response occurs more rapidly in patients than in control subjects[62] thus ensuring perpetuation of the disease process. A greater percentage of patients than controls on psychiatric evaluation are found to have mental illness in need of treatment. Most commonly this is in the form of obsessive–compulsive perfectionism, unacceptable but unconscious anger, and depression; although some patients exhibit alexithymia (where there is an impoverished inner life, and failure to develop a language in which to describe emotion), severe personality disorders are less commonly represented. In those patients whose intractable disease had its onset in infancy, much clinical evidence supports a significant developmental contribution from a dysfunctional mother–child dyad; the particular quality of this relationship contributes to the heightened anxiety so characteristic of atopic children, and reinforces scratching behavior.[63,64]

Psoriasis. In controlled studies patients with psoriasis score higher both for anxiety and depression than do medically ill controls.[65,66] It has been noted above that both of these affective states may be associated with pruritus.

While not all psoriatic patients experience pruritus, and ambient conditions, treatment regimens, and genetic make-up may contribute to this sensation, Gupta and colleagues have correlated pruritus with depression in psoriatics; the severity of the depression determines the severity of pruritus, and indeed this intrapsychic state was a more significant correlate than were external psychosocial, or dermatologic factors.[67]

PSYCHOBIOLOGIC AND PSYCHOTHERAPEUTIC TREATMENT OF PRURITUS

Psychobiologic Treatment[68]

Psychotropic drugs derive their action from an ability to potentiate or block chemical neurotransmitters in the interneuronal synaptic cleft. It has been noted in previous pages that in some cases specific neurotransmitters have been associated with specific clinical syndromes. This information is a useful guide in selecting the drug of choice. Readers who prescribe psychotropic medications should consult additional references for important information on side-effects and interactions. (See Table 25-1.)

Depressive disorders. Because both norepinephrine and serotonin pathways have been implicated in the pruritus of depression, either of two classes of antidepressant drug may be used.

1. Tricyclic (or heterocyclic) antidepressants. These drugs block the re-uptake of norepinephrine and to a variable extent serotonin by axon terminals, thus increasing the pool of available catecholamine. Doxepin (Sinequan®, Adapin®) blocks primarily norepinephrine; in addition, however, it has strong antihistamine action, which makes it specifically the drug of choice. The dosage schedules vary depending on whether its primary function is to be antipruritic or antidepressant.

   a. Antipruritic dosage. Doses range from 10 to 25 mg. at bedtime to 10 mg. three times daily, or 10 mg. in the morning and 25 to 50 mg. at bedtime, depending on the severity of itching and the response. A 5 percent doxepin topical cream is also reportedly an effective antipruritic.

   b. Antidepressant dosage. Treatment is started with a divided dose to allow gradual adjustment to the drug; this is converted to a single dose at bedtime to minimize side effects.

   A dosage of 25 mg. two to three times daily can be gradually increased to a total daily dose of 150 to 200 mg. over the first week. If within 3 weeks there is no effect, another drug of the same class may

Table 25-1 Psychobiologic treatment of pruritus

Psychiatric diagnosis	Dermatologic diagnosis	Relevant neurotransmitters	Blocker for neurotransmitter	Dosage schedules (see text for details)
Depression (overt or masked)	Generalized pruritus, Pruritus vulvae, Pruritus ani, Aquagenic pruritus, Any pruritic dermatosis	Norepinephrine	Tricyclic Antidepressant	Antipruritic 10 mg tid, 10 mg am, 20–25 mg hs to 25–50 mg hs, Antidepressant 75–200 mg hs
		Serotonin	Fluoxetine	20–40 mg od am
		Opioids	Pimozide	1.0–4.0 mg od am
Obsessive–Compulsive Disorders	Neurotic excoriations	Serotonin	Clomipramine	75–200 mg od hs
		Opioids	Pimozide	1.0–4.0 mg od am
Delusional Disorders	Delusions of Parasitosis, etc.	Dopamine, Opioids	Pimozide	1.0–10.0 mg od am
Anxiety	Generalized pruritus, Pruritus vulvae, Pruritus ani, Cholinergic pruritus, Any pruritic dermatosis	γ-aminobutyric	Benzodiazepines	Brief acute episodes only. Varies with each drug.
Phobic anxiety, Anxiety with depression			Tricyclic antidepressants	25–200 mg od hs

be substituted. For maintenance 25 to 50 percent of the therapeutic dose may be adequate; elderly patients require only 50 percent of the usual adult dose. An attempt at gradual withdrawal can be made after 6 symptom-free months.

2. Atypical (nontricyclic) antidepressants

   a. Fluoxetine (Prozac®) is a selective inhibitor of serotonin re-uptake. An effective drug for depression and pruritus, it is minimally sedating and neither cardiotoxic nor an appetite stimulant. An initial morning dose of 20 mg. can be increased to 40 mg. in 2 to 3 weeks if necessary; it may take as long as 6 weeks to achieve maximal benefit.

   b. Sertraline (Zoloft®) has a profile very similar to Fluoxetine. A more rapid therapeutic effect, sometimes within 1 week, and a lower incidence of restlessness are advantages, while the occasional early nausea usually wears off within 1 or 2 weeks. The dose range is from 25 mgm to 200 mgm daily, but 50 to 100 mgm in most cases proves effective.

3. Pimozide (Orap®). Because pimozide, a high potency, low dose neuroleptic, blocks opioid pathways, it is often effective in controlling pruritus, either when prescribed alone, or together with an antidepressant.

   An initial morning dose of 2.0 mg. can be titrated up or down over several days, according to response, to a maximum of 8 or 10 mg. daily.[50] Many patients respond within 1 to 2 weeks, and are controlled with as little as 1.0 to 2.0 mg. daily. If there is no response within 6 weeks the drug should be abandoned. Attempts at gradual withdrawal can be made after 6 symptom-free months.

Obsessive–compulsive syndromes. Obsessive–compulsive symptomatology has been associated with serotonin pathways. The tricyclic antidepressant clomipramine (Anafranil®) selectively blocks serotonin re-uptake, and improves symptoms in 50 percent of cases. Clomipramine is prescribed as described for doxepin earlier. Fluoxetine or Sertraline are also often effective.

Delusional syndromes. Opioid pathways have been implicated in the pruritus associated with hallucinatory or delusional syndromes. Because pimozide blocks opioid as well as dopamine receptors, it is the drug of choice when these syndromes are characterized by pruritus.

Anxiety

1. The majority of tranquilizers in current usage are benzodiazepines, and appear to modulate γ-aminobutyric acid, the major inhibitory neurotransmitter. All are habit-forming and their use should be confined to transient acute episodes.

Alprazolam (Xanax®) has certain advantages over the other benzodi-azepines in that it has antidepressant as well as anxiolytic activity. Dosage schedules range from 0.25 mgm to 1.0 mgm at h.s. to four times daily depending on the severity of symptoms. The smallest effective dose should be prescribed for the shortest possible time.[68]

2. Buspirone (BuSpar®) is a nonbenzodiazepine anxiolytic; the tranquilizing properties are attributed to an effect on serotonin binding sites in the frontal cortex. Buspirone is less sedating than the benzodiazepines, and it is not habit-forming. Occasional use, however, is precluded by the fact that 3 weeks are required for a therapeutic effect. Dosage schedules range from 5 mgms three times daily, increased by increments of 5 mgm every 2 to 3 days to a maximum total daily dose of 60 mgms.

3. Anxiety associated with phobic states, and with depression is better treated with tricyclic antidepressants.[68]

Psychotherapeutic Treatment

Whenever psychotropic drugs are prescribed the therapeutic response is enhanced by concurrent psychotherapy.

Insight oriented psychotherapy or psychoanalysis are effective in patients with generalized or localized pruritus, or obsessive–compulsive syndromes, if the criteria for these modalities are otherwise met. Younger patients, those for whom the quality of life is significantly impaired, or who do not respond readily to the measures described above should therefore be offered psychiatric referral.[10pp67-71]

Other modalities that have been used with benefit include hypnosis, biofeedback,[69] behavior modification,[70] and acupuncture;[71] support groups may also be helpful.[72]

REFERENCES

1. Ader R (ed.): *Psychoneuroimmunology.* New York, Academic Press, 1981.
2. Spitz RA: *The First Year of Life.* New York, International University Press. 1965, pp 35–52.
3. Greenspan SI: *The Development of the Ego.* New York, International University Press. 1989.
4. Hofer NA: Hidden regulatory processes in early social relationships, in Bateson PPG, Klopfer PH (eds): *Perspectives in Ethology,* Vol. 3. New York, Plenum Press. 1978, pp 135–136.
5. Taylor GJ: *Psychosomatic Medicine and Contemporary Psychoanalysis.* International University Press. Madison, Conn. 1987, pp 283–286.
6. Schanberg SM, Evoniuk G, Kuhn CN: Tactile and nutritional aspects of maternal care: Specific regulators of neuroendocrine function and cellular development. *Proc Soc Exp Biol Med* 175:135–146, 1984.
7. Freud S: *The Standard Edition of the Complete Psychological Works of Sigmund Freud,* Vol 7. London, Hogarth Press. 1953, pp 40–42.
8. Mahler MS, Pine F, Bergman A: *The Psychological Birth of the Human Infant.* New York, Basic Books. 1975, pp 222–224.

9. Engel GL: A unified concept of health and disease. *Perspect Bio Med* 3:459–485, 1960.
10. Koblenzer CS: *Psychocutaneous Disease.* Orlando, Fla, Grune and Stratton. 1987.
11. Lipowski ZJ: Psychosomatic medicine: An overview, in Hill O (ed): *Modern Trends in Psychosomatic Medicine* 3. London, Butterworths. 1976, pp 4–13.
12. Ciaranello RD: Neurochemical aspects of stress, in Garmezy N, Rutter M (eds): *Stress, Coping and Development in Children.* New York, McGraw Hill. 1983, pp 85–99.
13. Solomon GF: Psychoneuroimmunology: Interactions between central nervous system and immune system. *J Neurosci Res* 18:1–9, 1987.
14. Wiedermann CJ: Shared recognition molecules in the brain and lymphoid tissues: The polypeptide mediator network of psychoneuroimmunology. *Immunol Lett* 16:371–378, 1987.
15. Foreman JC: Neuropeptides and the pathogenesis of allergy. *Allergy* 42:1–11, 1987.
16. Camaro EG, Danao TC: The brain and the immune system. A psychosomatic network. *Psychosomatics* 30:140–146, 1989.
17. Cormia FE: Experimental histamine pruritus: Influence of physical and psychological factors on threshold reactivity. *J Invest Dermatol* 19:21–34, 1952.
18. Cormia FE, Kuykendall V: Experimental histamine pruritus. *J Invest Dermatol* 20:429–446, 1953.
19. Chapman LF, Goodell H, Wolff HG: Structures and processes involved in the sensation of itch, in Montagna N (ed): *Advances in Biology of the Skin,* Vol 1. New York, Pergamon Press. 1960, pp 99–105.
20. Morley JE: Neuroendocrine effects of endogenous opioid peptides in human subjects. *Psychoneuroendocrinology* 8:361–379, 1983.
21. Thornton JR, Losowsky MS: Opioid peptides and primary biliary cirrhosis. *BMJ* 197:1501–1504, 1988.
22. Solomon GF, Fiatarone MA, Benton D, et al: Psychoimmunologic and endorphin function in the aged. *Annals N Y Acad Sci* 521:43–58, 1988.
23. Hokfelt T, Johansson O, Kellerth J-O, et al: Immunohistochemical distribution of Substance P, in von Euler US, Pernow B (eds): *Substance P.* New York, Raven Press. 1977, pp 117–145.
24. Lightman SL, Jacobs HS: Naloxone: Non-steroidal treatment for post-menopausal flushing. *Lancet,* 2:1071, 1979.
25. Musaph H: *Itching and Scratching.* Philadelphia, FA Davis. 1964, pp 1–9.
26. Robertson IM, Jordan JM, Whitlock FA: Emotions and skin II—The conditioning of scratch responses in cases of lichen simplex. *Br J Dermatol* 92:407–412, 1975.
27. Calnan CD, O'Neill D: Itching in tension states. *Br J Dermatol* 64:274–280, 1952.
28. Cornbleet T: Scratching patterns: Influence of site. *J Invest Dermatol* 20:105–110, 1953.
29. Edwards EA, Shellow WVR, Wright ET, et al: Pruritic skin disease, psychological stress and the itch sensation. *Arch Dermatol* 112:339–343, 1976.
30. Werth GR: The hives dilemma. *Am Fam Physician* 17(5):139–143, 1978.
31. Fjellner B, Arnetz BB, Eneroth P, et al: Pruritus during standardized mental stress. Relationship to psychoneuroendocrine and metabolic parameters. *Acta Derm Venereol* (Stockh) 65:199–205, 1985.
32. Fjellner B, et al: Influence of grenz rays and psychological factors on experimental pruritus induced by histamine and compound 48/80. *Arch Dermatol Res* 281:111–115, 1989.
33. Whitlock FA: *Psychophysiological Aspects of Skin Disease.* Philadelphia, Saunders. 1976, pp 110–114.
34. Lyell A: The itching patient: A review of the causes of pruritus. *Scott Med J* 17:334–347, 1972.
35. Beare JM: Generalized pruritus. A study of 43 cases. *Clin Exp Dermatol* 1:343–359, 1976.
36. Kantor GR, Lookingbill DP: Generalized pruritus and systemic disease. *J Am Acad Dermatol* 9:375–382, 1983.
37. Rosenbaum M: Pruritus of unknown origin. *Hosp Pract* 23:(10)19–26, 1988.

38. Bernhard JD: Clinical aspects of pruritus, in Fitzpatrick TB, et al (eds): *Dermatology in General Medicine*, 3d Ed. New York, McGraw-Hill. 1987, pp 78–90.
39. Gupta MA, Gupta AK, Kirkby S, et al: Pruritus associated with nocturnal wakenings: Organic or psychogenic? *J Am Acad Dermatol* 21:479–484, 1989.
40. Edwards KCS: Pruritus in melancholia. *BMJ* Vol II:1527–1529, 1954.
41. Rodin G, Voshard K: Depression in the medically ill. *Am J Psychiatry* 143:696–705, 1986.
42. Eisenberg L: Sounding Board. Treating Depression and Anxiety in Primary Care. *N Engl J Med* 326:1080–1084, 1992.
43. Prange AJ, Loosen PT: Peptides in depression, in Usdin E, et al (eds): *Frontiers in Biochemical and Pharmacological Research*. New York, Raven Press. 1984, p 137.
44. Robinson P, Szewczyk M, Haddy L, et al: Outbreak of itching and rash. Epidemic hysteria in an elementary school. *Arch Intern Med* 144:1959–1962, 1984.
45. Berth-Jones J, Graham-Brown RAC: Cholinergic pruritus, erythema and urticaria: A disease spectrum responding to danazol. *Br J Dermatol* 121:235–237, 1989.
46. Kallrell JN: Aquagenic pruritus. *J Am Acad Dermatol* 20(6):1123, 1989.
47. Duke EE: Clinical experience with pimozide: Emphasis on its use in post-herpetic neuralgia. *J Am Acad Dermatol* 8:845–850, 1983.
48. Cotterill JA: Dermatologic non-disease: A common and potentially fatal disturbance of cutaneous body-image. *Br J Dermatol* 104:611–619, 1981.
49. Spitzer RL, Chair. *Diagnostic and Statistical Manual of Mental Disorders* (3d ed, revised). Washington, D.C., American Psychiatric Assoc. 1987, pp 200–201.
50. Munro A: Monosymptomatic hypochondriacal psychosis. *Br J Psychiatry* (Suppl.2)153:37–40, 1988.
51. Uehara M, Ofuji S: Primary eruption of prurigo simplex subacuta. *Dermatologica* 153:49–56, 1976.
52. Musaph H: Psychodynamics in itching states. *Int J Psychoanal* 49:336–339, 1968.
53. Vaalastia A, Suomalainen H, Rechardt L: Calcitonin gene-related peptide immunoreactivity in prurigo nodularis: A comparative study with neurodermatitis circumscripta. *Br J Dermatol* 120:619–623, 1989.
54. Greenberg HR, Sarner CA: Trichotillomania—symptom and syndrome. *Arch Gen Psychiatry* 12:482–489, 1965.
55. Obermayer ME: *Psychocutaneous Medicine*. Springfield, Ill, Charles C. Thomas. 1955, pp 187–196.
56. Menz J: Pruritus ani: A practical approach. *Aust Fam Physician* 17:963–966, 1988.
57. Rumpianski R, Shiskin J: Pruritus vulvae: A five year survey. *Dermatologica* 131:146, 1965.
58. Jeffcoate TNA: Pruritus vulvae. *BMJ* ii:1197, 1949.
59. Garrie EV, Garrie SA, Mote T: Anxiety and atopic dermatitis. *J Consult Clin Psychol* 42:742, 1974.
60. Faulstich M, Williamson DA, Duchman EG, et al: Psychophysiological analysis of atopic dermatitis. *J Psychosom Res* 29:415–417, 1985.
61. Faulstich M, Williamson DA: An overview of atopic dermatitis: Toward a bio-behavioral integration. *J Psychosom Res* 29:647–654, 1985.
62. Jordan JM, Whitlock FA: Atopic dermatitis, anxiety and conditioned scratch responses. *J Psychosom Res* 18:297–299, 1974.
63. Gil KM, Sampson HA: Psychological and social factors of atopic dermatitis. *Allergy* (44 suppl) 9:86–89, 1989.
64. Koblenzer CS, Koblenzer PJ: Chronic intractable atopic eczema. *Arch Dermatol* 124:1673–1677, 1988.
65. Lyketsos CG, Lyketsos GC, Richardson SC, et al: Dysthmic states and depressive syndromes in physical conditions of presumably psychogenic origin. *Acta Psychiatr Scand* 76:529–534, 1987.
66. Gupta MA, Kirby S, Gupta AK, et al: A psychocutaneous profile of psoriasis patients who are stress reactors. *Gen Hosp Psychiatry* 11:166–173, 1989.

67. Gupta MA, Gupta AK, Kirby S, et al: Pruritus in psoriasis. A prospective study of some psychiatric and dermatologic correlates. *Arch Dermatol* 124:1052–1057, 1988.
68. Bernstein JG: *Handbook of Drug Therapy in Psychiatry,* 2d ed. Littleton, Mass. Year Book Medical Publishers, 1988.
69. McMenamy CJ, Katz RC, Gipson M: Treatment of eczema by EMG biofeedback and relaxation training: A multiple baseline analysis. *J Behav Ther Exp Psychiatry* 19:221–227, 1988.
70. Allen KE, Harris FR: Elimination of a child's excessive scratching by training the mother in reinforcement procedures. *Behav Res Ther* 4:79–84, 1966.
71. Belgrade MJ, Solomon LM, Lichter EA: Effect of acupuncture on experimentally induced itch. *Acta Derm Venereol* (Stockh.) 64:129–133, 1984.
72. Cole WC, Roth HL, Sach LB: Group psychotherapy as an aid in the medical treatment of eczema. *J Am Acad Dermatol* 18:286–291, 1988.

TREATMENT

GENERAL PRINCIPLES, OVERVIEW, AND MISCELLANEOUS TREATMENTS OF ITCHING*

Jeffrey D. Bernhard

The foundation for appropriate treatment of itching is correct diagnosis, but symptomatic treatment is often required.[1,2] The irony is that we have nothing so simple and effective for itching as aspirin is for pain, a sad deficiency partly redressed by the substantial efficacy of placebos in treating this highly subjective and variable symptom.[3] A further cornerstone of management is understanding the nature of the disease. To take a simple but telling example, head lice feed and breed on the scalp; a short and simple application of an effective topical agent to the scalp, along with some attention to local epidemiology, will eradicate the infestation. Body lice, on the other hand, only feed on the body and then retreat to the patient's clothing; the clothes have to be treated as well. In the same vein, a diagnosis of dermatitis herpetiformis permits dramatically effective treatment with oral dapsone and a gluten-free diet. Diagnosis and treatment of Hodgkin's disease may eliminate the patient's itch and save his life. The diagnosis of a specific steroid responsive disorder, such as bullous pemphigoid, permits treatment with systemic corticosteroids and steroid-sparing agents such as azothioprine. For the most part, systemic corticosteroids have no role in the treatment of pruritus of undetermined origin (P.U.O.). Although they are sometimes used as a last

---

* Small parts of this chapter are based on parts of reference 1, (Chapter 8 of *Dermatology in General Medicine,* 3d ed, 1987; T.B. Fitzpatrick, et al, eds.) by kind permission of McGraw-Hill, Inc., New York. Material has been updated, expanded, and partially rearranged. Some short passages have been reproduced unchanged.

resort, the amount of information that can be gained from the use of systemic corticosteroids as a therapeutic or diagnostic trial is very limited at best. Treatment of itching in many specific disorders is discussed in the pertinent chapters of this book. Certain treatment modalities with wide applicability to a variety of disorders, such as phototherapy, are discussed in the remaining chapters of this section.

When a cause for itching cannot be determined, or is determined but cannot be eliminated, symptomatic treatment is required. This chapter will cover some general symptomatic measures and some miscellaneous treatments for itching. Other general reviews on treatment of itching are listed in the references.[4–6]

Symptomatic treatment of itching falls into six main categories, which will be discussed in successive sections of this chapter:

1. patient education
2. elimination of provocative factors
3. nonspecific topical preparations and skin hydration
4. chemical treatment, topical and systemic
5. physical modalities, such as phototherapy and electronic or thermal counterstimulation
6. drastic measures such as plasmapheresis
7. understanding support from physicians and family or friends.

PATIENT EDUCATION

The patient should be given a clear explanation of the diagnosis and of factors that are known to provoke or worsen itching. This is especially important in order to prevent misguided treatment or treatment with home remedies that may be momentarily soothing but harmful in the long run, such as rubbing with alcohol (or drinking it). Other home remedies and over-the-counter products may contain irritating or allergenic substances such as topical antihistamines and topical anesthetics.

The patient should also be taught that breaking the itch–scratch cycle is critical in situations in which it is playing a role, as in atopic dermatitis. An entire program, including symptomatic measures and medication, may be directed toward this end. When the urge to scratch comes, a cool washcloth, gentle pressure, or will power may be helpful instead. It is not helpful for the doctor or relatives to say "don't scratch." Such indignant commands are virtually always counterproductive. The patient must know that others realize how difficult, if not impossible, it is to resist scratching. Self-righteous injunctions without empathy and explanation do not help and invariably create additional stress on the patient.

Stress can make anything worse, and itching is no exception.[7,8] In addition, the discomfort, loss of sleep, anxiety, and fear of serious illness provoked by prolonged itching are major stresses in themselves. This is compounded by the fear, discomfort, and expense of investigations undertaken to evaluate pruritus, and by the barrier that an itchy skin condition can raise between the patient and loved ones. If all that were not bad enough, patients are plagued and humiliated by the conscious and subconscious psychologic "meanings" of skin disease, namely, that they are "dirty" and cannot control themselves.[9,10] Every effort to reduce or eliminate any aspect of stress that can be identified is therefore essential. Psychiatrists, social workers, and counselors can all be helpful in addressing stress in the personal and working life of the patient and in coping with the problems created by itching itself. It is too easy for patient and physician to blame itching on stress and "nerves": the role of itching in creating stress should not be underestimated. Although "neurodermatitis" may be a reasonable term to describe some cases of lichen simplex chronicus, it has been so often used imprecisely and dismissively that it is probably best avoided. In my own experience, the "diagnosis" of "neurodermatitis" makes the doctor feel better and the patient feel worse.

ELIMINATION OF PROVOCATIVE FACTORS

Every effort to eliminate or reduce the factors listed in Table 26-1 should be made. It is not necessary to curtail bathing unless the patient is overdoing it or finds it irritating. Hints on bathing and bath oils are given in the next section. It is important to recognize that some "bland" emollients, such as petrolatum, are soothing to some patients but irritating to others.

Table 26-1 Some external factors that cause or worsen itching

Dryness of the skin, excessive bathing, low ambient humidity
Contact with irritating fabrics such as wool[12] and certain synthetic fabrics
Contact with formaldehyde resins in permanent press clothing (causes allergic contact
    dermatitis in sensitive persons)[13]
Contact dermatitis from allergens or irritants in medicaments and home remedies
Alcohol ingestion; other causes of vasodilation
Hot foods and liquids (cause vasodilation)
Excessive ambient temperature; too many blankets
Stress, anxiety
Misguided treatment such as alcohol rubs, topical sensitizers
Certain laundry products intended to eliminate static
Certain medications (see Chap. 23)
Contact with dust, dust mites
Contact with certain plant products such as cactus spicules
Contact with certain animal products such as airborne moth hairs, threads, and shed skins
Fiberglass

Dryness of the air, and consequently of the skin, is particularly trouble-some in heated environments in winter: Not only is the air outside relatively dry, but heating it lowers the humidity even more. Forced hot air heating is the worst in this regard, and even many normal people begin to itch when subjected to it. The skin loses moisture to the air whenever ambient relative humidity drops below about 40%. Humidifiers, plants, and open basins of evaporating water may be helpful. Dessication of the air, and consequently of the skin, can even occur in the summer because of air conditioning.[11]

NONSPECIFIC TOPICAL AGENTS: EMOLLIENTS, BATH ADDITIVES, COOLING LOTIONS

Nonsteroidal topical agents such as lotions containing menthol, camphor, eugenol, phenol, tars, and salicylic acid are discussed in Chap. 27. Many of these act as counterirritants or relieve itching through their cooling effect. Phenol anesthetizes cutaneous nerve endings; it must be avoided in pregnant women and children under 6 months of age. Topical corticosteroids are not indicated for symptomatic treatment unless a steroid responsive disorder is diagnosed.

Whatever the cause of itching, dryness of the skin can be an exacerbating factor, so hydration or moisturization is often important. A wide variety of moisturizers is available over the counter.[14] Several more recently developed moisturizers, such as those containing lactic acid[15] or ammonium lactate[16] may be particularly effective for some patients. As xerosis is a frequent cause of or contributor to itching in the elderly, emollients, in conjunction with other measures designed to reduce drying and irritation of the skin, are often the initial treatment of choice.[17] Failure to respond to this approach indicates that further evaluation is required.

Bathing in moderation helps to maintain adequate hydration of the skin. Some patients find that the addition of commercially available colloidal oat-meal, with or without oil, is soothing. I usually tell my patients to bathe for no fewer then 10 and no more than 20 minutes. Sulzberger's household bath oil—2 teaspoons of olive oil plus one large glass of milk added to the bathtub—is still appealing to many patients. Baking soda added to the bath helps some patients as well.[18] Only mild soaps or cleansers should be used.[19] Many patients find that "Japanese style" bathing is helpful so long as the water is not too hot: a quick cleansing shower or bath during which a gentle cleanser is used is followed by a soothing, no-soap bath. Bath oils or bland emollients applied *after* bathing are soothing and can hydrate the skin.

Aloe vera is a popular favorite.[20] It may have some bactericidal and antifungal effects but has not been carefully investigated as an antipruritic. Some preparations may also cause contact sensitization. Careful studies on topical vitamin E, also a popular home remedy, are lacking as well, and it, too, can cause allergic contact dermatitis.[21]

CHEMICAL TREATMENT (TOPICAL AND SYSTEMIC)

For the most part, specific chemical treatments are discussed in the separate chapters concerned with the particular disorders for which they are helpful. Topical corticosteroids are, of course, helpful in the treatment of specific steroid-responsive disorders and will not be discussed here. A large variety of nonsteroidal topical approaches are discussed in Chap. 27. A brief overview of some of these is provided here as well.

Topical Anesthetics

Most of the older over-the-counter topical anesthetic preparations are not effective.[22] They do not penetrate the stratum corneum very well and some, such as benzocaine, can cause allergic reactions themselves.

Some topical agents contain local anesthetics such as pramoxine[23] and are helpful in providing short-term relief to some patients.[24(pp 205–208)]

The eutectic mixture of local anesthetics lignocaine and prilocaine (EMLA®) is effective in reducing experimental histamine and papain-induced pruritus,[25] and may be helpful in the treatment of certain localized itches, such as notalgia paresthetica.[26] Aside from the fact that it has a slow onset and limited duration of action, it is not known how practical or safe this approach might be for prolonged use over larger areas of the skin.

Topical Capsaicin Cream

This may be particularly helpful in the treatment of certain localized itches such as notalgia paresthetica (see Chap. 12). Capsaicin is a naturally oc-curring alkaloid found in hot peppers; it is the active principle that makes them hot and that produces erythema, pain, and inflammation when applied to mucous membranes. Application of capsaicin cream depletes the ner-uopeptide substance P from type C sensory neurons, which are unmyelinated, slowly conducting fibers involved in the sensations of cutaneous pain and pathological itch.[27] Depletion of Substance P interferes with the transmission of certain painful and itchy stimuli from the periphery to the central nervous system (CNS).[28] Topical capsaicin is effective in relieving the itch associated with some cases of post-herpetic neuralgia (its primary indication).[29,30] It has also been used to treat small numbers of patients with itchy psoriasis,[31,32] prurigo nodularis, and neurodermatitis circumscripta.[33] Preliminary evidence suggests that it may be helpful in treating post-burn pruritus and in treating localized areas of hemodialysis-related itching in some patients, but it is not clear how useful this approach might be over larger areas over a longer time frame.[34] In a patient with generalized pruritus, however, local treatment of the most aggravating "trigger" spots can sometimes produce more wide-spread relief. Topical capsaicin may find its most important application as an antipruritic in the treatment of particularly well-localized itches such as notalgia paresthetica.[35,36] Most patients experience at least some burning, irritation, or pain during the initial phase of treatment; eventually this response "burns out" if application is continued. Pretreatment with topical anesthetics such as 5% xylocaine ointment may ameliorate this response, and we have had some success using pretreatment with EMLA cream in this situation.

Topical Crotamiton

Topical crotamiton is used as an antiscabetic and has been the subject of some clinical interest as an antipruritic, but it is not clear that its antipruritic effect goes any further than the emollient and soothing effect of its lotion vehicle.[37,38]

Tricyclic Antidepressants (Oral and Topical); Other Psychotropic Drugs[39–41]

Doxepin and amitriptyline bind strongly to the H1-histamine receptor and have potent antihistaminic effects. Doxepin is often used in relatively low dosage for that reason alone. Aside from their antihistaminic effects, antidepressants may have other effects on the nervous system that may have some role in the treatment of psychogenic and neurogenic itching. Tricyclic agents may turn out to be effective when administered topically as well.[42] CNS-active agents may provide a logical treatment for some cases of so-called "senile pruritus."[43]

Topical Antihistamines

These have not found wide usage because of unimpressive efficacy and because of concerns about topical sensitization. Research in this area is still underway, and it is hoped that newer antihistamines will be effective topically without as much risk of contact sensitization.[44,45] Recent work with topical doxepin, a tricyclic medication with very potent antihistaminic effects, is particularly encouraging.[46]

Oral Antihistamines

Antihistamines are discussed in detail in Chap. 29 and their use in atopic dermatitis is discussed in Chap. 3. They are helpful *in disorders in which histamine plays a central role,* such as urticaria.[48] They are *not* particularly helpful in disorders in which histamine does not play a central role, except for their sedative, soporific, and placebo effects. Their lack of efficacy in so many pruritic disorders is one of the proofs that histamine cannot be the only important mediator of itching. Certain other CNS-active drugs may also be helpful in treating pruritus because of their sedative or other effects.[49]

Ketotifen is a mast cell blocker. It has antihistamine effects and also inhibits the release of certain mediators such as slow-reacting substance of anaphylaxis.[50] It may be helpful when other antihistamines are not. It has been used to relieve itching in chronic uremia[51] and to relieve the symptoms of various forms of mastocytosis.[52] Based on positive results in an initial study, oral ketotifen may also be effective in reducing pain, itching, and tenderness associated with neurofibromas.[53,54] Ketotifen was not available in the United States at the time this book went to press.

Considering that certain "idiopathic" itching states may be diminutive variants of certain histamine-mediated urticarial disorders,[55] it is hard to fault a therapeutic trial of oral antihistamines as part of the overall approach to the diagnosis and treatment of the itchy patient.

Cholestyramine and Other Ion-Binding Approaches

Oral cholestyramine may be helpful in relieving pruritus associated with renal failure, cholestasis, cholestasis of pregnancy, and polycythemia vera.[56–60] It presumably acts by binding and removing pruritogenic substances in the gut. Plasma perfusion through bilirubin- and bile acid-adsorbing resin columns is a more aggressive means to the same end.[61] Oral-activated charcoal has been used to treat itching in patients undergoing maintenance hemodialysis.[62] For further discussion, see Chap. 15, 16, and 17.

Opiate Antagonists

In 1979, Bernstein and Swift reported that intractable pruritus in a patient with primary biliary cirrhosis could be blocked by naloxone.[63] Summerfield demonstrated that naloxone relieved itching in some patients but not in others.[64] Subsequently, Bernstein and colleagues demonstrated that naloxone could block butorphanol-induced itching[65] and experimental histamine-induced pruritus,[66] although results in experimental systems may vary.[67]

Bergasa and colleagues have also demonstrated the efficacy of opiate antagonists in the treatment of pruritus in chronic cholestasis,[68,69] and believe that it may work because the unidentified pruritogens in cholestatic states may have opiate-like structures or activity.

Nalmefene is an oral opiate antagonist. It has been explored in the treatment of itching associated with atopic dermatitis and chronic urticaria.[70,71] Although it may be effective, it has severe side effects comparable to those of the opiate withdrawal syndrome. Bergasa and colleagues have also used oral nalmefene in the treatment of cholestatic pruritus.[72]

The specific blocking of enkephalen and endorphin opiate receptors in the CNS is not yet clinically practical for routine treatment of pruritus, but it is an exciting approach that holds considerable promise. The use of opiate antagonists in the full spectrum of itching of diverse etiologies remains to be explored.

Aspirin

Because of the presumed relation between itching and pain, aspirin has been suggested as a remedy for itching and is alleged to be symptomatically helpful in some patients. Salicylates were helpful in 15 of 17 patients with polycythemia treated in a carefully controlled clinical trial, perhaps because of blocked prostaglandin and serotonin release from platelets.[73] Under other circumstances, however, aspirin may worsen itching, perhaps by increasing the amount of certain prostaglandins.[74,75] Sensitivity to aspirin should also be considered as a possible cause of drug-induced P.U.O.

Daly and Shuster gave nightly oral doses of aspirin to 13 patients with pruritic dermatoses and were unable to demonstrate a beneficial effect.[76] Whether a larger sample, selection of different disorders, or different dosage schedule may have been effective remains an open question. Aside from their action in affecting peripheral inflammation, nonsteroidal antiinflammatory drugs may exert an independent effect (at least for pain, and perhaps for itch), on spinal processing in the central nervous system.[77]

Oral Cromalyn

Oral cromalyn is effective in the treatment of systemic mast cell disease.[78] It has also been tried in treating pruritus in Hodgkin's disease.[79]

Oral Hydroxyethylrutosides

These were helpful in the treatment of itching in six patients with primary biliary cirrhosis.[80]

Miscellaneous Chemical Treatment and Metabolic Interventions

Thalidomide has been used to treat prurigo nodularis[81] and actinic prurigo.[82] Oral evening primrose oil was used to treat refractory biliary pruritus in one trial involving 9 patients, 6 of whom improved.[83] Epomediol, a terpenoid compound, has been assessed in a small study of itching in intrahepatic cholestasis of pregnancy.[84] Propofol is an intravenous, hypnotic anesthetic agent. Borgeat and colleagues have reported that it relieves pruritus induced by epidural and intrathecal morphine,[85] and they have also found that subhypnotic doses were effective in a small study of 10 patients with cholestatic pruritus.[86] The intravenous route of administration limits its utility, but continuous infusion may be helpful in some patients in whom acute, short-term symptomatic management of itching is required.

PHYSICAL MODALITIES

Ultraviolet Phototherapy and PUVA Photochemotherapy

Ultraviolet phototherapy and PUVA photochemotherapy may be useful in a wide variety of pruritic states, ranging from pityriasis rosea to mastocytosis, renal itch, polycythemia-vera and myelofibrosis.[87-92] Ultraviolet B phototherapy may also be used in combination with certain other agents, such as oral cholestyramine.[93] Phototherapy and PUVA photochemotherapy are discussed in detail in Chap. 28.

Thermal Stimulation (Heating or Cooling the Skin)

Thermal counterstimulation with heat or with cold is effective in reducing both clinical and experimental itching.[94,95] Thermal stimulation may act directly on peripheral itch receptors or through a counterstimulatory effect in the CNS. In general cooling produces a more consistent inhibitory effect; heating actually increases itching in some patients and experimental subjects.

The value of applying heat or cold to an itchy spot has been known to generations of grandparents. As early as 1933, Sir Thomas Lewis determined that immersion of the skin at 40 to 41 degrees celsius would quickly abolish itch but intensify burning pain.[96] Sulzburger and Wolf noted that "substituting some other sensation, such as that of cold or heat" reduces itching, and that agents that cool by evaporation are often useful.[97] The Medical Letter notes that when hot water is used, it must be sufficiently hot (about 120 to 130 degrees fahrenheit) to be slightly painful, and that the required temperature "is much too high to be used safely in a bath or shower."[98]

Fruhstorfer and colleagues studied the effects of immersion in a water-bath at either 10 or 45 degrees celsius in 18 patients with atopic dermatitis and in 40 normal subjects with experimental itching induced by topical histamine application. They found that cooling "abolished itch in all patients and in most of the normal subjects," but that the effect of heating was less consistent. Heating aggravated itching in about one third of both patients and normal subjects, but reduced or eliminated it in two thirds of both groups.

Acupuncture, Transcutaneous Electrical Nerve Stimulation (TENS), and Vibration

Based on the analogy implicit in the argument that scratching may reduce itching by counterstimulation or by stimulating inhibitory pathways, a number of physical stimuli have been assessed for their effects in reducing itch. Vibration at certain frequencies, transcutaneous electrical nerve stimulation, acupuncture, and electro-acupuncture can reduce itching in both clinical and experimental settings.[99-105] Different treatment protocols, electrical frequencies, and amplitudes have been used in different studies. Some investigators find that intrasegmental stimulation is more effective than extrasegmental stimulation.[106] Wright and McMahon found that noxious stimuli (radiant heat, high intensity TENS, and large transdermal constant current) reduced experimental histamine-induced itch but that non-noxious stimuli (vibration, low-intensity TENS) did not.[107] One of the most interesting effects of TENS is that relief of itching is not confined to the area of skin stimulated, suggesting some level of action in the CNS. The difficulties in evaluating TENS in itching are comparable to those entailed in the treatment of low-back pain, in which it produces some relief in over 30% of patients.[108] Efficacy beyond the undeniable placebo effect has been demonstrated. In some clinical situations TENS seems to lose its efficacy after getting off to a brilliant start; Fjellner and Hägermark attribute this to a strong initial placebo effect.[99] Nonetheless, it probably deserves to be tried in clinical practice more often than it is. Monk has suggested that TENS may be useful in the treatment of idiopathic generalized pruritus of the elderly.[109]

DRASTIC MEASURES

Severe itching can completely destroy the quality of life. Although an extensive array of options is now available to treat itching in most cases, drastic measures such as partial external diversion of bile[110] and plasmapheresis have been tried and have been effective in certain specific situations.[111,112]

UNDERSTANDING SUPPORT FROM PHYSICIANS AND FAMILY OR FRIENDS

This is obviously good for anybody, whether they itch or not. But it is worth mentioning here because its absence can have such deleterious effects, further isolating the itchy patient, increasing his stress level (thereby lowering the itch threshold), and contributing to further self-aggression directed at the skin through scratching.[113,114]

REFERENCES

1. Bernhard JD: Clinical aspects of pruritus, in Fitzpatrick TB, Eisen AZ, Wolff K, et al. (eds.): *Dermatology in General Medicine*, 3d ed. New York, McGraw-Hill. 1987, pp 78–90.
2. Bernhard JD: Pruritus: Pathophysiology and clinical aspects, in Moschella SL, Hurley HJ (eds.): *Dermatology*, 4th ed. Philadelphia, Saunders, 1992, pp 2042–2047.
3. Epstein E, Pinski JB: A blind study. *Arch Dermatol* 89:548–549, 1964.
4. Winkelmann RK: Pharmacologic control of pruritus. *Med Clin N Am* 66:1119–1133, 1982.
5. Fransway AF, Winkelmann RK. Treatment of pruritus. *Sem Dermatol* 7:310–325, 1988.

6. Bernhard JD: Pruritus: Advances in treatment. *Adv Dermatol* 6:57–71, 1991.
7. Edwards AE, Shellow WVR, Wright ET, et al: Pruritic skin disease, psychological stress, and the itch sensation. A reliable method for the induction of experimental pruritus. *Arch Dermatol* 112:339–343, 1976.
8. Chrousos GP, Gold PW: The concepts of stress and stress system disorders. Overview of physical and behavioral homeostasis. *JAMA* 267:1244–1252, 1992.
9. Nadelson T: A person's boundaries: A meaning of skin disease. *Cutis* 21:90–94, 1978.
10. Lazare A: Shame and humiliation in the medical encounter. *Arch Intern Med* 147:1653–1658, 1987.
11. Chernosky ME: Pruritic skin disease and summer air conditioning. *JAMA* 179:1005–1010, 1962.
12. Wahlgren CF, Hagermark O, Bergstrom R: Patients' perception of itch induced by histamine, compound 48/80 and wool fibres in atopic dermatitis. *Acta Derm Venereol* (Stockh) 71:488–494, 1990.,
13. Fowler JF, Kinner SM, Belsito DV: Allergic contact dermatitis from formaldehyde resins in permanent press clothing: An underdiagnosed cause of generalized dermatitis. *J Am Acad Dermatol* 27:962–968, 1992.
14. Anonymous: All-purpose moisturizers. *Consumer Reports.* November, 1986, pp 733–738.
15. Baden HP: Management of scaly skin with Epilyt. *Sem Dermatol* 6:55–57, 1987.
16. Dahl MV, Dahl AC: Twelve percent lactate lotion for the treatment of xerosis. A double-blind clinical evaluation. *Arch Dermatol* 119:27–30, 1983.
17. Fleischer, AB Jr: Pruritus in the elderly: Management by senior dermatologists. *J Am Acad Dermatol* 28:603–609, 1993.
18. Rajatanavin N, Withers A, Bernhard JD: Baking soda and pruritus. *Lancet* 2:977, 1987.
19. Frosch PJ, Kligman AM: The soap chamber test: A new method for assessing the irritancy of soaps. *J Am Acad Dermatol* 1:35–41, 1979.
20. Shelton RM: Aloe vera. Its chemical and therapeutic properties. *Int J Dermatol* 30:679–683, 1991.
21. Bernhard JD: Aloe vera and vitamin E as dermatologic remedies. *JAMA* 259:101, 1988.
22. Dalihi H, Adrianc J: The efficacy of local anesthetics in blocking the sensation of itch, burning and pain in normal and "sun-burned" skin. *Clin Pharmacol Ther* 12:913–919, 1971.
23. Fisher AA: Allergic reactions to topical (surface) anesthetics with reference to the safety of tronothane (pramoxine HCl). *Cutis* 25:584–591, 1980.
24. Arndt KA: *Manual of Dermatologic Therapeutics with Essentials of Diagnosis,* 4th ed. Boston, Little, Brown, 1989.
25. Shuttleworth D, Hill S, Marks R, et al: Relief of experimentally induced pruritus with a novel eutectic mixture of local anaesthetic agents. *Br J Dermatol* 119:535–540, 1988.
26. Layton AM, Cotterill JA: Notalgia paresthetica—report of three cases and their treatment. *Clin Exp Dermatol* 16:197–198, 1991.
27. Lynn B: Capsaicin: Actions on c fibre afferents that may be involved in itch. *Skin Pharmacol* 5:9–13, 1992.
28. Bernstein JE: Capsaicin and substance P. *Clin Dermatol* 9:497–503, 1992.
29. Bernstein JE, Korman NJ, Bickers DR, et al: Topical capsaicin treatment of chronic postherpetic neuralgia. *J Am Acad Dermatol* 21:265–270, 1989.
30. Srebrnik A, Brenner S: Capsaicin in the relief of postherpetic neuralgia. *J Dermatol Treat* 2:147–148, 1992.
31. Bernstein JE, Parish LC, Rapaport M, et al: Effects of topically applied capsaicin on moderate and severe psoriasis vulgaris. *J Am Acad Dermatol* 15:504–507, 1986.
32. Kurkcuoglu N, Alaybeyi F: Topical capsaicin for psoriasis. *Br J Dermatol* 123:549–550, 1990.

33. Tupker RA, Coenraads PJ, van der Meer JB: Treatment of prurigo nodularis, chronic prurigo and neurodermatitis circumscripta with topical capsaicin. *Acta Derm Venereol* (Stockh) 72:463–465, 1992.

34. Breneman DL, Cardone JS, Blumsack RF, et al: Topical capsaicin for treatment of hemodialysis-related pruritus. *J Am Acad Dermatol* 26:91–94, 1992.

35. Wallengren J: Treatment of notalgia paresthetica with topical capsaicin. *J Am Acad Dermatol* 24:286–288, 1991.

36. Leibsohn E: Treatment of notalgia paresthetica with capsaicin. *Cutis* 49:335–336, 1992.

37. Smith EB, King CA, Baker MD: Crotamiton lotion in pruritus. *Int J Dermatol* 23:684–685, 1984.

38. Tan CC, Wong KS, Thirumoorthy T, et al: A randomized, crossover trial of Sarna and Eurax lotions in the treatment of haemodialysis patients with uraemic pruritus. *J Dermatol Treat* 1:235–238, 1990.

39. Gupta MA, Gupta AK, Haberman HF: Psychotropic drugs in dermatology. *J Am Acad Dermatol* 14:633–645, 1986.

40. Koblenzer CS: *Psychocutaneous Disease.* Orlando, Grune & Stratton, 1987.

41. Koo JYM, Pham CT: Psychodermatology. Practical guidelines on pharmacotherapy. *Arch Dermatol* 128:381–388, 1992.

42. Bernstein JE, Whitney DH, Soltani K: Inhibition of histamine-induced pruritus by topical tricyclic antidepressants. *J Am Acad Dermatol* 5:582–585, 1981.

43. Bernhard JD: Phantom itch, pseudophantom itch, and senile pruritus. *Int J Dermatol* 31:586–587, 1992.

44. DeDoncker P, Cauwenbergh G: The use of topical oxatomide in pruritus, in Panconesi E (ed): *Dermatology in Europe.* Proceedings of the 1st congress of the European Academy of Dermatology and Venereology, Florence, Italy, 25–28 September 1989. Oxford, Blackwell Scientific Publications. 1991, p 911–913.

45. Althaus MA, Berthet P: Dimethindene maleate (Fenistil® Gel) in the control of itching due to insect bites and sunburns. *Agents Actions,* Special Conference Issue c425–c427, 1992.

46. Drake L, Breneman D, Greene S, et al: Effects of topical doxepin 5% cream on pruritic eczema. *J Invest Dermatol* 98:605, 1992.

47. Herman LE, Bernhard JD: Antihistamine update. *Dermatol Clin* 9:603–610, 1991.

48. Monroe EW: Chronic urticaria: Review of nonsedating H1 antihistamines in treatment. *J Am Acad Dermatol* 19:842–849, 1988.

49. Krause L, Shuster S: Mechanism of action of antipruritic drugs. *BMJ* 287:1199–1200, 1983.

50. Grant SM, Goa KL, Fitton A, et al: Ketotifen. A review of its pharmacodynamic and pharmacokinetic properties, and therapeutic use in asthma and allergic disorders. *Drugs* 40:412–448, 1990.

51. Francos GC, Kauh YC, Gittlen SD, et al: Elevated plasma histamine in chronic uremia. Effects of ketotifen on pruritus. *Int J Dermatol* 30:884–889, 1991.

52. Shear NH, Krafchik BR, MacLeod SM: Diffuse cutaneous mastocytosis. Treatment with ketotifen and cimetidine. *Clin Invest Med* 6:36, 1983.

53. Riccardi VM: A controlled multiphase trial of ketotifen to minimize neurofibroma-associated pain and itching. *Arch Dermatol* 129:577–581, 1993.

54. Meyer LJ: Drug therapy for neurofibromatosis? *Arch Dermatol* 129:625–626, 1993.

55. Bernhard JD: A theorem of pruritus and urticarial diminution. *J Am Acad Dermatol* 28:800, 1993.

56. Silverberg DS, Iaina A, Reisin E, et al: Cholestyramine in uremic pruritus. *BMJ* 1:752–753, 1977.

57. Tan JKL, Haberman HF, Coldman AJ: Identifying effective treatments for uremic pruritus. *J Am Acad Dermtol* 25:811–818, 1991.

58. Datta DV, Sherlock S: Cholestyramine for long term relief of the pruritus complicating intrahepatic cholestasis. *Gastroenterology* 50:323–332, 1966.
59. Laatikainin T: Effect of cholestyramine and phenobarbital on pruritus and serum bile acid levels in cholestasis of pregnancy. *Amer J Obstet Gynecol* 132:501–508, 1978.
60. Chanarin I, Szur L: Relief of intractable pruritus in polycythaemia rubra vera with cholestyramine. *Br J Haematol* 29:669, 1975.
61. Alarabi AA, Wikstrom B, Loof L, et al: Treatment of pruritus in cholestatic jaundice by bilirubin and bile acid-absorbing resin column plasma perfusion. *Scand J Gastroenterol* 27:223–226, 1992.
62. Pederson JA, Matter BJ, Czerwinski AW, et al: Relief of idiopathic generalized pruritus in dialysis patients treated with activated oral charcoal. *Ann Intern Med* 93:446–448, 1980.
63. Bernstein JE, Swift R: Relief of intractable pruritus with naloxone. *Arch Dermatol* 115:1366–1367, 1979.
64. Summerfield JA: Naloxone modulates the perception of itch in man. *Br J Clin Pharmacol* 10:180–183, 1980.
65. Bernstein JE, Grinzi RA: Butorphanol-induced pruritus antagonized by naloxone. *J Am Acad Dermatol* 5:227–228, 1981.
66. Bernstein JE, Swift RM, Soltani K, et al: Antipruritic effect of an opiate antagonist, naloxone hydrochloride. *J Invest Dermatol* 78:82–83, 1982.
67. Fjellner B, Hagermark O: The influence of the opiate antagonist naloxone on experimental pruritus. *Acta Derm Venereol* (Stockh) 64:73, 1984.
68. Bergasa NV, Jones EA: Management of the pruritus of cholestasis: Potential role of opiate antagonists. *Am J Gastroenterol* 86:1404–1412, 1991.
69. Bergasa NV, Talbot TL, Alling DW, et al: A controlled trial of naloxone infusions for the pruritus of chronic cholestasis. *Gastroenterology* 102:544–549, 1992.
70. Monroe EW: Efficacy and safety of nalmefene in patients with severe pruritus casued by chronic urticaria and atopic dermatitis. *J Am Acad Dermatol* 21:135–136, 1989.
71. Harrison PV: Nalmefene and pruritus. *J Am Acad Dermatol* 23:530, 1990.
72. Bergasa NV, Alling DW, Talbot TL, et al: Relief from the intractable pruritus of chronic cholestasis associated with oral nalmefene therapy, (abstract). *Hepatology* 14(2):154A, 1991.
73. Fjellner B, Hagermark O: Pruritus in polycythemia: Treatment with aspirin and possibility of platelet involvement. *Acta Derm Venereol* (Stockh) 61:505, 1979.
74. Hagermark O: Influence of antihistamines, sedatives, and aspirin on experimental itch. *Acta Derm Venereol* (Stockh) 53:363–368, 1973.
75. Boss M, Burton JL: Lack of effect of the antihistamine drug clemastine on potentiation of itch by prostaglandins. *Arch Dermatol* 117:208–209, 1981.
76. Daly M, Shuster S: Effect of aspirin on pruritus. *BMJ* 293:907, 1986.
77. Malmberg AB, Yaksh TL: Hyperalgesia mediated by spinal glutamate or substance P receptor blocked by spinal cyclooxygenase inhibition. *Science* 257:1276–1279, 1992.
78. Soter NA, Austen KF, Wasserman SI: Oral disodium cromoglycate in the treatment of systemic mastocytosis. *N Engl J Med* 301:465–469, 1979.
79. Leven A, Naysmith A, Dickens S, et al: Sodium cromoglycate and Hodgkin's pruritus. *BMJ* 2:896, 1979.
80. Hishon S, Rose JD, Hunter JO: The relief of pruritus in primary biliary cirrhosis by hydroxyethylrutosides. *Br J Dermatol* 105:457–460, 1981.
81. Doyle JA, Connolly SM, Hunziker H, et al: Prurigo nodularis: A reappraisal of the clinical and histologic features. *J Cutan Pathol* 6: 392–403, 1979.
82. Bernal JE, Duran MM, Londono F: Cellular immune effects of thalidomide in actinic prurigo. *Int J Dermatol* 31:599–600, 1992.
83. Thuluvath PJ, Triger DR, Manku MS, et al: Evening primrose oil in the treatment of refractory biliary pruritus. *Eur J Gastroenterol and Hepatol* 3:87–90, 1991.

84. Gonzalez MC, Iglesias J, Tiribelli C, et al: Epomediol ameliorates pruritus in patients with intrahepatic cholestasis of pregnancy. *J Hepatol* 16:241–250, 1992.
85. Borgeat A, Wilder-Smith OHG, Saiah M, et al: Subhypnotic doses of propofol relieve pruritus induced by epidural and intrathecal morphine. *Anesthesiology* 76:510–512, 1992.
86. Borgeat A, Wilder-Smith OHG, Mentha G: Subhypnotic doses of propofol releive pruritus associated with liver disease. *Gastroenterology* 104:244–247, 1993.
87. Rajatanavin N, Scharf MJ, Bernhard JD: Phototherapy and photochemotherapy in dermatologic diseases. *Comp Ther* 14:11–18, 1988.
88. Smith ML, Orton PW, Chu H, et al: Photochemotherapy of dominant, diffuse, cutaneous mastocytosis. *Ped Dermatol* 7:251–255, 1990.
89. Honigsman H, Stingl G: *Therapeutic Photomedicine.* Basel, Karger, 1986.
90. Morison WL: *Phototherapy and Photochemotherapy of Skin Disease,* 2d ed. New York, Raven Press, 1991.
91. Abel EA: *Photochemotherapy in Dermatology.* New York, Igaku-Shoin, 1992.
92. Morison WL, Nesbitt JA: Oral psoralen photochemotherapy (PUVA) for pruritus associated with polycythema-vera and myelofibrosis. *Am J Hemat* 42:409–410, 1993.
93. Cerio R, Murphy GM, Sladen GE, et al: A combination of phototherapy and cholestyramine for the relief of pruritus in primary biliary cirrhosis. *Br J Dermatol* 116:265–267, 1987.
94. Murray FS, Weaver MM: Effects of ipsilateral and contralateral counterirritation on experimentally produced itch in human beings. *J Comp Physiol Psych* 89:819–826, 1975.
95. Fruhstorfer H, Hermanns M, Latzke L: The effects of thermal stimulation on clinical and experimental itch. *Pain* 24:259–269, 1986.
96. Lewis T: *Pain.* New York, Macmillan Company, 1942, p 113.
97. Sulzberger MB, Wolf J: Dermatologic therapy in general practice, 2d ed. Chicago, Year Book Publishers, 1942, p 59.
98. Anonymous: Hot water for itching. *Medical Let Drug Ther* 13:52, 1971.
99. Fjellner B, Hagermark O: Transcutaneous nerve stimulation and itching. *Acta Derm Venereol* (Stockh) 58:131–134, 1978.
100. Ekblom A, Fjellner B, Hansson P: The influence of mechanical vibratory stimulation and transcutaneous electrical nerve stimulation on experimental pruritus induced by histamine. *Acta Physiol Scand* 122:361–367, 1984.
101. Belgrade MJ, Solomon LM, Lichter EA: Effect of acupuncture on experimentally induced itch. *Acta Derm Venereol* (Stockh) 64:129–133, 1984.
102. Ekblom A, Hansson P, Fjellner B: The influence of extrasegmental mechanical vibratory stimulation and transcutaneous electrical nerve stimulation on histamine-induced itch. *Acta Physiol Scand* 125:541–545, 1985.
103. Duo LJ: Electrical needle therapy of uremic pruritus. *Nephron* 47:179–183, 1987.
104. Bjrn H, Kaada B: Successful treatment of itching and atopic eczema by transcutaneous nerve stiumulation. *Acupunct Electrother Res* 12:101–112, 1987.
105. Ely H: Shocking therapy: Uses of transcutaneous electric nerve stimulation in dermatology. *Dermatol Clin* 9:189–197, 1991.
106. Lundeberg T, Bondesson L, Thomas M: Effect of acupuncture on experimentally induced itch. *Br J Dermatol* 117:771–777, 1987.
107. Wright E, McMahon S: The inhibition of itch by noxious, but not innocuous, sensory counterstimulation in man. *J Physiol* 446:480P, 1992.
108. Anonymous: TENS for chronic low-back pain. *Lancet* 337:462–463, 1991.
109. Monk BE: Transcutaneous electronic nerve stimulation in the treatment of generalized pruritus. *Clin Exp Dermatol* 18:67–68, 1993.
110. Whitington PF, Whitington GL: Partial external diversion of bile for the treatment of intractable pruritus associated with intrahepatic cholestasis. *Gastroenterology* 95:130–136, 1988.

111. Gomez RL, Griffin JW, Squires JE: Prolonged relief of intractable pruritus in primary sclerosing cholangitis by plasmapheresis. *J Clin Gastroenterol* 8:301–303,1986.
112. Kohan AI, Findor JA, Igartua EB, et al: Intensive plasmapheresis as an alternative therapy for intractable pruritus of primary biliary cirrhosis. *Transfus Sci* 12:197–200, 1991.
113. Calnan CD, O'Neill D: Itching in tension states. *Br J Dermatol* 64:274–280, 1952.
114. Musaph H: Psychodynamics in itching states. *Int J Psychoanal* 49:336–340, 1968.

TWENTY-SEVEN

TOPICAL TREATMENT OF ITCHING WITHOUT CORTICOSTEROIDS

Jerome Z. Litt

INTRODUCTION

What if topical steroids, for one reason or another, were not available? How would the younger generation of dermatologists, the resident, the family physician, and the pediatrician treat pruritic disorders?

According to Maddin,[1] the ideal topical antipruritic agent should be effective, neither irritating nor toxic, cosmetically acceptable, stable, inexpensive, and should possess low sensitizing potential.

Why, then, should we even bother with nonsteroidal topical agents, if the steroids are readily available and fulfill almost all of Maddin's criteria? Topical steroid preparations are obviously beneficial in ameliorating pruritus when itching is a consequence of a steroid-responsive dermatosis. There are, however, many situations in which itching is not caused by a steroid-responsive dermatosis: renal failure, Hodgkin's disease, and fiberglass dermatitis, among others. In addition, there are situations in which the anti-inflammatory effect of the steroids is helpful, but not sufficient to completely relieve the itching.

Thus, there are many reasons for knowing about, and using, nonsteroidal products.

- They are useful when it is necessary to cover large areas of the body, or parts of the body such as the face and groins, where potent steroids are contraindicated.
- They are safer and cause fewer adverse side effects with prolonged use.

- They can be used in infants and children without the inherent absorptive dangers of topical steroids.
- They can be tailor-made to suit each condition and each patient. The vehicle, the concentration of active ingredient, and the quantity can be carefully chosen and controlled.
- Some pharmacies or pharmaceutical supply houses can make up large batches of these compounds, and they can be dispensed easily from the pharmacy or office (in states that permit office dispensing).
- Such products are often significantly less expensive than topical corticosteroids.
- They work not only when other products have failed but also as "first lines of defense."

There are many ways in which itching can be relieved. The following is a brief outline of some of the agents and products that are known to have a salutary effect on pruritus.

SOME WAYS THAT ITCHING CAN BE RELIEVED

I. Substituting some other sensation for the itching.[2] This can be accomplished by:
  A. Cooling. Cooling seems to act directly on the sensory receptors mediating itch. Eighteen patients with atopic dermatitis rated the intensity of spontaneous itch on one of their forearms before, during, and after immersion in a waterbath of 10°C. In 40 normal subjects, itch was elicited by topically applied histamine to the volar forearm. Cooling abolished itch in all atopic patients and in most of the normal subjects.[3]
    1. Physical Methods of Cooling
      a. Direct means
        i. Ice (cubes, packs, bags)
        ii. Cold compresses with water, milk, or Burow's solution (when impetiginized). Compresses act by virtue of evaporation which, of itself, is a cooling process.
        iii. Liquid nitrogen. Prurigo nodularis of 8 years duration was treated successfully in a 55-year-old black woman with blistering cryotherapy.[4]
      b. Other means
        i. Medicated Baths—A medicated bath is a convenient way to apply medication to the entire skin surface. It is indispensable in the management of acute, widespread eruptions and generalized pruritus. Baths soothe, soften, reduce inflammation, and relieve itching and dryness. The optimum temperature for a medicated bath is 40° to 44°C. (104°–112°F.)

(a) Colloid baths: Hydrolyzed starch (Linit); oatmeal (Aveeno); bran.

(b) Bath Oils: Bath oils generally consist of a mineral or vegetable oil plus a surfactant. Mineral oil products are adsorbed better than vegetable oil products.[5] Adsorption onto and absorption into the skin increases with increases in temperature and oil concentration. Examples of these bath oils are Alpha Keri Therapeutic Shower and Bath Oil (Westwood); Jeri Bath (Dermik); Nutraderm Bath Oil (Owen). (Caution! Guard against slipping in the tub!) Some bath oils can be patted on the wet skin after a shower. When applied as wet compresses, or after the bath, bath oils can be used to treat dry, pruritic skin.[6]

(c) Tar baths: Useful for chronic, pruritic, and generalized atopic dermatitis, psoriasis, lichen planus, and lichen simplex chronicus. Balnetar (Westwood); Lavatar (Doak); Polytar (Stiefel); and Zetar (Dermik) are examples. (Tar also acts in other ways [q.v.].) Nota bene: While these tar baths usually stain bathtubs, the stain is a result of the tar substances adhering to grime, dirt, or debris already present in the tub. To prevent this, have the patient scour the tub thoroughly with either Clorox or a scouring powder to remove the dirt and grime before adding the tar preparation.

(d) Potassium permanganate. For pruritic, eczematized atopic dermatitis and generalized moniliasis. Dissolve six 5-grain tablets in a 20-gallon tub (about 8 inches high) of warm water. (This is, roughly, a 1:40,000 solution.) Tablets must be completely dissolved!

(e) Baking soda. A "generous sprinkling" of baking soda (sodium bicarbonate) in tepid bath water has been found beneficial in aquagenic pruritus[7] and atopic eczema.[8]

ii. Wet Dressings—Wet dressings help reduce inflammation, remove crusts and debris, and allay itching of localized acute and eczematized patches such as found in atopic dermatitis and poison ivy dermatitis. The proper method to apply compresses or wet dressings is as follows: Use either a folded cotton handkerchief or pieces of bed linen folded eight layers thick. Dip this into the prepared solution (see following section) and gently wring it out so that the cloth is sopping wet. Pat this on the affected area—on and off, on and off—remoistening the cloth when necessary. Do this for 10 or 15 minutes every hour or so until the eruption has cooled down and has begun to dry up, or until the crusts have been removed. After compressing, pat the area dry, then apply the appropriate cream or lotion. (If you plan to use the same cloth for future compresses, make sure to rinse it out in plain water to avoid any chemical build-up.)

Repeat this procedure every hour or so until the oozing, weeping, or crusting has begun to dry up.

(a) Milk. Apply cool, whole milk to affected areas for 10 to 20 minutes every hour until symptoms subside (see previous section).

(b) Burow's solution—aluminum acetate. Available as Bluboro Powder (Herbert) or Pedi-Boro Soak Paks (Pedinol). One packet dissolved in a pint of water will yield a 1:40 dilution. This solution is soothing, drying, antipruritic, and antiseptic (see previous section).

(c) Potassium permanganate. Dissolve one 5-grain tablet in two quarts of warm water. This is, roughly, a 1:6,000 solution. The tablet must be completely dissolved! This solution can be used for impetiginized and localized areas of atopic dermatitis and contact dermatitis.

iii. "Shake" lotions—"Shake" lotions are suspensions of relatively inert powders in a liquid. They require shaking (to disperse the powders) before being applied. They are protective, soothing, and temperature-regulating. As the liquid portion of the lotion evaporates, it tends to cool and soothe, leaving a protective film of the powder on the skin. "Shake" lotions incorporating active medicinals (menthol, phenol, camphor, benzocaine [rarely]) are used to produce antipruritic effects. The classical shake lotion is calamine lotion. The official USP Calamine Lotion is as follows:

Calamine	9.6 gm
Zinc Oxide	9.0 gm
Glycerine	2.0 ml
Bentonite Magma	30.0 ml
Calcium Hydroxide (Lime Water Solution) q.s. ad	120.0 ml

iv. Alcoholic solutions. While alcoholic solutions provide transient relief by rapid evaporation, in the end, they have a drying effect on the skin, thus aggravating the itching (see the solutions in the following sections).

2. Chemical methods
   a. Phenol (1/8 to 2%)—a distillation product of coal tar or it may be synthesized from benzene. Acts directly on the cold recep-

tors to cause a feeling of coolness. It is found in many over-the-counter products, as well as in Panscol Lotion and Ointment, Dodd's Lotion, Schamberg's Lotion, and Zemo Lotion. Phenol also acts by its anesthetic and counterirritant actions (q.v.). Nota bene: do not use over wide areas, use with care in infants and children, and do not use in pregnant women.

  b. Menthol (1/8 to 1%)—an alcohol obtained from mint oil or it can be prepared synthetically. Acts directly on the cold receptors of the skin to cause a feeling of coolness.[9] Mentholated products can be found in a variety of o-t-c compounds; also in Sarna Lotion and Foam (Stiefel), Schamberg's Lotion, Topic Gel, Wibi Lotion, and Zemo Ointment. Menthol also acts by its anesthetic and counterirritant actions [q.v.].

  c. Camphor (0.1 to 3%)—a ketone obtained from the camphor tree, Cinnamomum camphora, an evergreen of eastern Asia, or produced synthetically from the fractional distillation of turpentine. This can be found in Sarna Lotion, Topic Gel, and various o-t-c products. Camphor also acts by its anesthetic and counterirritant actions [q.v.].

  d. Thymol (0.5 to 1%)—a crystalline phenol that occurs naturally in thyme oil or is prepared synthetically.

  e. Salicylic acid (1 to 5%)—May prevent itching as a result of its keratoplastic (building up of the horny layer of the skin) and anesthetic effect. (Salicylic acid is not soluble in lotions.)

  f. By various agents whose mode of action is unclear.

    i. Tars. Tars are dark-colored liquids containing mixtures of hydrocarbons and aromatic compounds obtained through the destructive distillation of the wood of various trees of the family Pinaceae. Some believe that the antipruritic effect of tar is a result of the phenolic substances present.

      (a) Crude coal tar (1 to 10%)

      (b) Liquor carbonis detergens (1 to 20%)

      (c) Ichthammol (1 to 20%)

      (d) Juniper tar (oil of cade; 1 to 20%)

      (e) Birch tar (1 to 20%)

      (f) Pine tar (1 to 20%)

    ii. Resorcinol (2 to 5%)

    iii. Iodochlorhydroxyquin (Vioform; Clioquinol)

    iv. Urea (2 to 10%). Urea increases water uptake in the stratum corneum and thus relieves dry, xerotic skin as well as the itching that accompanies the asteatotic condition.

    v. Ammonium lactate (Lac-Hydrin). Symptomatic relief of dry, itchy skin is provided by hygroscopic substances (humectants) that increase skin moisture. Lactic acid and other alpha-hydroxy acids are effective humectants.

   vi. Sulfur, precipitated (5 to 10%). Sulfur probably got its antipruritic reputation from its effectiveness in the treatment
   of scabies. Sulfur relieves the itching of chigger bites. Sodium thiosulfate is useful in the treatment of tinea versicolor.

B. Heat.
  1. Hot Baths. Very hot baths give momentary relief by substituting
   another sensation and perhaps by evoking dilatation. Afterwards a
   rebound phenomenon may supervene. "Application of heat in the
   form of very hot water . . . is often the most effective measure to
   relieve itching."[10] The temperature should be between 120° and
   130°F.
  2. Hot Water Bottle.

C. Counterirritation. Counterirritants reduce itching by stimulating cutaneous sensory receptors to provide a feeling of coolness, warmth, or
  slight pain which obscures the itch sensation. The activity of these
  agents is dependent on the concentration. (In low concentrations, they
  may depress the cutaneous receptors and result in an anesthetic effect.
  See following.)
  1. Phenol (1/8 to 2%)
  2. Menthol (1/8 to 1%)
  3. Camphor (3 to 11% acts as a counterirritant.) "Camphor is a relatively weak sensory irritant that may have a modest excitatory effect
   on thermosensitive cutaneous fibers."[11]

II. Anesthesia of Sensory Nerve Endings. Local anesthetics affect sensation
by interfering with the transmission of impulses along the sensory nerve
fibers.

A. Direct
  1. Benzocaine (0.5 to 20%). Available as Americaine, Calamatum,
   Ivarest, Ivy Dry Cream, Lanacane, Solarcaine, Unguentine, among
   others.
  2. Benzyl Alcohol (5 to 33%). Available as Topic, Rhulihist, and Rhu-
   ligel.
  3. Butamben Picrate (1%). Available as Butesin Picrate.
  4. Cyclomethycaine (0.5%). Available as Surfadil.
  5. Dibucaine (0.25 to 1%). Available as Nupercainal.
  6. Diperodon HCl (0.25%). Available as Dalicote.
  7. Tetracaine HCL (0.5–1%). Available as Pontocaine.
  8. EMLA Cream (acronym for Eutectic Mixture of Local Anesthetics).
   The eutectic mixture of the local anesthetics lignocaine and prilocaine has been successful in relieving artificially induced pruritus
   in 20 volunteers. Having a slow onset of action, EMLA was effective
   in reducing, but not abolishing, pruritus induced by histamine and
   the artificial pruritogens cowhage and papain.[12] Although it may
   not be suitable for chronic itching over large areas, it may be of

some value in the treatment of localized pruritus. (See, for example, notalgia paresthetica in Chap. 12.)

    9. Lidocaine (0.5 to 4%). Lidocaine preparations can be used effectively for the itching that accompanies insect bites and stings, for poison ivy dermatitis, and also for the itching and pain of mild sunburn. Available as Bactine First Aid Spray, Medi-Quick, Unguentine Plus, Xylocaine.

    10. Pramoxine HCl (0.5 to 2.5%). Pramoxine is a surface anesthetic that has a low index of sensitization and toxicity. It is structurally unrelated to the procaine-type drugs.[13] Available as PRAX, Tronothane HCl, Tronolane, and Itch-X.

  B. Products that exert a topical anesthetic action by depressing cutaneous sensory receptors.

    1. Phenol (1/8 to 2%)

    2. Menthol (1/8 to 1%)

    3. Camphor (0.1 to 3%)—camphor has "an irritant effect and probably a benumbing influence upon the peripheral sensory nerves. It acts as a local anesthetic."[14]

    4. Topical Antihistamines. Antihistamines also relieve itching by depressing cutaneous sensory receptors. Occasionally effective in stubborn, recalcitrant itching, as in cases of pruritus vulvae and pruritus scroti, they are often sensitizing and, therefore, infrequently used. (See also Chap. 29.)

      a. Diphenhydramine HCl (1 to 2%). Available as Caladryl, Surfadil, Ziradryl, and others.

      b. Phenyltoloxamine citrate (0.5–1%). Available as Hista-Calma Lotion.

      c. Pyrilamine maleate (1%). Available as Calamox, Dalicote, Ivarest, and others.

      d. Tripelennamine (0.5 to 2%). Available as Pyribenzamine.

III. Depletion of Substance P. Capsaicin, the pungent agent of hot pepper, acts by depleting neuropeptides—especially Substance P (a known inducer of mast cell degranulation)—from peripheral nerves and leads to a selective and long-lasting depression of C-polymodal nociceptors. Itching is therefore reduced in capsaicin-treated skin.[15,16] (Supplied as Zostrix Cream 0.025% [GenDerm]). It has been used successfully in cases of notalgia paresthetica,[17] in histamine-induced pruritus,[18] in pruritus related to hemodialysis,[19] in pruritic psoriasis,[20] and in the itching of prurigo nodularis.[21]

IV. Reducing Inflammation of the Skin

  A. Adrenocorticosteroid Preparations. Unavailable to dermatologists just a quarter of a century ago, perhaps the single most important step in dermatologic therapeutics has been the development of topical corticosteroids. These products modify or eliminate many common and uncommon diseases in a very effective manner. The functions of topical corticosteroids include anti-inflammatory, vasoconstrictive, and antimitotic activities. Once applied to the skin, they begin to work almost instantaneously. Classified according to their strength, corticosteroids tend to fall into groups of low, medium, and high potency effect. This is measured by vasoconstriction assays that usually correspond to actual function. In general, fluorinated corticosteroids are more potent than the non-fluorinated varieties. Delivery systems include ointments, creams, gels, lotions, solutions, aerosols, and impregnated tapes. Occlusion of these agents will increase their penetration and strength. Different areas of the skin require different steroids. The thin skin of the face, the genital areas, and the intertriginous regions require low potency preparations, whereas the thicker skin areas respond well to the higher potency varieties. Topical corticosteroids may be used in addition to many of the nonsteroidal remedies discussed in this chapter.

V. Destroying the Organisms That Have Prompted the Itching in Various Diseases. Many cutaneous infections and infestations, such as those caused by dermatophytes, yeast organisms, viruses, bacteria, and parasites induce pruritus. Appropriate antifungal, anticandidal, antiviral, antibacterial, and parasiticidal medications, where indicated, by eradicating the infection or infestation, will often terminate the itching. Until these specific remedies work, however, it may be necessary to offer some early symptomatic relief of the attendant pruritus with some of the methods described above.

VI. Unproven Methods

    A. Folklore

        In all civilizations people have placed a high value on the medicinal properties of herbs and plants, and physicians of all ages have advised their students not to turn their backs on successful folk medicines. What we know today as "folk medicine" has a long and honorable history dating back as far as 50 centuries of recorded experience.

        The regimens of folk medicines are by no means the product of scientific research. Rather, they evolved in early times in the absence of it and were usually the result of trial and error experimentation in the nonprofessional community. Paracelsus said that he acquired his most effective remedies from various sources, including barbers, surgeons, midwives, monks, hangmen, gypsies, and herb-collecting old women.

        A folklore remedy for itching: One part of sulfur to two parts of inner lard of pork, thoroughly combined, should be rubbed into the affected parts.[22]

        A remedy for insect bites: "Run fast and find three kinds of leaves, one jagged (like the dandelion), one round, and one long. Crush them in your hand and rub them hard over the bitten place. Rub rub rub."[23]

For poison ivy dermatitis: Use equal parts of apple cider vinegar and vinegar. Dab on the affected parts and allow to dry on the skin.[24]
B. Anecdotal remedies for itching abound: Break a vitamin E capsule and apply; rub an aspirin on insect bites;[25] for rectal and vaginal itching, I, personally, recommend yogurt applications every 2 or 3 hours.
C. Herbals. Some herbal remedies include the juice of the milkweed plant for poison ivy dermatitis and chickweed poultices for hives.[25]

EXAMPLES OF ANTI-PRURITIC COMPOUNDED MEDICATIONS

Shake Lotions

"Shake" lotions are suspensions of relatively inert powders in a liquid. They require shaking (to disperse the powders) before being applied. Lotions are very easy to apply and dressings are not required. They are particularly suited for subacute, widespread, and intertriginous dermatoses. Shake lotions incorporating active medicinals (menthol, phenol, camphor, benzocaine [rarely]) are used to produce antipruritic effects.

Best dispensed in wide-mouthed bottles, shake lotions should be applied every 3 or 4 hours using a small, flat varnish paint brush. They should be applied coat over coat, and wet-dressed off every 24 hours. The classical shake lotion is calamine lotion. The official USP Calamine Lotion is as follows:

Calamine	9.6 gm
Zinc Oxide	9.0 gm
Glycerine	2.0 ml
Bentonite Magma	30.0 ml
Calcium Hydroxide (Lime Water Solution) q.s. ad	120.0 ml

Any, or a combination of, antipruritics such as phenol, menthol, camphor, thymol, and the like can be added in appropriate percentages to calamine lotion to make it an effective and inexpensive antipruritic remedy.

Menthol	0.3 gm	[0.25%]
Phenol	0.6 gm	[0.50%]
Calamine Lotion	q.s. ad 120.0 ml	

Indications: The above is a basic soothing lotion for pityriasis rosea, poison ivy dermatitis, and other acute and subacute pruritic dermatoses.

Menthol	0.3 gm	[0.25%]
Phenol	0.6 gm	[0.50%]
Liquor Carbonis Detergens	6.0 ml	[5.00%]
Calamine Lotion	q.s. ad 120.0 ml	

This is excellent for subacute contact and atopic dermatitis, as well as for intertriginous eruptions.

Creamy-type Lotions

Creamy-type lotions (water-in-oil and oil-in-water emulsions)—are preparations that are soothing, less drying, smoother, and more elegant in appearance than shake lotions. They are useful in the more chronic types of eczematous eruptions, such as contact dermatitis, pityriasis rosea, and extensive insect bites. Creamy-type lotions are best applied in a thin film every 3 or 4 hours by rubbing in gently with the fingertips. Examples of creamy-type lotions are: Keri Lotion, Nivea Lotion, Nutraderm Lotion, WIBI, and Mi-Fine-Skin Lotion. Menthol and/or phenol can be added to creamy lotions as follows:

> Menthol .... 0.3 gm [0.25%]
> Phenol .... 0.6 gm [0.50%]
> Creamy-type Lotion   q.s. ad 120.0 ml

Schamberg's lotion (C&M Pharmacal; Syosset Labs). Schamberg's Lotion contains menthol 0.15 percent, phenol 1.0 percent, zinc oxide, peanut oil, lime water, and dispersant.

Sarna lotion (Stiefel Laboratories). Sarna Lotion contains menthol 0.5 percent and camphor 0.5 percent in an emollient base. Sarna also comes in a Foam.

Indications: These three lotions are often effective in relieving the pruritus associated with pityriasis rosea, chronic contact dermatitis, extensive insect bites, lichen planus, and chronic atopic dermatitis. (Note: Use only sparingly in infants and young children.)

Creams

Creams are semisolid (non-pourable) soft to moderately firm, water-washable emulsions, generally of the oil-in-water type. The main difference between lotions and creams is that lotions contain greater proportions of water, while creams contain greater proportions of fats and oils. Creams are not nearly as messy as ointments or pastes and are, therefore, more cosmetically agreeable. They are useful in delivering small amounts of active ingredients to the skin. They cannot, however, carry the higher concentrations of active ingredients as ointments or pastes can. Creams are generally employed for relatively localized dermatoses, and should be applied with the fingertips, one coat over the other, every 3 or 4 hours. Example of creams are Nutraderm Cream, Lubriderm Cream, Hydrophilic Ointment, Mi-Fine-Skin Cream and Moisturel Cream.

> Menthol .... 0.15 gm [0.25%]
> Phenol .... 0.30 gm [0.50%]
> Cream   q.s. ad 60.0 gm

Indications: This is good for localized pruritic, subacute or chronic eczematous dermatoses; insect bites; urticaria; lichen planus; contact dermatitis; atopic dermatitis; and lichen simplex chronicus.

Vioform cream 3 percent (Ciba). Indications: A good preparation for seborrheic dermatitis, tineas, and moniliasis of intertriginous areas (stains yellowish).

```
Salicylic Acid ........................1.8 gm [3.0%]
Precipitated Sulfur ...................3.0 gm [5.0%]
Purified Water .......................6.0 ml [10.0%]
Hydrophilic Ointment USP      q.s. ad  60.0 gm
```

Indications: The above is an effective cream for pruritic seborrheic dermatitis of the face and chest.

Ointments

Ointments are semisolid, soft to very firm, greasy preparations that can carry active ingredients in concentrations of up to 40 percent. They are occlusive, macerating, and are for the most part not miscible with water and messy to use. They lubricate, help in the removal of crusts and scales, and are useful in softening dry, flaky skin. They are also used as protective coverings not only to prevent contact of the skin surface with noxious agents, but also to reduce heat loss. Unlike creams, they are not water-washable, and are, therefore, rarely used in hairy areas. Ointments can be removed by washing with soap and hot water. Ointments, per se, have no antipruritic properties. When combined, however, with agents such as menthol, phenol, and various tars, they allay itching. Ointments should be rubbed into the skin with the fingertips 3 or 4 times daily. Examples of ointments include Cold Cream, Hydrophilic Petrolatum and White Petrolatum.

```
Menthol ...........................0.3 gm [0.25%]
Phenol ............................0.6 gm [0.50%]
Mineral Oil .......................1.2 ml [1.00%]
Cold Cream                    q.s. ad 120.0 gm
```

Indications: This is an excellent preparation for chronic pruritic dermatoses: chronic atopic dermatitis, chronic contact dermatitis, hypertrophic lichen planus, and insect bites.

Whitfield's ointment half-strength. Indications: This is a time-honored proprietary medication that is very effective for pruritic tinea pedis.

Menthol . . . . .0.030 gm [0.10%]
Phenol . . . . .0.075 gm [0.25%]
Mineral Oil . . . . .0.3   ml   [1.00%]
Cold Cream   q.s. ad 30.0   gm

Indications: This is occasionally effective in chronic, stubborn pruritus ani. Apply 2 or 3 times daily and after each bowel motion.

Pastes

Pastes are preparations that have about 50 percent powdered ingredients in a greasy base, such as petrolatum. Pastes help protect the skin from outside forces, such as rubbing and scratching; they absorb moisture; and they help to dry up weeping and oozing lesions. Because they tend to "stay put," they help carry active medicated constituents to the areas where they are needed.

They usually require bandaging; they are slightly messy; and they can be difficult to remove, although it is neither necessary nor desirable to remove all the paste in cleansing. The best way to apply pastes is with a wooden applicator such as a tongue depressor. Pastes should be left on all day. To remove them, use a vegetable oil or a light mineral oil.

Burow's Solution .10.0 ml
Aquaphor . . . . .20.0 gm
Paste of Zinc Oxide   q.s. ad 60.0 gm

Indications: Known familiarly as "1–2–3 paste," this modification, substituting Aquaphor for the original lanolin, is a superb preparation for bland therapy as in severe cases of pruritic hand eczema, erosions, and ulcerations, as well as in acute and subacute dermatoses of the feet.

Vioform (iodochlorhydroxyquin) Powder . . . . 0.6 gm [1%]
"1–2–3 Paste" [see above]   q.s. ad 60.0 gm

Indications: This is a fine paste for moniliasis of the groin, umbilicus, and corona of the penis, as well as for subacute, pruritic tinea pedis.

Menthol . . . . .0.030 gm [0.10%]
Phenol . . . . .0.075 gm [0.25%]
Mineral Oil . . . . .0.300 ml   [1.00%]
"1–2–3 Paste" (see above)   q.s. ad 30.000 gm

Indications: This is a good preparation for subacute and stubborn pruritus ani. Apply twice daily and after each bowel motion. It's somewhat messy, but when it works, it's like a miracle.

Solutions

Solutions are clear liquids in which the solvent is one or more of the following: water, alcohol, acetone, ether, or mineral oil. Solutions can carry one or more active ingredients. Alcoholic or hydroalcoholic solutions of medicinals are called tinctures. Suspensions are turbid preparations in which the active ingredients are physically dispersed rather than dissolved. They often require shaking before application. While alcoholic solutions provide transient relief by rapid evaporation, in the end, they have a drying effect on the skin, thus aggravating the itching.

One percent Aqueous Gentian Violet USP. Indications: Gentian Violet is a marvelous preparation for pruritic moniliasis of the groins, penis, inframammary, umbilical, and diaper areas. It is a good, nonstinging antiseptic and fungistatic agent that has the advantage of a startling color and the disadvantage of a stain that is difficult to remove. Specific antifungal agents such as the imidazoles are of course helpful as well. Directions: Apply twice daily using a cotton-tipped applicator.

Castellani's paint (Carbol Fuchsin Solution). Indications: This is probably the best preparation for pruritic tinea cruris and moniliasis of intertriginous areas. Directions: Apply to affected areas with cotton-tipped applicator twice daily. This preparation stains. (Note: Do not use full strength in infants and small children. Try one-quarter strength dilution when all other therapies have failed.) Available as Castaderm and Neo-Castaderm.

> Menthol . . . . .0.15 gm [0.5%]
> Salicylic Acid . . . . .1.50 gm [5.0%]
> 70% Alcohol   q.s. ad 30.00 ml

Indications: This can be used for dyshidrosis (pompholyx) of the palms and soles.

Directions: Apply with cotton-tipped applicator to vesicles twice daily.

Undiluted liquor carbonis detergens. Indications: This is good for lichen simplex chronicus of the scrotum. Directions: Paint on affected areas with cotton-tipped applicator 2 or 3 times daily.

Varnishes

Varnishes are solutions or suspensions of active materials in a vehicle with a rapidly evaporating solvent containing a film-forming solute that leaves an adherent film on the skin.

```
Acetone ...........................10.0 ml  [16.7%]
Collodion .........................10.0 gm  [16.7%]
Crude Coal Tar              q.s. ad  60.0 gm
```

This varnish, known as "Black Cat," is good for stubborn pruritic lichen simplex chronicus; nummular eczema; and hypertrophic lichen planus.

Directions: Apply to affected areas with a tongue depressor. Dust over with baby powder. Leave on for 3 days. Remove with Vaseline. Repeat.

Nota bene: Tar preparations used on the scrotum are potential carcinogens. Use sparingly and infrequently.

```
Phenol ............................  0.3  [1%]
Benzocaine ........................  3.0  [10%]
Flexible Collodion         q.s. ad  30.0
```

Dispense in an applicator bottle.

Indications: Use this for chigger and insect bites. Directions: Apply two or three times daily. Do not use phenol on infants or pregnant women.

Powders

Powders are used principally in the management of intertriginous eruptions. They absorb moisture, prevent maceration, allay itching, soothe, protect mechanically, and reduce friction. The following is known as Prehn's Dusting Powder:

```
Fluffy Tannic Acid
Bentonite
Kaolin                     aa q.s. ad  60.0
```

Dispense in a sifter-top can.

Indications: Use this for hyperhidrosis of the feet and contact dermatitis of the feet due to shoe contactants.

Directions: Dust into shoes and socks daily.

Zeasorb Powder [Stiefel]
Indications and Directions: Follow the directions as above.

REFERENCES

1. Maddin S, Dodd W: Current Dermatologic Therapy, Philadelphia, Saunders, 1991.
2. Sulzberger MB, Wolf J, Witten VH, et al: *Dermatology: Diagnosis and Treatment,* 2d ed. Chicago, Year Book Publishers. 1961, pp 73–81.
3. Fruhstorfer H, Hermanns M, Latzke L: The effects of thermal stimulation on clinical and experimental itch. *Pain* 24:259–269, 1986.

4. Waldinger TP, Wong RC, Taylor WB, et al: Cryotherapy improves prurigo nodularis. *Arch Dermatol* 120:1598–1600, 1984.
5. Taylor, EA: Oil adsorption: A method for determining the affinity of skin to adsorb oil from aqueous dispersions of water-dispensable oil preparations. *J Invest Dermatol* 37:69, 1961.
6. Lubowe II: Treatment of pruritus and xerosis of various dermatoses: Evaluation of a bath oil. *West J Med* 1:45, 1960.
7. Bayoumi A-HM, Highet AS: Baking soda baths for aquagenic pruritus. *Lancet* 2:464, 1986.
8. Rajatanavin N, Withers A, Bernhard JD: Baking soda and pruritus. *Lancet* 2:977, 1986.
9. Aioardi C, Dost FH: Menthol and menthol-containing external remedies. International symposium on menthol and menthol-containing external remedies; use, mode of effect and tolerance in children. International symposium, Paris, April 1966; proceedings, edited by Do FH, Leiber B; contributors: Aioardi C, et al. Stuttgart, Thieme, 1966.
10. Anonymous: Hot water for itching. *Medical Lett Drug Ther* 13:52, 1971.
11. Green BG: Sensory characteristics of camphor. *J Invest Dermatol* 94:662–666, 1990.
12. Shuttleworth D, Hill S, Marks R, et al: Relief of experimentally induced pruritus with a novel eutectic mixture of local anaesthetic agents. *Br J Dermatol* 119:535–540, 1988.
13. Osol A (ed): *Remington's Pharmaceutical Sciences,* Easton, Penn, Mack Publishing. 1970, #16.
14. Lerner MR, Lerner AB: *Dermatologic Medications,* 2d ed. Chicago, Year Book Publishers, 1960.
15. Lynn B: Capsaicin: A probe for itching and related sensation. *Skin Pharmacol* 2:220, 1989.
16. Cappugi P, Lotti T, Tsampau D, et al: Capsaicin treatment of different dermatological afflictions with itching. *Skin Pharmacol* 2:230, 1989.
17. Wallengren A: Treatment of Notalgia paresthetica with capsaicin (Zostrix). *Skin Pharmacol* 2:229, 1989.
18. Toth-Casa I, et al: Capsaicin prevents histamine-induced itching. *Int J Clin Pharmacol Res* VI(2):163–169, 1986.
19. Breneman DL, et al: Topical capsaicin for treatment of pruritus related to hemodialysis. *Clin Pharmacol Ther* 45:2, 188, 1989.
20. Berberian B, Bernstein JE, Dodd WA, et al: Double-blind evaluation of capsaicin cream in pruritic psoriasis. *Clin Res* 38(2):664A, 1990.
21. Vaalasti A: Poster Exhibit at the Clinical Dermatology in the Year 2000. World Congress, London, May, 1990.
22. Kourennoff PM: *Russian Folk Medicine.* New York, Pyramid Books, 1971.
23. Fisher MFK: *A Cordiall Water.* London, Faber & Faber, 1961.
24. Jarvis DC: *Folk Medicine.* Greenwich, Conn. Fawcett Publications, 1965.
25. Tkac D (ed): *The Doctors Book of Home Remedies,* Emmaus, Penn, Rodale Press, 1990, p 572.

GENERAL REFERENCES

Arndt KA: *Manual of Dermatologic Therapeutics.* Boston, Little Brown and Company, 4th ed, 1988.
Bernhard JD: Pruritus: Advances in Treatment. *Advances in Dermatology,* 6, 1990.
Litt JZ: Alternative topical therapy, in Ely H, Thiers BH (eds): *Dermatologic Therapy II* (in Dermatologic Clinics), Philadelphia, Saunders, 1989, pp 43–52.
Reynolds JFF: *Martindale: The Extra Pharmacopoeia,* 28th ed. London, Pharmaceutical Press, 1982.
The Merck Index, llth ed. Rahway, N.J., Merck & Company, 1989.

TWENTY-EIGHT

PHOTOTHERAPY OF PRURITUS

Mark Lebwohl

PHOTOTHERAPY OF PRURITUS

The beneficial effects of sunlight on a number of skin conditions have been known for centuries, and psoriasis, one of the most light-responsive dermatoses, can be pruritic in a significant proportion of patients. In a study of 200 hospitalized psoriasis patients, pruritus was a prominent complaint in 80 percent.[1] As the pruritus of psoriasis responds to phototherapy along with the skin lesions, it may not be surprising that many pruritic conditions are also responsive to ultraviolet therapy (Table 28-1).

Ultraviolet therapy was first incorporated into a systematic in-hospital regimen by William Goeckerman in 1925.[2] That regimen consisted of daily quartz lamp exposures and crude coal tar applications. Subsequent modifications of the original regimen have eliminated the need for tars and decreased the frequency of treatment to three times per week, enabling patients to be treated on an outpatient basis. The increasing ease of administration of phototherapy has lead to its routine use in the treatment of many pruritic conditions, most notably uremic pruritus.

PUVA, also called photochemotherapy, has been a dramatically effective therapy for psoriasis since 1974. Modified forms of what we now call PUVA have been in use for the treatment of vitiligo for decades. PUVA is a very effective treatment, not only for psoriasis, but for numerous other pruritic dermatoses as well (Table 28-2). It is useful for several conditions, such as psoriasis and atopic dermatitis, which also respond to ultraviolet B (UVB).

Table 28-1 Administration of ultraviolet B[3]

1. Calculate the minimal erythema dose (MED).
2. Begin exposures with approximately 70 percent of the MED.
3. Increase 0 to 17 percent at each successive treatment, depending on patient response.
4. Determine holding dose based on skin type and response.
5. Maintenance treatments may be required.

For disorders that require concomitant administration of UVA, add approximately 1 J/cm^2 of UVA for every 10 mJ/cm^2 of UVB administered.

PUVA is often more effective in these conditions than UVB and patients who fail UVB can appropriately be started on PUVA. Several conditions, such as urticaria pigmentosa, appear to be uniquely responsive to PUVA, and others, such as solar urticaria and actinic reticuloid, are variably responsive and can easily be made worse by overaggressive administration of PUVA.

The aim of this chapter is to discuss the phototherapy of pruritus. What is known of the mechanisms by which phototherapy and photochemotherapy improve pruritus will be reviewed as will pruritic disorders that respond to phototherapy with UVB, UVA and UVB together, UVA (ultraviolet A) alone, or PUVA. The mechanisms of phototherapy are also presented briefly. As a lengthy discussion on the administration of phototherapy and photochemotherapy is beyond the scope of this chapter, the reader is referred to more detailed references for a more in depth review of the mechanics of phototherapy.[3,4] These are summarized in Tables 28-1 and 28-2.

Table 28-2 Administration of PUVA[3]

1. Appropriate blood tests and eye examinations should be obtained.
2. Patients must be given instructions about sun protection and ingestion of oral methoxsalen.
3. The appropriate dosage of methoxsalen (Oxsoralen) is 0.6 mg/kg p.o. 2 hours before exposure to UVA. A new liquid form of methoxsalen (Oxsoralen-ultra) is better absorbed and is prescribed in a dosage of 0.4 mg/kg p.o. 60–75 minutes before exposure to UVA.
4. Initial UVA dose depends on skin type and ranges from 0.5 J/cm^2 for skin type I patients up to 3.0 J/cm^2 for skin type VI. Provided patient has not burned, exposures for fair skinned patients are increased by 0.5 J/cm^2 at each visit. For black patients exposure may be increased by up to 1.5 J/cm^2 at each visit.
5. Patients are treated two to three times per week at least 48 hours apart and increments range from 0.5 to 1.5 J/cm^2 per visit depending on patient skin type and response.
6. Determine holding dose based on skin type and treatment response.
7. Maintenance treatments after clearing may be required.

UVB Phototherapy and Pruritus: Mechanism of Action

Despite substantial effort to determine how UVB improves pruritus, the precise mechanism has remained elusive. A systemic effect of UVB on pruritus was first demonstrated by Gilchrest and co-workers.[5] Patients with uremic pruritus were treated on one-half of their bodies with UVB and the other half with placebo consisting of low doses of UVA. All patients improved on both sides of the body indicating a systemic benefit resulting from UVB to half of the body. This has lead to the hypothesis that in patients with chronic renal failure, ultraviolet B somehow inactivates itch-inducing substances that Bernhard has called the "I factors".[6]

Over the years various investigators have attempted to pinpoint the nature of those factors responsible for uremic pruritus. (See Chap. 15.) Alteration of calcium metabolism as a cause of uremic pruritus has been suggested by several different lines of evidence. Several series have demonstrated rapid relief of uremic pruritus following subtotal parathyroidectomy in patients with renal failure and secondary hyperparathyroidism.[7,8] Recurrence of the uremic pruritus following infusion of calcium strongly suggests a role for calcium in the etiology of pruritus.[7] Blachley and colleagues[9] have demonstrated elevation of calcium, magnesium, and phosphorus in the skin of patients with uremic pruritus.[9] Treatment with UVB results in a reduction of cutaneous phosphorus, but not calcium or magnesium. These authors hypothesize the "microprecipitation" of calcium or magnesium phosphate as a cause of uremic pruritus. A role for divalent cations in the development of uremic pruritus is further supported by the observation that uremic pruritus can disappear after lowering of the concentration of magnesium in the dialysate.[10] It should be pointed out, however, that not all patients with renal failure and secondary hyperparathyroidism complain of itching and parathyroidectomy does not always relieve uremic pruritus.[11,12]

An increase in numbers of mast cells in the spleens and bone marrows of some patients with renal failure and a concomitant increase in serum histamine levels in some of those patients has lead to the hypothesis that uremic pruritus is histamine mediated.[13] A reduction in the itch response to histamine following exposure to UVB has been demonstrated by Fjellner and Hagermark.[14] Direct effects of ultraviolet radiation on mast cells have also been demonstrated.[15] Most recently, erythropoietin has been used successfully in the treatment of uremic pruritus and this therapy has resulted in a reduction in plasma histamine.[16]

Peripheral nerve dysfunction has also been suggested as a cause of uremic pruritus. Kumakiri and colleagues[17] have demonstrated profound effects of ultraviolet radiation, especially UVA, on cutaneous nerves. While a reduction in cutaneous nerve terminals has been demonstrated in patients with chronic renal failure, this abnormality does not correlate with the presence of uremic pruritus, and it is not clear that the benefit of phototherapy is related to a direct effect on cutaneous nerves.[18]

Elevation of epidermal vitamin A levels has also been demonstrated in patients with uremic pruritus and phototherapy with UVB results in a reduction of epidermal vitamin A levels to the normal range, a reduction that parallels the reduction in severity of uremic pruritus.[19] Although this has lead the authors to suggest that UVB reduces uremic pruritus by a mechanism that involves photoconversion of epidermal vitamin A, other authors have failed to show an association between serum vitamin A levels and uremic pruritus.[20]

Atrophy of sebaceous glands[21] and of eccrine sweat glands[22] in uremic skin have also been noted and the severity of uremic pruritus has been positively correlated with a degree of xerosis.[23] As UVB can result in xerosis, its beneficial effect on uremic pruritus suggests that another mechanism is at work. Whether UVB has a direct effect on the "itch factors" of uremic pruritus or an indirect beneficial effect on the symptom of itching remains to be determined. It should be noted that UVA has been used successfully in the treatment of uremic pruritus.[24] The authors reporting success of UVA in the treatment of uremic pruritus, however, also noted a similar reduction in itching in placebo-treated control patients, suggesting a placebo response.[25,26]

The mechanisms of action of ultraviolet light in the treatment of other forms of pruritus have been less well studied. Phototherapy results in marked improvement in the pruritus of primary biliary cirrhosis.[27] In some patients there is concomitant reduction in serum bile acids. At least one author has found that UVA is more effective than UVB in the treatment of cholestatic pruritus.[28] Nonspecific effects of ultraviolet light on an "itch receptor" have been suggested by one group of authors[27] while another group has suggested that phototherapy reduces cutaneous bile acid levels resulting in relief of itching.[29] Naloxone, an opioid antagonist, can improve the pruritus of primary biliary cirrhosis, suggesting that opioid activity is involved in cholestatic pruritus, but this does not explain the beneficial effects of phototherapy.[30] Perhaps UVB exerts an effect on the peripheral or central metabolism of opioid molecules.

PUVA and Pruritus: Mechanism of Action

Orally ingested or topically applied psoralens intercalate between DNA base pairs. Exposure to UVA results in the formation of monofunctional and bifunctional adducts of pyrimidine bases in DNA. This results in cross linkage of DNA strands and suppression of DNA synthesis and cell division. This has been presumed to be the main mechanism of benefit in psoriasis. However, other mechanisms may be at work in pruritic skin diseases benefited by PUVA. Formation of reactive oxygen species, free radicals, and reactive photoexcited psoralens affect DNA, RNA, proteins, and cell membranes.[31] Phototoxic effects of PUVA on circulating lymphocytes and on immune function may also play a role in the beneficial effects observed in some pruritic dermatoses. Stimulation of melanogenesis also occurs and may account for some benefit seen in photosensitivity disorders.

In contrast to the systemic benefit of UVB in the treatment of uremic pruritus, PUVA appears to have a local effect for many of the conditions for which it is beneficial. Polymorphous light eruption, for example, will only benefit in exposed areas. Areas shielded during PUVA therapy remain photosensitive. Similarly, in atopic dermatitis Morison and co-workers[32] demonstrated that PUVA therapy only has a local beneficial effect on treated areas. In a bilateral paired comparison trial in which half the body was shielded from UVA, only the side exposed to PUVA showed an improvement in atopic dermatitis.

While some of the local protective effect of PUVA may be due to increased pigmentation and epidermal thickening, other factors must be at work as well. Photosensitive eczema, for example, responds to PUVA therapy with a reduction in photosensitivity that is so great that it cannot be explained only on the basis of tanning and epidermal thickening. Solar urticaria is another condition in which patients with exquisite sun sensitivity can be effectively made sun-tolerant by treatment with PUVA and occasionally with UVA phototherapy. Both treatments cause degranulation of mast cells and repeated exposures to UVA can maintain this degranulated state. PUVA ultimately stabilizes mast cell membranes, producing mast cells that are less likely to degranulate and cause urticaria.[33]

Administration of UVB

Several different regimens exist for the administration of UVB, but most have some features in common. Starting doses depend on the patient's Fitzpatrick skin type. Initial doses usually range from under 10 mJ per cm^2 for patients with type I skin (always burn, never tan) to 50 mJ per cm^2 or more for black patients with type VI skin. As energy output is determined by radiometers that are easily miscalibrated, determinations may be inaccurate. Starting doses are therefore often determined by the phototherapist's previous experience using the same phototherapy unit. Alternatively, UVB can be started at 50 to 80 percent of the minimal erythema dose. Increments again depend on the patient's skin type and whether or not the patient has developed erythema. Increments usually range from 0 to 100 percent of the initial treatment dose. Patients can be treated from three to five times per week. Some conditions, such as uremic pruritus, may respond to treatment regimens as infrequent as once or twice per week (see Table 28-1).

Administration of PUVA

Methoxsalen must be ingested either 2 hours (Oxsoralen) or roughly 1 hour and 15 minutes (Oxsoralen-ultra) before exposure to UVA. Methoxsalen dosages range from 0.6 to 0.8 mg/kg body weight for Oxsoralen and 0.3 to 0.4 mg/kg for Oxsoralen-ultra. Starting doses of UVA can be determined by minimal phototoxicity dose testing as is widely done in Europe or by the Fitzpatrick skin type. The number of joules/cm^2 administered by the latter method is the skin type multiplied by one half. Thus, for a patient with skin type III (sometimes burns but always tans), 1.5 J/cm^2 would be administered. Increments are similarly based on the skin type or minimal phototoxicity dose. Patients should be treated two or three times per week, preferably on alternate days as burns caused by PUVA may only begin to be apparent at 24 hours (see Table 28-2).

DISORDERS TREATED WITH ULTRAVIOLET LIGHT

Uremic Pruritus

With the introduction of hemodialysis, the longevity of patients with chronic renal failure has increased dramatically and, not surprisingly, there has been a concomitant increase in the prevalence and duration of uremic pruritus. (See Chap. 15.) UVB was first used for uremic pruritus in 1975.[34] Shortly thereafter, Gilchrest and colleagues[5] examined three phototherapy schedules varying from one to three treatments per week. The percentage of patients responding to treatment was not influenced by the frequency of UVB exposure, although patients treated three times weekly tended to respond more quickly. In that study, 32 of 38 patients improved after six or eight exposures to UVB. Fifteen of the patients experienced a recurrence of pruritus after a mean remission of 3 months. Sixteen of the patients were free of pruritus for a mean of at least 10.6 months at the time of that report. When relapses were again treated with UVB phototherapy, improvement occurred even more quickly than during the initial treatment.

Primary Biliary Cirrhosis

The mechanism of itching in primary biliary cirrhosis is discussed in Chap. 16. Traditional treatment has been with oral cholestyramine. Phototherapy for this condition was first attempted following a British patient's observation that her itching disappeared while sunbathing in Italy. Based on that observation, Hanid and Levi[27] treated six women with primary biliary cirrhosis and severe pruritus. Exposure to gradually increasing ultraviolet light from a mercury vapor lamp over 10 days resulted in resolution of itching in five of the six patients within 1 week. A reduction in serum-bile acid was noted in four of these five responding patients. The sole nonresponding patient had an increase in serum bile acids. When phototherapy was discontinued the pruritus returned within 2 weeks. One of the patients continued ultraviolet light treatment twice weekly for over 2 years and remained free of itching during that time except during periods when she missed her treatments.

Anecdotal reports further support a beneficial role for UVB in the treatment of primary biliary cirrhosis. One author claims success when only UVA is used.[28] It has been our practice to treat patients with a combination of UVA and UVB using a regimen similar to that used for psoriasis. For every 10 mJ of UVB administered, we simply add approximately 1 J of UVA. The combination of phototherapy with oral cholestyramine for the treatment of pruritus in patients with primary biliary cirrhosis has also been advocated.[29]

Atopic Dermatitis

Many patients with atopic dermatitis note improvement of their symptoms after exposure to summer sun or after vacationing in sunny climates. It would therefore be reasonable to expect that phototherapy would be beneficial. In fact, the Goeckerman regimen combining ultraviolet light and tars for psoriasis has also been used successfully for atopic dermatitis. Most recently, Midelfart and co-workers[35] have suggested the combination of UVB and UVA for the treatment of atopic dermatitis. They treated 23 patients with a combination of UVB and UVA and 33 patients with UVB alone. In the combination treatment group, 48 percent of patients cleared completely and another 48 percent noted good improvement. In the UVB group only 27 percent completely cleared and 58 percent achieved good results. Thus, the combination of UVA and UVB was found to be better than UVB alone. Most recently, high dose UVA #1 alone has shown promise in the treatment of atopic dermatitis.[36] (UVA #1 consists of the portion of UVA radiation greater than 340 nanometers.) UVA #1 was administered daily at a dose of 130 joules/cm². Significant improvement was noted in 1 week.

PUVA has also been found to be effective in the treatment of atopic dermatitis and, in one study, was found to be much more effective than UVB alone. Morison and co-workers treated 15 patients with severe atopic dermatitis uncontrolled by topical and oral steroids. The patients were divided into three groups: whole body PUVA (5 patients), PUVA on one side of the body and only lubricants on the other side (5 patients), and PUVA on one side of the body with UVB to the other side (5 patients). The results showed an unequivocal dramatic local response to PUVA. In the whole body PUVA group, patients experienced 99 percent clearance in 20 to 58 treatments. In patients treated with PUVA on one side only, there was 95 percent clearance on the PUVA treated side but no change on the untreated side. Finally, in patients treated with PUVA on one side and UVB on the other, eczema cleared by 95 percent in 7 to 12 treatments compared to an exacerbation of eczema in four patients out of five on the UVB treated side. Unfortunately, the beneficial effects of PUVA were short lived. Weekly maintenance treatments were required in most of the treated patients and most of the patients experienced exacerbations during the maintenance phase that followed clearing. The exacerbations generally occurred when a reduction in the frequency of maintenance treatments was attempted. Fortunately, the flares of eczema again responded to a clearing regimen of PUVA with two or three treatments per week and a higher dose of UVA. Also noteworthy was the dramatic response of blepharitis to 4 to 10 exposures of PUVA in which patients did not wear goggles and simply kept their eyes closed during treatment.[32] As ocular toxicity is of concern in patients treated with PUVA, it is noteworthy that UVA does not penetrate through the eyelids.[37] Thus, treatment of the eyelids can be undertaken in patients with atopic blepharitis.

Photosensitivity Disorders

Phototherapy and photochemotherapy can be easily performed for some photosensitive conditions such as polymorphous light eruption. Other conditions such as actinic reticuloid, chronic photosensitive eczema, and solar urticaria are treatable with PUVA but the treatment of these conditions is difficult, fraught with risk, and best performed in a center experienced in the treatment of these disorders.

Solar urticaria is characterized by the abrupt onset of pruritus and hives within minutes following sun exposure. Phototesting should be performed on small areas of skin to determine the responsible wavelength of light, as UVB, UVA, or even, rarely, visible radiation can elicit the reaction. Exposure of small areas of skin to small increments in dose of the appropriate light source should be performed to establish the minimum urtication dose. If UVA does not cause the urticaria, patients can be treated three times a week with a PUVA schedule similar to that used in psoriasis. When solar urticaria is caused by UVA, patients are started at a dose that is 80 percent of the minimum urtication dose. Because of the risks of eliciting urticaria with the treatment, only one part of the body should be treated at a time. The dose of UVA can be increased by 0.1 to 0.5 Joules/cm^2, three times per week. Patients are exposed to sunlight once a week and after 4 to 10 weeks of treatment, they are usually able to tolerate at least 1 hour of sun exposure. To maintain tolerance, patients should expose themselves to sunlight for at least 1 or 2 hours every week. Occasionally UVA therapy without oral psoralens can desensitize patients. Alternatively, gradually increasing exposure to the responsible wavelength of light will result in solar urticaria but repeating the exposure at hourly intervals may cause degranulation of mast cells so that the skin becomes tolerant to light. Once tolerance is achieved, patients must expose themselves to light on a daily basis to maintain the tolerance.[3,33]

PUVA therapy of chronic photosensitive eczema, photosensitivity associated with atopic dermatitis, persistent light reaction, and actinic reticuloid is particularly risky because these symptoms can be severe and are often triggered by exposure to UVA. Consequently, patients with these disorders are often treated in the hospital and are first started on high doses of prednisone. The minimum photosensitizing dose of UVA is first determined. This must be done with great care as some patients are so exquisitely sensitive to UVA that even small amounts of UVA penetrating clothing are able to elicit a reaction. Patients are then started on oral prednisone at dosages that may be as high as 100 mg per day and some centers then start patients on a PUVA regimen similar to that used for psoriasis.[3,38] Because severe flair-ups can occur, it has been our practice to repeat minimum photosensitivity dose testing while on prednisone and start PUVA at a UVA dosage less than the minimum photosensitivity dose. Patients are treated three times per week and prednisone can be tapered off over approximately 4 to 6 weeks. Once patients are tolerant of sunlight, weekly maintenance treatments are continued. Oral azathioprine is sometimes used alone or in combination with PUVA in these settings.

Lichen Planus

This very pruritic eruption can be effectively treated with photochemotherapy. In an early trial of PUVA for lichen planus, Ortonne and co-workers[39] treated seven patients with UVA doses starting at 1.5 to 2 J/cm^2 that were gradually increased to a maximum of 7 J/cm^2. Patients were started at three treatments per week but the number of treatments was gradually increased to five per week. Pruritus disappeared between the second and fifth week of treatment, and six of the seven patients experienced complete clearing. This was confirmed histologically with disappearance of the superficial dermal infiltrate. The total number of treatments to clearing ranged from 17 to 48 and the total dose of UVA administered ranged from 58 to 230 J/cm^2.

Gonzales and colleagues[40] performed a bilateral comparison study of 10 patients with lichen planus, treating only one half of the body. The duration of lichen planus in these patients ranged from 1 month to 2 years and many had been treated with systemic corticosteroids without complete resolution of the condition. A psoriasis protocol was followed in treating the patients with PUVA and 5 of the 10 patients cleared completely on both sides of the body, suggesting some systemic benefit. Three other patients had marked improvement but one of these relapsed and was considered a treatment failure as were two other patients. No maintenance treatments were administered and at the time of publication all patients in complete remission had remained free of the disorder for up to 4 years. Thus, PUVA therapy may cure lichen planus and because prolonged maintenance therapy is not necessary, the side effects of PUVA are minimized. It should be noted that some patients may experience a temporary exacerbation of lichen planus on start-ing PUVA. Also of interest was the observation that both black patients en-rolled in the latter study were among the treatment failures.[40] In our photo-therapy unit, however, we have successfully treated a black patient with lichen planus.

Miscellaneous Disorders

Small trials and anecdotal reports have supported the use of phototherapy and photochemotherapy for a number of other pruritic conditions. Eosino-philic pustular folliculitis associated with human immunodeficiency virus in-fection responds to ultraviolet B after only six to nine treatments.[41] PUVA has also been successfully used in the treatment of pruritus associated with AIDS.[42] Because of concern over possible immunosuppressive effects of PUVA, many patients are reluctant to undergo this treatment even though clinically significant immunosuppression does not occur. The immunosup-pressive effects of ultraviolet B have not been addressed in the treatment of this disorder, but they are also likely to be clinically insignificant.

Five patients with dermatitis herpetiformis who either did not respond to a gluten-free diet and dapsone or did not tolerate dapsone were suc-cessfully treated with PUVA. Skin lesions improved after only 3 weeks of treatment and immunoglobulin A (IgA) and C3 disappeared from the skin. In all patients symptoms recurred within 2 weeks to 2 months but mainte-nance PUVA again resulted in remission.[43] One patient with disabling pruritus associated with polycythemia vera responded to PUVA[44] as did a patient with Grover's disease (transient acantholytic dermatosis).[45] Three patients with diffuse granuloma annulare improved with PUVA including one patient who remained clear for at least $3\frac{1}{2}$ years after treatment.[46] A solitary patient with the hypereosinophilic syndrome also responded to PUVA[47] as did a patient with generalized lichen nitidus, which is not surprising considering the latter disorder's similarities to lichen planus.[48]

Fifteen patients with prurigo nodularis were treated with trioxsalen baths followed by UVA exposure. Of the 15 patients, 13 achieved good to excellent results,[49] and in our center we have observed some benefit with oral PUVA for this condition. Two patients with persistent pruritus due to insect bite reactions have also been successfully treated with PUVA.[50]

Macular amyloidosis has been successfully treated with both UVB and PUVA.[51] Both of these treatments are also successful for many patients with chronic idiopathic pruritus. All possible causes of pruritus must first be con-sidered including scabies and atopic dermatitis. Systemic disorders such as Hodgkin's disease, uremic pruritus, and cholestatic pruritus must also be ruled out. A thorough review of medications should be undertaken as well. In elderly patients early bullous pemphigoid can present with pruritus even in the absence of skin lesions. Once known causes of pruritus are eliminated, it is our practice to start patients on a course of treatment with UVB three times per week. If that regimen is ineffective within approximately 10 to 15 treatments, patients are switched to PUVA.

Chronic urticaria has also been successfully treated with PUVA.[3] Urticaria pigmentosa also responds to PUVA with relief of pruritus and resolution of skin lesions. Histologic examinations show a reduction in mast cell numbers in the papillary dermis and a lower histamine content of lesional skin. Remissions are unfortunately short lived and regular maintenance therapy is required.[52] PUVA is also effective in the treatment of aquagenic pruritus.[53]

REFERENCES

1. Newbold PCH: Pruritus in psoriasis, in Farber EM, Cox AJ (eds): *Psoriasis: Proceedings of the Second International Symposium.* New York, Yorke Medical Books. 1977, p 334.
2. Goeckerman WH: Treatment of psoriasis. *Northwest Med* 23:229–231, 1925.
3. Morison WL: *Phototherapy and Photochemotherapy of Skin Disease,* 2 ed. New York, Raven Press, 1991.
4. Epstein JH, Farber EM, Nall L, et al: Current status of oral PUVA therapy for psoriasis. *J Am Acad Dermatol* 1:106–117, 1979.
5. Gilchrest BA, Rowe JW, Brown RS, et al: Ultraviolet phototherapy of uremic pruritus: Long-term results and possible mechanism of action. *Ann Intern Med* 91:17–21, 1979.
6. Bernhard JD: Pruritus: Advances in Treatment. *Adv Dermatol* 6:57–71, 1991.
7. Hampers CL, Katz AI, Wilson RE, et al: Disappearance of "uremic" itching after subtotal parathyroidectomy. *N Engl J Med* 279:695–697, 1968.
8. Kleeman CR, Massry SG, Popovtzer MM, et al: The disappearance of intractable pruritus after parathyroidectomy in uremic patients with secondary hyperparathyroidism. *Trans Assoc Am Physicians* 81:203–212, 1968.
9. Blachley JD, Blankenship M, Menter A, et al: Uremic pruritus: Skin divalent ion content and response to ultraviolet phototherapy. *Am J Kidney Dis* 5:237–241, 1985.
10. Graf H, Kovarik J, Stummvoll HK, et al: Disappearance of uraemic pruritus after lowering dialysate magnesium concentration. *BMJ* 2:1478, 1979.
11. Young AW, Sweeney EW, David DS, et al: Dermatologic evaluation of pruritus in patients on hemodialysis. *N Y State J Med* 73:2670–2674, 1973.
12. Rosen T: Uremic pruritus: A review. *Cutis* 23:790–792, 1979.
13. Neiman RS, Bischel MD, Lukes RJ: Uraemia and mast-cell proliferation. *Lancet* 20:959, 1972.
14. Fjellner B, Hagermark O: Influence of ultraviolet light on itch and flare reactions in human skin induced by histamine and the histamine liberator compound 48/80. *Acta Derm Venereol* 62:137–140, 1982.
15. Fjellner B: Experimental and clinical pruritus: Studies on some putative peripheral mediators; the influence of ultraviolet light and transcutaneous nerve stimulation. *Acta Derm Venereol Suppl* 97:1–34, 1981.
16. DeMarchi S, Cecchin E, Villalta D, et al: Relief of pruritus and decreases in plasma histamine concentrations during erythropoietin therapy in patients with uremia. *N Engl J Med* 326:969–974, 1992.
17. Kumakiri M, Hashimoto K, Willis I: Biological changes of human cutaneous nerves caused by ultraviolet irradiation: An ultrastructural study. *Br J Dermatol* 99:65–75, 1978.
18. Fantini F, Baraldi A, Sevignani C, et al: Cutaneous innervation in chronic renal failure patients: An immunohistochemical study. *Acta Derm Venereol* 72:102–105, 1992.

19. Berne B, Vahlquist A, Fischer T, et al: UV treatment of uraemic pruritus reduces the vitamin A content of the skin. *Eur J Clin Invest* 14:203–206, 1984.

20. de Kroes S, Smeenk G: Serum vitamin A levels and pruritus in patients on hemodialysis. *Dermatologica* 166:199–202, 1983.

21. Rosenthal SR: Uremic dermatitis. *Arch Dermatol Syph* 23:934–945, 1931.

22. Cawley EP, Hoch-Ligeti C, Bond GM: The eccrine sweat glands of patients in uremia. *Arch Dermatol* 84:889–897, 1961.

23. Nielsen T, Hemmeloff Andersen KE, Kristiansen J: Pruritus and xerosis in patients with chronic renal failure. *Dan Med Bull* 27:269–271, 1980.

24. Hindson C, Taylor A, Martin A, et al: UVA light for relief of uraemic pruritus. *Lancet* 1:215, 1981.

25. Spiro JG, Scott S, MacMillan J, et al: Treatment of uremic pruritus with blue light. *Photodermatol Photoimmunol Photomed* 2:319–321, 1985.

26. Taylor R, Taylor AEM, Diffey BL, et al: A placebo-controlled trial of UV-A phototherapy for the treatment of uraemic pruritus. *Nephron* 33:14–16, 1983.

27. Hanid MA, Levi AJ: Phototherapy for pruritus in primary biliary cirrhosis. *Lancet* 2:530, 1980.

28. Person JR: Ultraviolet A (UV-A) and cholestatic pruritus. *Arch Dermatol* 117:684, 1981.

29. Cerio R, Murphy GM, Sladen GE, et al: A combination of phototherapy and cholestyramine for the relief of pruritus in primary biliary cirrhosis. *Br J Dermatol* 116:265–267, 1987.

30. Bergasa NV, Talbot TL, Alling DW, et al: A controlled trial of naloxone infusions for the pruritus of chronic cholestasis. *Gastroenterology* 102:544–549, 1992.

31. Honigsmann H, Wolff K, Fitzpatrick TB, et al: Oral photochemotherapy with psoralens and UVA (PUVA): Principles and practice, in Fitzpatrick TB, Eisen AZ, Wolff K, et al (eds): *Dermatology in General Medicine*, 3 ed. New York, McGraw-Hill. 1987, Chap 12, pp 1533–1538.

32. Morison WL, Parrish JA, Fitzpatrick TB: Oral psoralen photochemotherapy of atopic eczema. *Br J Dermatol* 98:25–30, 1978.

33. Bernhard JD, Jaenicke K, Momtaz-T K, et al: Ultraviolet A phototherapy in the prophylaxis of solar urticaria. *J Am Acad Dermatol* 10:29–33, 1984.

34. Saltzer EI: Relief from uremic pruritus: A therapeutic approach. *Cutis* 16:298–299, 1975.

35. Midelfart K, Stenvold S, Volden G: Combined UVB and UVA phototherapy of atopic eczema. *Dermatologica* 171:95–98, 1985.

36. Krutmann J, Czech W, Diepgen T, et al: High-dose UVA1 therapy in the treatment of patients with atopic dermatitis. *J Am Acad Dermatol* 26:225–230, 1992.

37. Prystowsky JH, Keen MS, DeLeo VA: Measurement of the transmittance of ultraviolet and visible radiation through human eyelids. *Photochem Photobiol* 51:35, 1990.

38. Morison WL, White HAD, Gonzalez E, et al: Oral methoxsalen photochemotherapy of uncommon photodermatoses. *Acta Derm Venereol* (Stockh) 59:366–368, 1979.

39. Ortonne JP, Thivolet J, Sannwald C: Oral photochemotherapy in the treatment of lichen planus (LP). *Br J Dermatol* 99:77–88, 1978.

40. Gonzalez E, Momtaz-T K, Freedman S: Bilateral comparison of generalized lichen planus treated with psoralens and ultraviolet A. *J Am Acad Dermatol* 10:958–961, 1984.

41. Buchness MR, Lim HW, Hatcher VA, et al: Eosinophilic pustular folliculitis in the acquired immunodeficiency syndrome: Treatment with ultraviolet B phototherapy. *N Engl J Med* 318:1183–1186, 1988.

42. Gorin I, Lessana-Leibowitch M, Fortier P, et al: Successful treatment of the pruritus of human immunodeficiency virus infection and acquired immunodeficiency syndrome with psoralens plus ultraviolet A therapy. *J Am Acad Dermatol* 20:511–514, 1989.

43. Kalimo K, Lammintausta K, Viander M, et al: PUVA treatment of dermatitis herpetiformis. *Photodermatol Photoimmunol Photomed* 3:54–55, 1986.

44. Swerlick RA: Photochemotherapy treatment of pruritus associated with polycythemia vera. *J Am Acad Dermatol* 13:675–677, 1985.

45. Paul BS, Arndt KA: Response of transient acantholytic dermatosis to photochemotherapy. *Arch Dermatol* 120:121–122, 1984.
46. Hindson TC, Spiro JG, Cochrane H: PUVA therapy of diffuse granuloma annulare. *Clin Exp Dermatol* 13:26–27, 1988.
47. Van den Hoogenband HM, van den Berg WHHW, van Diggelen MW: PUVA therapy in the treatment of skin lesions of the hypereosinophilic syndrome. *Arch Dermatol* 121:450, 1985.
48. Randle HW, Sander HM: Treatment of generalized lichen nitidus with PUVA. *Int J Dermatol* 25:330–331, 1986.
49. Vaatainen N, Hannuksela M, Karvonen J: Local photochemotherapy in nodular prurigo. *Acta Derm Venereol* (Stockh) 59:544–547, 1979.
50. Beacham BE, Kurgansky D: Persistent bite reactions responsive to photochemotherapy. *Br J Dermatol* 123:693–694, 1990.
51. Hudson LD: Macular amyloidosis: Treatment with ultraviolet. *Cutis* 38:61–62, 1986.
52. Kolde G, Frosch PJ, Czarnetzki BM: Response of cutaneous mast cells to PUVA in patients with urticaria pigmentosa: Histomorphometric, ultrastructural, and biochemical investigations. *J Invest Dermatol* 83:175–178, 1984.
53. Menagé HDP, Norris PG, Hawk JLM, et al: The efficacy of psoralen photochemotherapy in the treatment of aquagenic pruritus. *Br J Dermatol* 129:163–165, 1993.

ANTIHISTAMINES

Lori E. U. Herman

INTRODUCTION

Antihistamines are among the most widely used medications in the world.

A survey of American households conducted in 1984 suggested that more than 30 million people in the United States take antihistamines every year. In 1987, the combined sales of over-the-counter and prescription single-entity antihistamines totaled $211 million.

Histamine, a neurotransmitter widely distributed throughout the body, acts as a chemical messenger via interaction with three distinct histamine receptors, H_1, H_2, and H_3, each with a specific function. This interaction leads to a range of biologic actions, many of which were first described in a series of articles by Dale and Laidlaw.[1-3]

Receptors for these compounds have now been identified on virtually every tissue in the human body, although all three classes of antihistamine are not universally present on every tissue. H_1 receptors are located in the brain and act as an alerting mechanism for the central nervous system. Their blockade is responsible for the sedative effect of antihistamines. H_2 receptors mediate the secretion of gastric acid and various other hormones. H_3 receptors appear to be involved in vasodilation and/or vasoconstriction of blood vessels. Several comprehensive reviews on this subject have appeared in the literature in recent years.[4-6]

HISTORICAL BACKGROUND

The search for this class of compounds began after the role of histamine in the anaphylactoid reaction was postulated in 1929. In 1937 Bovet and Staub reported that one of a group of phenolic esters inhibited some of the actions of histamine, such as anaphylactic shock and smooth muscle contraction.[7] This substance, 2-isopropyl-5-methyl-phenoxyethyl-diethylamine, protected guinea pigs against a series of otherwise lethal doses of histamine. Early compounds were too toxic for human use but a dimethylamine derivative, Antergan, first researched by Halpern,[8] proved safe for clinical use.

Subsequently, various compounds including diphenhydramine[9] and tripelennamine,[10] were synthesized in the United States.[11] These original H_1 blockers were chemical alterations of the basic structure of histamine through substitution of the imidazole ring. By increasing the bulk of this structure, a number of antihistamines were synthesized.

Following the discovery of histamine antagonists, suspicion that histamine was acting through specific binding sites was confirmed first by Folkow and co-workers in 1948[12,12a] and later by Furchgott and colleagues in 1955.[12b] In 1966 the H_1 receptor was identified but blockade of this site by available antihistamines uniformly failed to inhibit gastric acid secretion.[13]

The discovery of H_2 receptors soon followed and led to the introduction by Black and colleagues in 1972 of a new class of drugs that selectively inhibits gastric acid secretion.[12] A third type of histamine receptor, H_3, has now been identified as participating in auto-inhibition of histamine release in the brain.[14]

PHARMACOLOGY

All histamine antagonists reversibly and competitively inhibit the interaction of histamine with its receptor. These agents can conveniently be divided into the classic sedating histamine blocking agents, the newer nonsedating histamine blocking agents and tricyclic antidepressants. These will each be discussed separately (Table 29-1).

Traditional Antihistamines

Mechanism of action. Antihistamines competitively inhibit the action of histamine on its receptors. Once histamine has been released and bound to its receptors, however, they are unable to reverse its actions. Thus antihistamines are used more effectively as preventive therapy rather than as treatment for the symptoms of allergy and anaphylaxis. Symptoms frequently improve but, as events lead to the release of histamine often also trigger release or synthesis of a variety of mediator substances, relief is often only partial. Histamine itself induces the liberation of proinflammatory chemicals such as Substance P.

Over the past decade much research has been done on the absorption, dispersion, metabolism and excretion of conventional H_1 antagonists. These

Table 29-1 Oral Antihistamines

Chemical Type	Generic Name	Brand Name	Usual Adult Dosage	Formulations
Carbon-Linked alkylamines	Brompheniramine maleate	Dimetane	4 mg q4–6h	4 mg tablet; liquid
	Extended-release	Dimetane Extentabs	8–12 mg q8–12h	8 mg, 12 mg tablet
	Chlorpheniramine maleate	Chlor-Trimeton	4 mg q 4–6h	4 mg tab; liquid
	Extended-release	Chlor-Trimeton Repetabs	8–12 mg q 8–12h	8 mg, 12 mg tab; cap
		Teldrin	12 mg q 12h	12 mg tablet
	Dexchlorpheniramine maleate	Polaramine	2 mg q 4–6h	2 mg tablet; liquid
	Extended release	Polaramine Repetabs	4–6 mg q 8–10h	4 mg, 6 mg tablets
Ethanolamines	Triprolidine HCl	Actidil	2.5 mg q 4–6h	2.5 mg tablet; liq
	Clemastine fumarate	Tavist	1.34–2.68 mg q 12h	2.68 mg tablet
		Tavist-1	1.34 mg q 12h	1.34 mg tablet
	Diphenhydramine HCl	Benadryl	25–50 mg q 4–6h (max 300 mg/day)	25 mg, 50 mg liquid, tablets, capsules
		Benadryl OTC		
	Carbinoxamine maleate	Rondec	4 mg q 6h	4 mg tab, syrup
	Extended release	Rondec-TR	8 mg q 12h	12 mg tablets
	Dimenhydrinate	Dramamine	50–100 mg q 4–6h	50 mg tabs, syrup
	Doxylamine succinate	Decapryn	25 mg	25 mg tablets
Ethylene diamines	Tripelennamine HCl	PBZ	25–50 mg q 4–6h (max 600 mg/day)	50 mg tablets
		PBZ-SR	100 mg q 8–12h	100 mg tablets
	Pyrilamine maleate	Fiogesic	25 mg q 6–8h	25 mg tablets

(continued)

Table 29-1 Continued

Chemical Type	Generic Name	Brand Name	Usual Adult Dosage	Formulations
Phenothiazines	Promethazine-HCl	Phenergan	12.5 mg q 12h or 25 mg qhs	12.5 mg, 25 mg tablets, liquid
	Methdilazine	Tacaryl	8 mg q 6–12h	8 mg tab; syrup
	Trimeprazine tartrate	Temaril	2.5 mg q 6h	2.5 mg tabs; syrup
	Extended release		5 mg q 12h	5 mg spansules
Piperazines	Buclizine HCl	Bucladin-S	50 mg q 8h	50 mg chewtabs
	Meclizine HCl	Bonine	25–50 mg q 24h	25 mg chewtabs
		Antivert	25–50 mg q 24h	12.5,25,50 mg tabs
Piperidines	Azatadine maleate	Optimine	1–2 mg q 12h	1 mg tablets
	Cyproheptadine HCl	Periactin	4 mg q 6–8h	4 mg tablets, liquid
	Terfenadine	Seldane	60 mg q 12h	60 mg tablets
	Astemizole	Hismanal	10 mg/day	10 mg tablets
	Loradadine	Claritin	10 mg/day	10 mg tablets
Tricyclic antidepressants	Doxepin HCl	Adapin or Sinequan	10–75 mg qhs	10–150 mg tablets
			10 mg q 8h	10 mg tablets
Miscellaneous	Hydroxyzine HCl	Atarax	10–50 mg q 6h	10,25,50 mg tabs, liquid
	Diphenylpyraline	Hispril	5 mg q 12h	5 mg spansule

This table includes examples from each class of antihistamines but is not intended to be all inclusive.

compounds are rapidly and well absorbed from the gastrointestinal tract following oral ingestion with beneficial effects developing within 15 to 30 minutes of administration.[15] Peak serum concentrations are attained within 1 to 3 hours[16] and physiological effects are maximal within 1 to 2 hours, persisting about 3 to 6 hours.[15] Exceptions to this include meclizine hydrochloride, the effects of which may last from 12 to 24 hours, and hydroxyzine, which has a half-life in adults of roughly 20 hours.[17]

Extensive studies of the metabolic fate of H_1 antagonists have been restricted to a few agents chiefly because preparations for intravenous administration are not available for most of these compounds. The two most extensively studied compounds from which most of the data are derived are diphenhydramine and chlorpheniramine.

Oral administration of diphenhydramine results in peak concentrations in the blood at about 2 hours post ingestion.[18] It persists at about this level for another 2 hours and then diminishes in concentration exponentially with a plasma elimination half-life varying between 3.4 and 9.3 hours.[18–20] Studies carried out on chlorpheniramine show a similar pattern.[21]

Classic H_1 antihistamines are extensively dispersed throughout the body, including the central nervous system (CNS), and studies suggest that minimal elimination of nonmetabolized antihistamine occurs. In man, most of the H_1 blockers undergo extensive biotransformation in the liver, frequently to active metabolites. It has therefore been difficult to determine the relationship between plasma antihistamine concentrations and therapeutic and undesired ill effects.[22] In the case of chlorpheniramine only about 11% of unchanged chlorpheniramine is recovered from the urine,[23] for diphenhydramine approximately 2% is recovered unchanged.[22]

New second- and third-generation antihistamines such as astemizole, terfenadine, and loratadine compete with histamine for receptors on various cell surfaces and have the added capability of inhibiting the release of a variety of inflammatory mast cell mediators.

Differences in chemical structure may account for these unique properties. Traditional antihistamines possess an ethylamine moiety that is similar in composition to histamine. New nonsedating antihistamines have a distinct tricyclic-ringed structure that may account, at least in part, for some of the properties attributed to these agents.

Azatadine, like other second-generation antihistamines, has the ability to selectively inhibit mediator release from mast cells, but like classic antihistamines, is still quite sedating. True third-generation H_1-receptor blockers, represented by astemizole and terfenidine, however, have the ability to stabilize mast cells while causing no more sedation than placebo. They are thus also referred to as the "nonsedating" antihistamines. Intermediate between these two classes in terms of sedative properties are loratidine, the breakdown product of azatadine, and cetirizine, the breakdown product of hydroxyzine.

Sedative effects are encountered only when high doses of these medications are administered.

Sedative effects. Traditional antihistamines may act either to stimulate or depress the CNS. The mechanism by which this occurs remains elusive. These agents, however, are very lipid soluble, readily cross the blood-brain barrier,[24] and bind with high affinity to cerebral H_1-receptors.[5] Symptoms of excitation usually indicate toxicity. Severe toxicity is most often observed in children and can lead to convulsions. Central depression is evidenced by diminished alertness, delayed reaction time, and somnolence.

Positron emission tomography studies indicate that the H_1 receptors in the brain are primarily located in the more primitive midbrain. The sedative effects of antihistamines, however, appear to be mediated in much higher functioning regions of the brain engaged in memory, alertness, and awareness of the environment.[25] Although antihistamines have been available for years, attempts at predicting the degree of sedative effects have been fraught with problems. Generally, the ethanolamine class, including diphenhydramine, is considered more sedating than agents of the piperazine class such as hydroxyzine and cyproheptadine.

Nonsedating Antihistamines

Mechanism of action. There has been a renewal of interest in antihistamine therapy during the past decade since the development of the class of H_1 blockers known as the nonsedating or "low sedative" antihistamines.[26] The best studied of these include terfenadine, loratadine, and astemizole. Each of these is different in origin, chemical structure, solubility, metabolic effects, and specificity of action. They have in common, however, the characteristic of not readily permeating the blood–brain barrier in usual therapeutic doses. The pharmacokinetic properties of these antihistamines have been thoroughly investigated.

Each of the three most commonly prescribed antihistamines of this class, terfenadine, loratadine, and astemizole, reach peak plasma concentrations approaching 1 to 2 hours after oral ingestion. Duration of action is ordinarily longer than that found in classic H_1 blockers with an elimination half-life of between 8 and 11 hours reported for loratadine,[27] from 16 to 23 hours for terfenadine, and approximately 104 hours for astemizole.[28]

Although the enzyme system responsible for metabolism of loratadine is not known, both terfenadine and astemizole are metabolized by the cytochrome P-450 enzyme P-450 3A4. Increased plasma levels of unmetabolized parent compound can be a result of an overdosage of the medication, administration of the medication to individuals with liver dysfunction, drug–drug interactions resulting in inhibition of cytochrome P-450 3A4, or delay in elimination of the parent compound.[29] Furthermore, cytochrome P-450

3A4 activity can be inhibited by flavenoids found naturally in grapefruit juice and perhaps in some nutritional supplements.[29–31] Increased levels of the parent compound can lead to inhibition of the cardiac potassium slow channel resulting in prolongation of the QT interval and potentially fatal arrhythmias such as torsades de pointes.

Rare cases of adverse cardiac events have been reported with doses of astemizole as low as 20 to 30 mg daily which is two to three times the recommended daily dose.[32] One case of cardiac toxicity was reported in a patient taking the recommended daily dose of terfenadine, 120 mg, with insufficient information to identify any other risk factors except perhaps age.[29]

As a result of this and other new information indicating potentially life-threatening drug interactions and adverse events with higher doses, labeling for the nonsedating antihistamines terfenadine and astemizole has been changed. The revised labeling contraindicates the coadministration of terfenadine and astemizole with either of the antifungal agents ketoconazole or itraconazole and with the macrolide antibiotics such as erythromycin, troleandomycin, clarithromycin, and azithromycin.[32] The recommended dose of astemizole remains 10 mg daily. The recommended daily dose of terfenadine should not exceed 120 mg given in two divided doses.[33,34]

The ability of terfenadine but not its metabolite to block potassium channels suggests that terfenadine carboxylate may be a good candidate for future research: it possess nonsedating properties yet does not appear to affect potassium currents.[29]

Sedative effects. This new class of anti-H_1 agents, classified as the nonsedating antihistamines, lacks any direct chemical relationship to histamine. Their elemental structures are more polar than the classic antihistamines, which limits their access to the CNS and reduces their sedative side effects. Included in this class are terfenadine, loratadine, cetirizine, and astemizole, all of which have great difficulty traversing the blood–brain barrier and a lower affinity for brain H_1 receptors compared with peripheral H_1 receptors.[35] While still capable of blunting the histaminergic response, they produce fewer undesired CNS side effects. They also typically have a lower affinity for cholinergic, alpha adrenergic, dopaminergic, and serotonergic receptor sites in the brain compared with classic H_1 antagonists.[25]

Tricyclic Antidepressants

Mechanism of action. Tricyclic antidepressants, although not considered antihistamines in the conventional sense, bind H_1 receptors with a high degree of affinity and to a lesser extent, H_2 receptors. Their significant therapeutic benefit in the treatment of chronic urticaria was first reported by Green and Green in 1967[36] and later laboratory data using H_1 receptor assays derived from cultured mouse neuroblastoma cells confirmed their competitive inhibition of histamine.[37,38]

Studies done on doxepin, a tertiary amine-type tricyclic, have demonstrated that it is 775 to 1000 times more potent than diphenhydramine and 56 times more potent than hydroxyzine at blocking histamine H_1 receptors. It is comparable to cimetidine in H_2-blocking ability and also possesses potent antimuscarinic, antiserotonergic, and anti-α-adrenergic activity.[39,40] The clinical efficacy of these compounds appears to result from the combined H_1, H_2, and muscarinic blocking activities these agents demonstrate.[39–42]

Side effects. Mild side effects commonly reported with doxepin include drowsiness and dry mouth. Dry eyes, blurred vision and increased appetite have also been reported, albeit much less frequently.[40,43,44] As with other tricyclic antidepressants, doxepin administered to normal subjects does not result in stimulation or mood elevation.[44] Doxepin in high doses may cause anticholinergic effects,[45] however, and care should be taken in the treatment of elderly patients with cardiac problems. Treatment with monoamine oxidase inhibitors should be discontinued at least 2 weeks prior to starting therapy with doxepin.[46]

APPLICATIONS IN CLINICAL PRACTICE

Urticaria

Blockade of histamine receptor sites is of significant therapeutic benefit in the treatment of seasonal allergic rhinitis, acute and chronic urticaria, and perhaps some cases of eczematous dermatoses.

In the absence of identification and removal of the causative agent, therapy with antihistamines is the treatment of choice for urticaria. Because of their blend of properties, the newer nonsedating H_1 blockers seem to be superior for patients with chronic idiopathic urticaria. Terfenadine, the first nonsedating antihistamine approved by the Food and Drug Administration, has been available since 1985. More than 800 patients with chronic urticaria have been evaluated in studies on clinical efficacy.

Two studies compared terfenadine with traditional sedating antihistamines. The first, reported from Scandinavia, found terfenadine superior to clemastine in overall effectiveness ($p < 0.02$) and in ability to reduce itching and hives ($p < 0.01$).[47] The second, a Japanese study, demonstrated the overall effectiveness of terfenadine and clemastine to be comparable.[48]

Astemizole has been shown to be as or more effective than the classic H_1 antihistamines such as chlorpheniramine and possibly superior to other nonsedating antihistamines. More than 400 patients in several clinical trials have been evaluated to assess the efficacy of astemizole in the treatment of chronic urticaria. Two clinical trials from Scandinavia and Great Britain have compared the efficacy of astemizole with chlorpheniramine. In the first study astemizole, 10 mg once a day, was compared with chlopheniramine, 6 mg twice a day. Astemizole proved more effective in relieving the signs and symptoms of urticaria when compared with chlorpheniramine.[49]

The second trial evaluated patients with dermatographism. Astemizole effectively reduced the frequency of dermatographism and the accompanying pruritus better than did chlorpheniramine.[50]

Loratadine, another nonsedating antihistamine available worldwide since 1988, and just released in the United States, has demonstrated excellent clinical efficacy with minimal side effects in the treatment of chronic urticaria. It was statistically more effective than placebo, clinically more beneficial than terfenadine, and was demonstrated to be comparable in clinical efficacy to the classic sedating antihistamine, hydroxyzine.[51-53] No significant disparity in the incidence of adverse effects, including sedation or dry mouth, or changes from baseline levels in vital signs or laboratory tests, were observed between loratadine as compared with placebo in a study of 548 patients, 224 of whom took loratadine.[53]

Ketotifen, a new class of antiallergic compound, combines the traits of mediator release inhibition and mediator antagonism.[54] While having no influence on the liberation of histamine, this agent inhibits the release of slow-reacting substance of anaphylaxis from mast cells and basophilic leukocytes.[55] Ketotifen has been successfully used to relieve the symptoms of diffuse cutaneous mastocytosis, urticaria pigmentosa, systemic mastocytosis, as well as bronchial asthma.[56]

Several investigators have compared the effectiveness of the newer nonsedating antihistamines to traditional H_1 antagonists in the treatment of allergic rhinitis. The nonsedating antihistamines appear to be as beneficial as the classic antihistamines in relieving the sneezing, rhinorrhea, and pruritus associated with seasonal allergic rhinitis.[57-59]

Overall, because of their combination of properties, the newer nonsedating antihistamines are emerging as the treatment of choice for chronic idiopathic urticaria. The clinical profile of this class of agents with respect to efficacy, safety, and convenience varies among individual drugs with loratadine appearing to have a slight edge over the others. As compared with classic antihistamines these new preparations represent a major advancement in the treatment of histamine-mediated allergic disorders.

The nonsedating antihistamines are also helpful in alleviating the symptoms of physical urticarias and may, in fact, be helpful in cases in which conventional antihistamines have failed. Rajatanavin and Bernhard found that terfenidine taken at slightly higher than the recommended dosage was effective in treating a patient whose solar urticaria failed to respond to conventional antihistamines, B-carotene, and PUVA treatment.[60,61] They observed that terfenidine effectively blocked the edema and pruritus but did not prevent the development of blotchy macular erythema. This dissociation of an initial agent (erythema) from subsequent events (wheal and itch) has also been observed in several other physical urticarias[62] treated with terfenidine.

Trials combining H_2-receptor blockaders with classic H_1 antihistamines have also demonstrated greater efficacy in the treatment of dermatographism than either given alone. In a double-blind, randomized crossover study of 20 dermatographism, patients combination therapy with cimetidine and chorpheniramine significantly reduced wheal size, flare size, and duration of wheal compared to placebo or either drug alone.[63] Individual cases demonstrating improvement in dermatographism have also been reported for ranitidine.[64]

Other Histamine-Mediated Disorders

H_1 blockers with low sedative profiles have also proved beneficial in the treatment of other histamine-mediated disorders.

Dermatitis

As therapy for pruritus associated with atopic and contact dermatitis, the newer nonsedating antihistamines have proven to be rather disappointing compared to results using traditional sedating antihistamines.

The few studies examining the efficacy of nonsedating antihistamines have produced conflicting results. Shuster and co-workers have provided evidence that antihistamines with a sedative action are superior to the newer nonsedating antihistamines in alleviating the itch of eczematous dermatitis. In a study of 23 patients with either atopic dermatitis or psoriasis neither terfenadine 60 mg twice daily nor astemizole 10 mg once daily influenced the itching evaluated subjectively on a linear visual analog scale or scratching measured objectively as nocturnal scratching of patients with atopic dermatitis. A significant ($p \leq 0.05$) diminution in pruritus was demonstrated for both the sedative benzodiazepine anxiolytic nitrazepam, 10 mg at bedtime, and for the classic H_1 blocker trimeprazine, 10 mg administered three times daily, but not for terfenidine.[65] From these results Kraus and Shuster propose that "sedation is more important than peripheral H_1 blockade in treating the itch of dermatoses such as eczema and psoriasis". A separate clinical trial of 25 adult patients with atopic dermatitis conducted by Wahlgren and colleagues compared terfenidine 60 mg twice daily with the sedative antihistamine clemastine administered 2 mg twice daily. They found that neither drug differed significantly from placebo in its antipruritic effect, supporting the notion that histamine is not important in the pathogenesis of itching in atopic dermatitis.[66] Berth-Jones and Graham-Brown's study also failed to demonstrate a beneficial effect from terfenidine in treatment of atopic dermatitis.[67]

Another recent report, however, lends support to the contention that nonsedating antihistamines may play a part in reducing the itch of some patients with atopic dermatitis. Doherty and co-workers[68] conducted a randomized double-blind, parallel, placebo-controlled study in which either acrivastine, terfenadine, or placebo was administered to 49 adult patients with atopic dermatitis. Results from a visual analog scale analyzed at 1 week indicated that terfenadine significantly reduced itching when compared with placebo. According to the patient's own assessments, both terfenadine and acrivastine were more beneficial in reducing symptoms than placebo alone. Although this was a parallel rather than a crossover study, it is difficult to ignore the positive finding.

The newer agents may play an important role in selected patients with atopic dermatitis and a history of contact urticaria. In a double-blind crossover study Hjorth investigated the effects of terfenadine in 30 patients with atopic dermatitis whose history implied contact urticaria.[69] Patients were randomly assigned to a 2-week course of treatment with either terfenadine 60 mg twice daily or placebo. Therapy with terfenadine reduced the severity of itching in approximately 52% of patients; 34% reported no change in their symptoms and 14% reported an increase in their pruritus.

Lendenmann and colleagues[70] similarly demonstrated in two randomized crossover double-blind studies of 28 atopic patients with sensitivity to an identified allergen that both terfenadine and cetirizine led to significant diminution of both histamine- and allergen-induced skin reactions at 2 and 5 hours after administration of medication.

Although these results suggest that therapy with nonsedative antihistamines may be helpful in selected patients with atopic dermatitis, perhaps on the basis of an urticarial component to their condition, further work in this area is still needed to resolve the issue.

Pruritus Associated with Systemic Disease

Several investigators have reported moderate-to-good results with nonsedative antihistamine therapy of nonurticarial pruritus but no large studies have been done. Duncan and co-workers[71] treated 8 patients with pruritus due to chronic obstructive liver disease in a single-blind randomized crossover trial comparing the antipruritic action of cholestyramine, chlorpheniramine, terfenadine, and placebo. Itching was recorded daily by each patient on a four-point scale. Patients received treatment for a total of 14 days. Mean cumulative pruritus scores were found to be lower in patients taking cholestyramine and terfenadine compared with patients taking placebo or chlopheniramine.

Nykamp[72] compared terfenidine with diphenhydramine and trimeprazine in 21 end-stage renal failure patients to determine whether terfenidine provided greater relief from uremic pruritus than other agents commonly prescribed. Patients were randomly assigned to receive either diphenhydramine

25 mg twice daily, trimeprazine 2.5 mg twice daily, terfenadine 60 mg twice daily, or placebo. Terfenidine was not more effective than either of the other agents or placebo in relieving symptoms of uremic pruritus in these patients.

Cimetidine is a potent H_2-receptor antagonist the primary use of which is in the treatment of disorders associated with gastric-acid hypersecretion. It has also been used with limited success, in the treatment of pruritus related to chronic renal failure,[73] cholestasis,[74] myeloproliferative disorders such as polythemia vera,[75] and Hodgkin's disease.[67,76] Although anecdotal reports have been encouraging, results from controlled studies with cimetidine have been disappointing. Limited success with cimetidine may be the result of its possible effects on the immune system separate from its antihistaminic effects. Furthermore, Davies and Greaves have shown that H_1 but not H_2 receptors are involved in itching provoked by histamine, so there is little reason to expect that H_2 antagonists should be helpful in the treatment of itching.[76a]

Harrison and co-workers[74] failed to demonstrate any improvement from cimetidine in a double-blind, crossover study of six patients, all with cholestasis and pruritus. Patients received either cimetidine, 300 mg four times daily or an identical placebo for a period of 3 days. Symptoms did not improve significantly with either cimetidine or placebo in three patients while two responded to placebo alone and only one reported improvement with cimetidine.

Likewise, there are several accounts in the literature of patients with severe generalized pruritus associated with Hodgkin's disease responding to treatment with cimetidine but this has not been substantiated with any large double-blind crossover studies.[67,76]

Additional Therapeutic Uses

It is generally agreed that mast cell-released histamine is one of the biologic mediators involved in psoriasis, degranulating mast cells being one of the first morphologic changes observed.

Recent studies suggest that long-term therapy with H_2-receptor antagonists, after initial worsening of the disease, may produce temporary improvement in cutaneous psoriatic lesions. It appears the improvement is not observed until approximately the third month of treatment.[77] Most of this work is preliminary, however, and follow-up with randomized, placebo-controlled studies is necessary. Cimetidine may also act as an immunomodulator. This may be an important aspect of its effectiveness in the treatment of psoriasis in the setting of AIDS, according to early reports.[77a]

Improvement of lichen nitidus after therapy with oral astemizole has recently been reported. Ocampo and Torne published two cases of widespread lichen nitidus that improved or cleared with astemizole alone over a 2-week period.[78] Subsequent reports have demonstrated similar results in conjunction with topical steroids.[79] Whether concurrent administration of topical steroids is essential, however, is not known.

Specific agents of this class also possess anti-motion-sickness properties, anti-Parkinsonian activity, and, when used in greater concentrations than necessary for their antihistaminic properties, local anesthetic effects.[80]

ADVERSE EFFECTS

H_1 blocking agents have a wide therapeutic-to-toxic ratio in adults and, in therapeutic doses, neither the classic nor the nonsedating H_1 antagonists routinely cause significant adverse effects. A significant group of patients, however, find it necessary to discontinue a particular preparation because of the severity of these side effects. In one study this ranged from 6 to 16%.[81] In addition, fatalities with overdosage have occurred, particularly in children.

Common side effects of conventional antihistamines have been well documented and include sedation, depression, or excitation of the CNS, anticholinergic effects, and gastrointestinal symptoms consisting of loss of appetite, nausea, and epigastric distress. Of these, drowsiness is by far the most prevalent adverse effect and reportedly to occurs in 20% to 60% of patients taking diphenhydramine.[82] With traditional antihistamines drowsiness will often disappear within a few days of continued use.[80] Tolerance to the sedative effects of antihistamines can also be accomplished by administering them as a single dose in the evening.[17]

Additional CNS effects include dizziness, fatigue, lassitude, incoordination, tinnitus, vertigo, and diplopia. Euphoria, insomnia, nervousness, irritability, tremors, and an increased susceptibility to convulsions may also occur, particularly in children.[80]

The next most frequent adverse effects involve the gastrointestinal tract. These may include anorexia, nausea, vomiting, abdominal discomfort, diarrhea, or constipation.

About 3% of patients experience anticholinergic symptoms such as dryness of the mucous membranes, dysuria, urinary retention, and increased intraocular pressure. Conventional antihistamines should be avoided, therefore, in patients with narrow angle glaucoma. Although anticholinergic effects are rare with the nonsedating antihistamines, the potential for these symptoms to develop still exists.

Astemizole-associated urinary retention has been reported in four patients who received 10-mg astemizole once daily for 2 to 8 days. Symptoms developed within 2 to 3 days of initiating therapy and resolved within 24 hours of discontinuation of the medication.[83] A case of blurred vision confirmed with a positive rechallenge is also on file with the manufacturer.

Rarely, phenothiazine antihistamines may exert alpha-adrenergic blocking activity which may interfere with or counteract the effects of adrenergic agents.[84]

Leukopenia and agranulocytosis appear to be reversible adverse effects of both H_1- and H_2-receptor antagonists. There are four specific antihistamines known to induce agranulocytosis: thenaldine, pyribenzamine, methaphenadene, and the over-the-counter antihistamine, brompheniramine.[85-88] Recently Hardin also published a case of fatal agranulocytosis occurring after administration of the widely used over-the-counter antihistamine chlorpheniramine.[89] Hemolytic anemia has been reported in two patients who ingested 150 to 200 mg/day of diphenhydramine for 3 to 5 months.[90]

Tardive dyskinesia can also be exacerbated or unmasked by oral or parenteral administration of antihistamines. This has been reported both with doxylamine and with diphenhydramine.[91,92] Acute dystonia has also been reported as an infrequent reaction to diphenhydramine.[93]

Weight gain has been reported as an adverse reaction to certain antihistamines. In the case of cyproheptadine and ketotifen this is a direct consequence of their antiserotonergic effects.[55] Weight gain is also a frequent unwanted effect of astemizole, occurring in approximately 3.6% of patients, but is independent of serotonin antagonism.[94]

Headache, generalized joint pains, blurred vision, drowsiness, depression, and extreme excitation have been reported with the use of terfenidine. Similar adverse effects have also been reported with astemizole.[95]

In cases of astemizole overdose serious ventricular arrhythmias such as prolonged QT-interval, and ventricular tachycardias including torsades de pointes, have been reported.[34] Terfenidine has also been associated with arrhythmias, especially in cases of reduced metabolism such as occurs with concomitant administration of ketoconazole and erythromycin.[31,96-98]

Hypersensitivity reactions to antihistamine preparations are comprised of both allergic and photoallergic dermatoses. Contact dermatitis has been reported in patients who have received diphenhydramine and photosensitivity dermatitis has been reported after ingestion of both promethazine and diphenhydramine.[99,100] Application of topical antihistamine preparations is therefore strongly discouraged. Vasculitis has also been documented after oral intake of diphenhydramine hydrochloride.[101,102]

Cutaneous reactions have also been reported with the nonsedating antihistamines. Terfenadine has caused both rashes and paradoxical urticaria according to case reports.[103]

Because antihistamines blunt the cutaneous histamine response, their withdrawal should precede any skin testing for allergies. In the case of astemizole the attenuating effect, that is, the suppression of skin test reactivity to histamine, may persist for as long as 6 to 14 weeks after cessation of the drug. Therefore astemizole therapy should be discontinued a minimum of 6 weeks prior to skin testing and some patients may require a longer drug-free interval.[17,104]

DRUG INTERACTIONS

Most classic antihistamines have additive effects with alcohol and CNS depressants leading to increased somnolence. Monoamine oxidase inhibitors sustain and intensify the anticholinergic effects of antihistamines.

In general, nonsedating antihistamines do not significantly differ from placebo in the incidence of anticholinergic side effects and therefore these agents are safe to use in patients taking monoamine oxidase inhibitors.[17,35,59] Moreover, no cases of worsening of glaucoma have been reported with either terfenadine[33] or astemizole.[34] Only four cases of urinary retention associated with ingestion of astemizole have been reported.[83] The effects of anticholinergic medications such as tricyclic antidepressants may be additive with those of antihistamines, especially in elderly patients.[105]

Serious ventricular arrhymias, including torsades de pointes, appear to be potentiated by the concomitant use of either terfenadine or astemizole with either of the antifungal agents ketoconazole or itraconazole and with the macrolide antibiotics exemplified by erythromycin. The mechanism appears to be reduced metabolism by the liver.[96] Co-administration of these medications is now contraindicated by the manufacturers of terfenadine and astemizole and the Food and Drug Administration.[32,106]

USES IN PREGNANCY AND BREASTFEEDING

The safety profile of most traditional antihistamines has not been established for use during pregnancy. In a large study conducted by the Collaborative Perinatal Project, no evidence was found to suggest a relationship between the use of classic H_1 antihistamines and the development of major or minor fetal malformations.[107] However, both adverse fetal effects and prenatal death have been reported in association with maternal ingestion of antihistamines. A report of Saxen noted a higher incidence of cleft palate defects with ingestion of diphenhydramine in the first trimester of pregnancy.[108] A case of perinatal mortality was reported by Kargas and co-workers[108a] less than 8 hours after the simultaneous ingestion by the mother of diphenhydramine and temazepam, a benzodiazepine hypnotic. Three hours after ingestion of 30 mg of temazepam and 4 1/2 hours after ingestion of 50 mg of diphenhydramine, violent intrauterine fetal movements were noted which ceased abruptly. Four hours later a stillborn infant was delivered with no gross or microscopic abnormalities. A synergistic effect on the fetus of diphenhydramine and temazepam was felt to be responsible for the death of the infant.[108a]

Antihistamines administered in the later stages of pregnancy have been infrequently associated with platelet dysfunction,[109] and phenothiazines taken late in pregnancy have been reported to induce jaundice[110] and possibly extrapyramidal effects[111] in infants born prematurely.

The effects of nonsedating antihistamines administered during pregnancy have not been sufficiently studied and are therefore contraindicated.

Very few studies on the influence of antihistamines in breast-fed infants are available. Most studies suggest, however, that the small amounts detectable in breast milk are of no clinical importance.[112]

In their statement regarding the safety of certain medications taken by mothers during breast-feeding, the American Academy of Pediatrics Committee on Drugs listed diphenhydramine as a maternal medication "usually compatible with breastfeeding."[113] They reported no adverse signs or symptoms in infants or effects on lactation.[114] Clemastine, however, was reported by Kok and co-workers[115] to cause drowsiness in a 10-week-old, previously well, exclusively breastfed infant who was exposed through her mother's milk.[115] Despite the endorsement of the American Academy of Pediatrics, the manufacturer still advises against the use of these medications, including diphenhydramine, during breast-feeding.

The influence of nonsedating antihistamines on breast-fed infants is even less well characterized. In a study by Hilbert and colleagues[116] of six nonpregnant lactating women, only 0.029% of the dose of loratidine administered to the mothers was excreted into breast milk during a 48-hour period as either loratidine or its active metabolite. Even in the estimated "worst-case" scenario of the mother receiving the maximal dose of loratidine that could be expected under any circumstance, the quantity of the drug and its metabolite transmitted to an infant was calculated to be only 1.1% of the adult dose on a mg/kg basis. The safety of loratidine in adults is well documented and it is unlikely that this dose would proffer a hazard to infants. The safety profile of the new nonsedating antihistamines has not been established for infants, however.

TOPICAL ANTIHISTAMINES

Topical antihistamine preparations are widely used products and readily available without prescription. In addition to their antipruritic effects, they are locally anesthetizing and limit vessel permeability.[117] Topical preparations including traditional H_1 antihistamines as well as topical tricyclic antidepressants have been shown to reduce the pruritus associated with common dermatoses as well as that associated with urticaria.[118–121]

Double-blind studies by Bernstein and colleagues as well as Drake and co-workers have shown that topically applied 5% doxepin cream can significantly reduce itching compared with placebo in patients with atopic dermatitis, lichen simplex chronicus, nummular eczema, and contact dermatitis.[118,118a,122] A significant number of patients in the study by Bernstein, however, complained of sedation and anticholinergic side effects associated with the topical treatment.[118]

The incidence of cutaneous reactions to topically applied antihistamines is difficult to assess. Diphenhydramine hydrochloride, an oxygen-linked ethanolamine antihistamine, is commonly found in many topical preparations. In a series reported by Vickers, 12 of 117 cases of contact dermatitis reported in 1 year were due to a lotion containing diphenhydramine and calamine. All 12 cases were confirmed with patch testing.[123] Diphenhydramine has also been reported as a cause of photoallergic contact dermatitis as have topical phenothiazine preparations such as promethazine.[124–126]

Topical preparations may also be a cause of systemic side effects. Significant systemic absorption may occur following topical application of an antihistamine especially to open skin areas. Several such cases have been reported in children in whom topical diphenhydramine was used to treat pruritus associated with varicella-zoster infection. Acute delirium developed in all cases that resolved with discontinuation of the offending agent.[127–129]

OPTIMIZING ANTIHISTAMINE TREATMENT

Classic H_1 antihistamines have both therapeutic efficacy and cost advantage compared to the newer nonsedating antihistamines. The obvious disadvantage is their sedative effects, which impede judgment and slow motor skills. One approach to overcoming this handicap is to make use of the differential pharmacokinetics between histamine antagonism and its unwanted side effects. The sedative effects of first-generation antihistamines are felt to correlate with drug serum concentration while histamine antagonism trails behind this and may persist for several hours despite low serum drug concentration.[130]

With this in mind, bedtime dosing is often useful in mitigating subjective symptoms while significantly lessening objective diminished alertness and delayed reaction time the following morning. In one study by Goetz and colleagues[131] administration of a single 50 mg bedtime dose of hydroxyzine eliminated the significant prolongation of two parameters, simple reaction time and choice reaction time, that had been observed with 25 mg of hydroxyzine given twice daily reported in a previous study. Daytime drowsiness, dry mouth, and irritability were not eliminated in this study.[132]

In clinical practice, however, these symptoms can be further improved by taking the nighttime dose either earlier or with dinner. If nighttime itching remains a problem, patients may benefit from combining a liquid formulation for immediate release with a spansule for delayed overnight action.

Although adverse effects of doxepin are considered to be less than those of classic H_1 antagonists such as diphenhydramine, drowsiness is still a frequent complaint and complaints of dry mouth are actually noted more often.[43] Given its long half-life of 19 hours, however, one can easily administer it in a single or double-dose regimen improving compliance and convenience while use of the liquid formulation allows for more accurate titration of the drug to the symptoms.[43]

Some antihistamines, such as cyproheptadine, are also reasonably effective serotonin antagonists. This may be helpful in some settings, such as polycythemia vera, in which serotonin is thought to play a role.

There are many formulations of antihistamines now available by prescription or over the counter that allow patients to more accurately tailor individual or combined products to their specific needs.

CONCLUSION

Although all antihistamines inhibit the different actions of histamine, they are a very diverse group of drugs. The antihistamines available today have a broad spectrum of therapeutic benefit with minimal side effects.

By their action at the histamine receptor as a competitive inhibitor, they can prevent the effects of histamine, but are unable to reverse these effects.

In the past 10 years, a new class of H_1 blockers has been developed. The sedative and anticholinergic effects associated with the older antihistamines are absent. This now allows clinicians to select a drug based on the profile of side effects as well as the profile of beneficial effects.

Used judiciously, the antihistamines available today have a broad application of therapeutic uses with very few significant side effects.

These compounds are extremely effective in ameliorating pruritus directly associated with histamine release and although not specific, traditional H_1 antagonists with their soporific side-effect, remain a mainstay in the treatment of itching associated with nonhistamine mediated disorders.

REFERENCES

1. Dale HH, Laidlaw PP: The physiological action of iminazolylethylamine. *J Physiol* 41(B):318–344, 1910.
2. Dale HH, Laidlaw PP: Further observations on the actions of beta-imidazolyl-ethyamine. *J Physiol* 43:182–195, 1911.
3. Dale HH, Laidlaw PP: Histamine shock. *J Physiol* 52:355–390, 1919.
4. Herman LE, Bernhard JD: Antihistamine update. *Derm Clin* 9(3):603–10, 1991.
5. Knowles S, Shear NH: Antihistamines. *Clin Dermatol* 7(3):48–59, 1989.
6. Sabbah A: The rebirth of the H1-antagonists. *Allergie et Immunologie* 24:224–230, 1992.
7. Bovet D, Staub AM: Action protective des ethers phenoliques au cours de l'intoxication histaminique. *C R Soc Biol* 124:547, 1937.
8. Halpern BN: Les antihistaminiques de synthèse. Essais de chimiothéapie des états allergiques, *Arch Int Pharmacodyn Ther* 68:339–408, 1942.
9. Loew ER, Kaiser ME, Moore V: Synthetic benzhydryl alkamine ethers effective in pre-

venting fatal experimental asthma in guinea pigs exposed to atomised histamine. *J Pharmacol Exp Ther* 83:120–128, 1945.

10. Yonkman FF, Chess D, Mathieson D, et al: Pharmacodynamic studies of a new antihistamine agent, N'-pyridyl-N'benzyl-N-dimethylethylene diamine HCL, pyribenzamine HCL. *J Pharmacol Exp Ther* 87:256, 1946.

11. Bovet D: Introduction to antihistamine agent and antergan derivatives. *Ann NY Acad Sci* 50:1089–1126, 1950.

12. Black JW, Duncan WAM, Durant CJ, et al: Definition and antagonism of histamine H_2 receptors. *Nature* 236:385–390, 1972.

12a. Black JW, Duncan WAM, Durant CJ, et al: Definition and antagonism of histamine H_2 receptors. *Nature* 236:385–390, 1972.

12b. Furgott RF, The pharmacology of vascular smooth muscle. *Pharmacol Rev* 7:183–265, 1955.

13. Ash ASF, Shild HO: Receptors mediating some actions of histamine. *Br J Pharmac Chemother* 27:427–439, 1966.

14. Arrang JM, Garbarg M, Schwartry JC. Autoinhibition of brain histamine release mediated by a novel class (H_3) of histamine receptor. *Nature* 302:832–837, 1983.

15. Douglas WW: Histamine and 5-hydroxytryptamine (serotonin) and their antagonists, in Gilman AG, Goodman LS, Gilman A, et al. (ed.): *Goodman and Gilman's The Pharmagological Basis of Therapeutics.* 7th ed. New York: Macmillan, 1985, chap. 26, 618–627.

16. Simons FE, Simons KJ, Chung M, Yeh J: The comparative pharmacokinetics of H1-receptor antagonists. *Ann Allergy* 59(6):20–24, 1987.

17. Drouin MA: H_1 antihistamines: Perspective on the use of the conventional and new agents. *Ann Allergy* 55:747–752, 1985.

18. Carruthers SG, Shoeman DW, Hignite CE, et al: Correlation between plasma diphenhydramine level and sedative and antihistaminic effects. *Clin Pharmacol Ther* 23:375–382, 1978.

19. Berlinger WG, Goldbert MJ, Spector R, et al: Diphenhydramine: Kinetics and psychomotor effects in elderly women. *Clin Pharm Therapeutics* 32:387–391, 1982.

20. Spector R, Choudhury AK, Chiang CK, et al: Diphenhydramine in orientals and caucasians. *Clin Pharm Therapeutics* 28:229–234, 1980.

21. Simons FER, Simons KJ: H1 receptor antagonists: *Clinical Ped Clin N Amer* 30(5):899–915, 1983.

22. Paton DM, Webster DR: Clinical pharmacokinetics of H1-receptor antagonists (the antihistamines). *Clin Pharm* 10:477–497, 1985.

23. Simons KJ, Simons FER, Luciuk GH, et al: The urinary excretion of chlorpheniramine and its metabolites in children. *J Pharm Sci* 73:595–599, 1984.

24. Knight A: Astemizole-a new, non-sedating antihistamine for hayfever. *J Otolaryn* 14(2):85–88, 1985.

25. Gengo, FM: How antihistamines act on the central nervous system. Symposium, All Council of America, New York, NY Feb 21, 1990.

26. Mann KV, Crowe JP, Tietze KJ: Nonsedating histamine H1-receptor antagonists. *Clin Pharm* 8:331–344, 1989.

27. Hilbert J, Radwanski E, Weglein R, et al: Pharmkokinetics and dose proportionality of loratidine. *J Clin Pharm* 27:694–698, 1987.

28. Brandon ML: Newer non-sedating antihistamines will they replace older agents? *Drugs* 30:377–381, 1985.

29. Woosley RL, Yiwang C, Freiman JP, et al: Mechanism of the cardiotoxic actions of terfenidine. *JAMA* 269(12):1532–1536, 1993.

30. Peck CC, Temple R, Collins JM: Understanding consequences of current therapies. *JAMA* 269(12):1550–1552, 1993.

31. Honig PK, Wortham DC, Zamani K, et al: Terfenidine-ketoconazole interaction: Pharmacokinetics and electrocardiographic consequences. *JAMA* 269(12):1513–1518, 1993.
32. Kessler DA, ed. Reports of dangerous cardiac arrhythmias prompt new contraindications for the drug Hismanal. *FDA Med Bull* 23(1):2, 1993.
33. *Physicians Desk Reference*, Oradell, NJ: Medical Economics Company, 44:1477, 1990.
34. *Physicians Desk Reference*, Oradell, NJ: Medical Economics Company, 44:1082, 1990.
35. Monroe EW: Chronic urticaria: Review of nonsedating H1 antihistamines in treatment. *JAAD* 19(5):842–849, 1988.
36. Green MA, Green RC: Psychotropic adjuvant in allergen disorders. *Psychosomatics* 8:29–32, 1967.
37. Richelson E: Histamine H1 receptor-mediated guanosine 3″5′-monophosphate formation by cultured mouse neuroblastoma cells. *Science* 201:69–71, 1978.
38. Richelson E: Tricyclic antidepressants block H1 receptors of mouse neuroblastoma cells. *Nature* 274:176–177, 1978.
39. Figueirado A, Fontes Ribeiro CA, Goncalo M, et al: Mechanism of action of doxepin in the treatment of chronic urticaria. *Fundam Clin Pharm* 4:147–158, 1990.
40. Goldsobel AB, Rohr AS, Siegel SC, et al: Efficacy of doxepin in the treatment of chronic idiopathic urticaria. *J All Clin Immun* 78(5):867–873, 1986.
41. Green JP, Maayani S: Tricyclic antidepressant drug block histamine H2 receptor in brain. *Nature* 269:163–165, 1977.
42. Kanof PD, Greengard P. Brain histamine receptors as targets for antidepressant drugs. *Nature* 272:329–333, 1978.
43. Greene SL, Reed CE, Schroeter AL: Double-blind crossover study comparing doxepin with diphenhydramine for the treatment of chronic urticaria. *J Am Acad Derm* 12:669–675, 1985.
44. Harto A, Sendagorta E, Ledo A: Doxepin in the treatment of chronic urticaria. *Dermatologica* 170:90–93, 1985.
45. Arnold SE, Kahn RJ, Faldetta LL, et al: Tricyclic antidepressants and peripheral anticholinergic activity. *Psychopharm* 74:325–328, 1981.
46. Neittaanmaki H, Myohanen T, Fraki JE: Comparison of cinnarizine, cyproheptadine, doxepine, and hydroxyzine in the treatment of idiopathic cold urticaria: Usefulness of doxepin. *J Am Acad Dermatol* 11:483–489, 1984.
47. Fredriksson T, Hersle K, Hjorth N, et al: Terfenidine in chronic urticaria: A comparison with clemastine and placebo. *Cutis* 38:128–130, 1986.
48. Harada S: Clinical investigation of terfenidine on chronic urticaria. (Abst) *Ann Allergy* 55:284, 1985.
49. Mobacken H, Faergeman J, Gisslen H, et al: Astemizole in chronic idiopathic urticaria. A comparison with chlopheniramine. (Abst). *Ann Allergy* 55:254, 1985.
50. Krause LB, Shuster S: A comparison of astemizole and chlorpheniramine in dermographic urticaria. *Br J Derm* 112:447–453, 1985.
51. Bruttmann G, Belaich S, DrGreef H, et al: Comparative effects of loratidine and terfenidine in the treatment of chronic idiopathic urticaria. Seventeenth World Congress of Dermatology, West Berlin, May 1987.
52. Monroe EW: Efficacy and safety of loratindine in the management of idiopathic chronic urticaria. Presented at the Claritine Symposium, Brussels, February 1988.
53. Monroe EW, Fox RW, Green AW, et al: Efficacy and safety of loratidine in the management of chronic idiopathic urticaria. Presented at the Seventeenth World Congress of Dermatology, West Berlin, May 1987.
54. Wilhelms OH: Antagonism of picumast and ketotifen against histamine, acetylcholine, LTC_4, slow-reacting substance of anaphylaxis and barium chloride in the guinea pig ileum bioassay. *Int Arch All Appl Immun* 82:544–546, 1987.
55. El-Hefny A: Treatment of wheezy infants and children with ketotifen. *Pharmatherapeutica.* 3:388, 1983.

56. Shear NH, Krafchik BR, MacLeod SM: Diffuse cutaneous mastocytosis: Treatment with ketotifen and cimetidine. *Clin Invest Med* 6:36, 1983.

57. Carpio JD, Kabbash L, Turenne Y, et al: Efficacy and safety of loratidine (10 mg once daily), terfenidine (60 mg twice daily), and placebo in the treatment of seasonal allergic rhinitis. *J Allergy Clin Immunol* 84:741–746, 1989.

58. Irander K, Odkvist LM, Ohlander B: Treatment of hayfever with loratidine—a new non-sedating antihistamine. *Allergy* 45:86–91, 1990.

59. Sorkin EM, Heel RC: Terfenidine—A review of its pharmacodynamic properties and therapeutic efficacy. *Drugs* 29:34–56, 1985.

60. Rajatanavin N, Bernhard JD: Solar urticaria: Treatment with terfenidine. *J Am Acad Dermatol* 18:574, 1988.

61. Bernhard JD: Treatment of solar urticaria with terfenadine. *JAAD* 28:668, 1993.

62. Cox NH, Higgins EM, Farr PM: Terfenidine inhibits itch and wheal, but not abnormal erythema, in physical urticarias. *J Am Acad Dermatol* 21;586–587, 1990.

63. Kaur S, Greaves M, Eftekhari N: Facticious urticaria (dermographism): treatment by cimetidine and chlorpheniramine in a randomized double-blind study. *Br J Derm* 104:185–190, 1981.

64. Deutsch PH: Dermatographism treated with hydroxxyzine and cimetidine and ranitidine. *Ann Int Med* 101(4):569, 1984.

65. Krause L, Shuster S: Mechanism of action of antipruritic drugs. *Br Med J* 287:1199–1200, 1983.

66. Wahlgren CF, Hagermark O, Bergstrom R: The antipruritic effect of a sedative and a non-sedative antihistamine in atopic dermatitis. *Br J Derm* 122:545–551, 1990.

66a. Berth-Jones J, Graham-Brown RAC: Failure of terfenidine in relieving the pruritus of atopic dermatitis. *Br J Dermatol* 121:635–637, 1989.

67. Aymard JP, Lederlin P, Witz F, et al: Cimetidine for pruritus in Hodgkin's disease. *Br Med J* 280(6208):151–152, 1980.

68. Doherty V, Sylvester DGH, Kennedy CTC, Harvey SG, et al. Treatment of atopic eczema with antihistamines with a low sedative profile. *Br Med J* 298:96, 1989.

69. Hjorth N: Terfenidine in the treatment of chronic idiopathicc urticaria and atopic dermatitis. *Cutis* 42:29–30, 1988.

70. Lendenmann B, Wuthrich B, Tarral A: Pharmacological control of histamine- and allergen-induced skin reactions: A comparison between terfenidine and cetirizine in two randomized cross-over double-blind studies. *Dermatologica* 181:177, 1990.

71. Duncan JS, Kennedy HJ, Triger DR: Treatment of pruritus due to chronic obstructive liver disease. *Br Med J* 289:22, 1984.

72. Nykamp D: Comparison of H1-antihistamines for pruritus in end-stage renal disease. *Drug Intelligence Clin Pharm* 20:806, 1986.

73. Zappacosta AR, Hauss D: Cimetidine doesn't help pruritus of uremia. *NEJM* 300:1280, 1979.

74. Harrison, AR: Littenberg G, Goldstein L, Kaplowitz N: Pruritus, cimetidine and polycythemia. *NEJM* 300:433–434, 1979.

75. Weick JK, Donovan PB, Najean Y, Dresch C, et al: The use of cimetidine for the treatment of pruritus in polycythemia vera. *Ann Int Med* 142:241–242, 1982.

76. Staubli M, Graf W, Straub PW. Pruritus in Hodgkin's disease responding to cimetidine. *J Suisse Med* 111(20):723–724, 1981.

76a. Davies MW, Greaves MW: Sensory responses of human skin to synthetic histamine. *Br J Clin Pharmacol* 9:461, 1980.

77. Nielson HJ: Histamine and histamine type-Z receptor antagonists in psoriasis. *Dan Med Bull* 38:478–480, 1991.

77a. Stashower ME, Yeager JK, Smith KJ, et al: Cimetidine as therapy for treatment-resistant psoriasis in a patient with acquired immunodeficiency syndrome. *Arch Dermatol* 129:848–850, 1993.

78. Ocampo J, Torne R: Generalized lichen nitidus: Report of two cases treated with astemizole. *Int J Dermatol* 28:49–51, 1989.
79. Vaughn RY, Smith JG Jr: The treatment of lich nitidus with astemizole. *JAAD* 23:4(1), 757, 1990.
80. Pearlman DS: Antihistamines: Pharmacology and clinical use. *Drugs* 12:258–273, 1976.
81. Cited in Wyngaarden JB and Seevers MH: The toxic effects of antihistaminic drugs. *JAMA* 145(5):277–282, 1951.
82. Connell JT: Methods of studying antihistamines. *NER All Proc* 7(4):346–355, 1986.
83. Lin AYF, Zahtz G, Myssiorek D: Astemizole-associated urinary retention. *Otolaryngol Head Neck* 104(6):893–894, 1991.
84. Legge DA, Tiede JJ, Peters GA, et al: Death from tension pneumothorax and chlorpromazine cardiorespiratory collapse as separate complications of asthma. *Ann Allergy* 27:23–29, 1969.
85. Adams DA, Perry S: Agranulocytosis associated with thenalidine tartrate therapy. *JAMA* 167:1207–1210, 1958.
86. Chaen AM, Meilman E, Jacobson BB: Agranulocytosis following pyribenzamine. *NEJM* 241:865–866, 1949.
87. Drake TG: Agranulocytosis during therapy with the antihistamine agent methaphenadene (Diatrin). *JAMA* 142:477–478, 1950.
88. Hardin AS, Padilla F: Agranulocytosis during therapy with a brompheniramine medication. *J Arkansas Med Soc* 75:206–208, 1978.
89. Hardin AS: Chlopheniramine and agranulocytosis. *Ann Int Med* 108(5):770, 1988.
90. Swanson M: Drugs, chemicals and hemodialysis. *Drug Intell Clin Pharm.* 7:6–24, 1973.
91. Brait KA, Zagerman AJ: Dyskenesias after antihistamine use. *NEJM* 296(2):111, 1977.
92. Favis GR: Facial dyskinesia related to antihistamine? *NEJM* 294:730, 1976.
93. Lavenstein BL, Cantor FK: Acute dystonia: An unusual reaction to diphenhydramine. *JAMA* 236(3):291, 1976.
94. Wilson JD, Hillas JL: Astemizole: A new long-acting antihistamine in the treatment of seasonal allergic rhinitis. *Clin All* 13:131–140, 1983.
95. Ontario Medical Association. Terfenidine and astemizole: Adverse effects. Drug Report No: 17, 1985.
96. Kaliner MA: Nonsedating antihistamines: pharmacology, clinical efficacy and adverse effects. *Am Fam Phys* 45(3):1337–1342, 1992.
97. Leor J, Harman M, Rabinowitz B, et al: Giant U waves and associated ventricular tachycardia complicating astemizole overdose: successful therapy with intravenous magnisium. *Am J Med* 91:94–97, 1991.
98. MacConnell TJ, Stanners AJ: Torsades de Pointes complicating treatment with terfenidine. *BMJ* 302(6790):1469, 1991.
99. Coskey RJ: Contact dermatitis caused by diphenhydramine hydrochloride. *JAAD.* 8:204–206, 1983.
100. Takeshi H: Allergic and photoallergic dermatitis from diphenhydramine. *Arch Derm* 112:1124–1126, 1976.
101. Davenport PM, Wilhelm RE: An unusual vasculitis due to diphenhydramine. *Arch Derm* 92:577–580, 1965.
102. Winkelman RK, Winston BC: Cutaneous and visceral syndromes of necrotizing or allergic angiitis: A study of 38 cases. *Medicine* 43:59–89, 1964.
103. Strickler BHE, Van Dijke CPH, Isaacs AJ, et al: Skin reactions to terfenidine. *Br Med J* 293:586, 1986.
104. Welch MJ: New-generation antihistamines. *West J Med* 154(4):455, 1991.
105. *Physicians Desk Reference,* Oradell, NJ: Medical Economics Company, 44:1582, 1990.
106. *HHS News,* Food and Drug Administration P92-25, July 20, 1992.

107. Hernonen OP, Sloan D, Shapiro S: *Birth defects and drugs in pregnancy*. Littleton, MA: Publishing Sciences Group, 1977, pp 323–337.

108. Saxen I: Cleft palate and meternal diphenhydramine intake. *Lancet* 1:407–408, 1974.

108a. Kargas GA, Kargas SA, Bruyere HJ, et al: Perinatal mortality due to interaction of diphenhydramine and temazepam. *NEJM* 313(22):1417, 1985.

109. Pockedly C, Ente G: Adverse hematologic effects of drugs. *Ped Clin N Amer* 19:1095–1111, 1972.

110. Done AK: Developmental pharmacology. *Clin Phar Therapeutics* 5:432–479, 1964.

111. Hill RM, Desmond MM, Kay JL: Extrapyramidal dysfunction in an infant of a schizophrenic mother. *J Ped* 69:589–595, 1966.

112. Catz CS, Giacoia GP: Drugs and breast milk. *Ped Clin N Amer* 19(1):151–166, 1972.

113. Pruitt AW, Anyan WR, Hill RM, et al: The transfer of drugs and other chemicals into human breast milk. *Pediatrics* 72(3):375–383, 1983.

114. Knowles JA: Excretion of drugs in milk-a review. *J Ped* 66:1068, 1965.

115. Kok THHG, Taitz LS, Bennett MJ, et al: Drowsiness due to clemastine transmitted in breast milk. *Lancet* 1:914–915, 1972.

116. Hilbert J, Radwanski E, Affrime MB, et al: Excretion of loratidine in human breast milk. *J Clin Pharmacol* 28:234–239, 1988.

117. Stuttgen G, Blitstein-Willinger E, Rudolph R: The therapeutical value of antihistamines today. *Z Hautkr* 59(6):355–366, 1984.

118. Bernstein JE, Whitney DH, Soltani K: Inhibition of histamine-induced pruritus by topical tricyclic antidepressants. *J Am Acad Derm* 5(5):582–585, 1981.

118a. Bernstein JE, Gillenwater GE: Relief from eczema-associated pruritus by doxepin hydrochloride. *J Invest Derm* 86(4):463, 1986.

119. Lever LR, Hill S, Dykes PJ, et al: Efficacy of topical dimetindene in experimentally induced pruritus and weal and flare reactions. *Skin Pharm* 4:109–112, 1991.

120. Locci F, Del Giacco GS: Treatment of chronic idiopathic urticaria with topical preparations: Controlled study of oxatomide gel versus dechlorpheniramine cream. *Drugs Exp Clin Res* 17(8):399–403, 1991.

121. Rampini E, Oberhauser V, Nunzi E: Evaluation of the local antihistaminic activity of dimetindene maleate by a quantitative method. *Dermatologica* 157:105–109, 1978.

122. Drake L, Breneman D, Greene S, et al: Effects of topical doxepin 5% cream on pruritic eczema. *J Invest Derm* 98:605, 1992.

123. Vickers CFH: Dermatitis medicamentosa. *Br Med J* 1:1366, 1961.

124. Emmett EA: Diphenhydramine photoallergy. *Arch Dermatol* 110:249, 1974.

125. Pan CV, Quintela AG, Anuncibay PG, et al: Topical promethazine intoxication. *Ann Pharm* 23:89, 1989.

126. Shawn DH, McGuigan MA: Poisoning from dermal absorption of promethazine. *Can Med Assoc J* 130:1460–1461, 1984.

127. Bernhardt DT: Topical diphenhydramine toxicity. *Wis Med J* 90(8):469–471, 1991.

128. Chan CY, Wallander KA: Diphenhydramine toxicity in three children with varicalla-zoster infection. *Ann Pharm* 25:130–132, 1991.

129. Filloux F: Toxic encephalopathy caused by topically applied diphenhydramine. *J Ped* 108(6):1018–1020, 1986.

130. Simons FER, Simons KJ: H1 receptor antagonist treatment for chronic rhinitus. *J All Clin Immun* 81:975–980, 1988.

131. Goetz DW, Jacobson JM, Murnane JE, et al: Prolongation of simple and choice reaction times in a double-blind comparison of twice daily hydroxyzine versus terfenidine. *J All Clin Immun* 84:316–322, 1989.

132. Goetz DW, Jacobson JM, Apaliski SJ, et al: Objective antihistamine side effects are mitigated by evening dosing of hydroxyzine. *Ann Allergy* 67:448–454, 1991.

INDEX

Page numbers followed by *f* indicate illustrations.
Page numbers followed by *t* indicate tables.